E. Biemer · W. Duspiva

Reconstructive Microvascular Surgery

With Forewords by
Ursula Schmidt-Tintemann and Dieter Buck-Gramcko

With 315 Figures, some in Color

Springer-Verlag
Berlin Heidelberg New York 1982

Priv.-Doz. Dr. EDGAR BIEMER
Priv.-Doz. Dr. WOLFGANG DUSPIVA
Klinikum rechts der Isar der Technischen Universität München,
Ismaninger Straße 22, 8000 München 80,
Federal Republic of Germany

Translator: MYRA SOUTAR, PH.D.
Language Editor: DAVID SOUTAR, F.R.C.S.,
Glasgow and West of Scotland Plastic and Maxillo-Facial Surgery
Service, Canniesburn Hospital, Bearsden,
Glasgow G61 1QL, Great Britain

Translation of the German edition:
Rekonstruktive Mikrogefäßchirurgie

ISBN-13: 978-3-642-68456-2 e-ISBN-13: 978-3-642-68454-8
DOI: 10.1007/978-3-642-68454-8

Library of Congress Cataloging in Publication Data
Biemer, E. (Edgar), 1940 Reconstructive microvascular surgery. Translation of: Rekonstruktive Mikrogefäßchirurgie. Includes bibliographies and index. 1. Blood-vessels–Surgery. 2. Microsurgery. 3. Surgery, Plastic. 4. Transplantation of organs, tissues, etc. I. Duspiva, W. (Wolfgang), 1941 II. Title. [DNLM: 1. Hand injuries–Surgery. 2. Microsurgery–Methods. 3. Replantation–Methods. 4. Transplantation–Methods. 5. Vascular surgery–Methods. WG 170 B587r] RD598.5.B5413 617'.413059 81-23276

Reproduction of figures: Gustav Dreher GmbH, Stuttgart

2124/3130-543210

Foreword to the German Edition

The importance of a new operating technique is not judged by the success of one individual case. Only careful observation of the results of numerous operations can show whether the technique may be practised widely and whether the effort expended is justified by the results. Only then, can a new technique take its place in the repertoire of an operative discipline.
The time has come for plastic surgery to avail itself of microvascular surgical techniques and, where there is sufficient experience, the results are good.
Clinical experience has shown that the replantation of amputated extremities can be rewarding when the criteria governing the indications for such surgery are followed rigorously. It is necessary to convey patients quickly to a medical centre which has a clinical organisation specialising in microvascular surgery. Follow-up investigations of the initial successes in replantation of fingers, hands and toes have shown us that such operations are of great importance, not only for the subjective wellbeing of the patients, but for their increased competence to return to work.
Microvascular surgical techniques have also stood the test with regard to free transplantation of tissue, the fundamental advantages being the variable donor-site and a reduced hospital stay.
Indeed, plastic surgery has developed microvascular surgery to an extent where the possibilities offered by this operative technique are inestimable. Certainly, in years to come, the technique will offer new paths for surgeons in many other areas of surgery. One needs little imagination to project the possible rôle of the technique in organ transplantation.
The knowledge and experience of microvascular surgical techniques may belong to every surgeon, but for the plastic surgeon the theory and practice of these techniques are indispensible.
It is to the authors' credit that in this book they not only reproduce their results, but more important, impart their personal experiences and thoughts. Their untiring surgical activity in this field has led to many new discoveries and their book includes everything from improvements in instrumentation and operative strategy to post-operative management and after-care. This book therefore, constitutes a piece of medical history and I am proud that colleagues from my own department have accomplished something so outstanding.

Munich — Prof. Dr. URSULA SCHMIDT-TINTEMANN

Foreword to the German Edition

The major breakthrough in microsurgery followed the clinical application of microvascular surgical techniques: the resulting success brought universal recognition. Many years previously, experimental studies had demonstrated the basic requirements of this technique and microsurgery of the peripheral nerves was practised in many clinics. The pioneers in in this new field of plastic surgery in Australia, China, Japan and the U.S.A. had a difficult and onerous start. There then followed, in the first half of the 1970's, increasing disseminated clinical activity which acted as a proving ground for the preceding experiments, and led to countless new possibilities for the application of microsurgical techniques.

Edgar Biemer and Wolfgang Duspiva played a crucial rôle in the development of microvascular surgery in Europe. Through their initiative, a replantation centre was established in Munich in November 1975, alongside the already existing replantation services in Vienna, at the two University Clinics for Plastic and Reconstructive Surgery (from June 1974), and in Hamburg at the "Berufsgenossenschaftliches Unfallkrankenhaus" (from April 1975). The Munich centre soon accumulated a remarkably high number of replantation cases, surpassing the other centres. The authors stand unrivalled with an accumulation of 300 replantations in two years, and a healing rate of 86%. Nevertheless, microvascular surgery is not simply the activity of one or two surgeons. Success requires a team of well skilled microsurgeons, whose unflagging commitment, in conjunction with theatre sisters and anaesthetists, helps to bring these long operations to a successful conclusion. The overall organisation of a unit is strongly influenced by the introduction of microsurgical operations and must adjust to the altered circumstances. Through good collaboration, these problems were happily solved in Munich and the high standard, to which this book testifies, became possible.

Alongside replantation, free tissue transfer with microvascular anastomosis is the realm of the microvascular surgeon. Such operations require planning, and, although not emergency operations like replantations, they are, nonetheless, largescale. Careful attention to the indications for surgery combined with the surgeon's manual dexterity can offer many a patient significant help in his return to a professional working life. Publications in this new field of surgery are essential and the authors, despite their continuing work load, have provided the first comprehensive presentation on microvascular techniques in Germany. In the near future, microsurgical techniques will gain entry into all surgical disciplines, and thereby unleash new methods of treatment.

Hamburg — Prof. Dr. Dieter Buck-Gramcko

Preface to the German Edition

For many years, the operative manipulation of the most minute structures was frustrated by the limitations of the human eye. With the introduction of the operating microscope by Nylen (1921), fine detailed anatomy was made visible, so that structures could be prepared, presented and manipulated. Nylen used the microscope for treating diseases of the middle ear. In 1946 Perrit in the U.S.A. introduced the operating microscope into the field of ophthalmic surgery. In 1964, Smith, Kunze and Mitchen published reports on their clinical experience using the operating microscope in nerve surgery. Using this technique, it was possible to divide a peripheral nerve into individual fascicle bundles and reapir each bundle precisely.

Following on from these developments, the term "microsurgery" was introduced to cover that branch of surgery which was carried out using the "equiped" eye – either by using loupe spectacle magnification or, more commonly, the operating microscope. The term "microvascular surgery" developed for the operative treatment of small vessels below 2 mm in diameter. Experimental studies for the use of microsurgery in the clinical situation developed alongside its use on small research animals for transplantation models in immunological study. Microsurgical techniques were used in the transplantation of rat liver, kidneys, pancreas, heart and other organs. The clinical application of these microsurgical techniques is nowadays called "reconstructive microvascular surgery". Microvascular surgery, like microsurgery, is not an independent operative discipline, but is purely a technique which may be applied to different specialties, and its use in the future is thereby reinforced. Animal experimental work is an essential prerequisite for the mastery of microvascular surgical technique. In addition to the technical aspects, such experimentation increases the experience of the surgeon by enabling research into suturing and the testing of new developments. Furthermore, regular training is imperative to maintain an optimum standard of safety and confidence for use in the clinical situation.

The first part of the book deals with operating microscopes, instrumentation and microsurgery of vessels commonly used for practice. Methods, documentation and recording of results are presented, and the experimental basis of the techniques involved in microvascular suturing is explained in detail in specific cases. The second part of the book deals with the clinical application of microvascular surgery in replantation and transplantation surgery. The presentations are based on the experience of over 500 clinical cases. The detailed descriptions of the techniques and, in particular, the operating microscopes, instruments and suture materials, do not present a complete picture of all the operative procedures, nor all the available products, but are those with which the authors have had considerable experience.

Preface to the German Edition

Acknowledgements

The authors wish to record their special thanks to the many people who supported them and enabled them to gain the experimental and clinical experience on which this book is based. The preliminary work and subsequent laboratory investigations were made possible and encouraged by the support of the Director of the Institute for Experimental Surgery of the "Technische Universität", Munich – Herr Professor Dr. G. Blümel. The countless organisational problems following the clinical application of this new technique, especially in the area of replantation surgery, were expertly handled by the Director of the Surgical Clinic and Outpatients Dept. of the T.U. in Munich – Herr Professor Dr. Georg Maurer.

Frau Professor Dr. Ursula Schmidt-Tintemann, Head of the Department for Plastic and Reconstructive Surgery of the T.U., Munich, especially deserves our thanks for her continual support and encouragement throughout our work.

Herr Professor Dr. E. Kolb and his colleagues from the Institute for Anaesthesiology and Herr Professor Dr. H. Anacker and the Radiological Institute were most helpful throughout the clinical application of microsurgery. The introduction of Xeroangiography by Herr Dr. Kramann has proved of great value in assessing the late results of replantation surgery. The authors wish to express their thanks to Herr Professor Dr. Dieter Buck-Gramcko, Senior Surgeon of the Department of Hand Surgery and Plastic Surgery at the "Berufsgenossenschaftliches Unfallkrankenhaus", Hamburg – Bergedorf for providing the Foreword, and in showing great interest in their work.

The clinical application of microsurgery, particularly in the field of replantation surgery, was only made possible by inaugurating a 24 hour stand-by service. The willingness of our colleagues in the replantation team was of immeasurable importance; in addition to their duties in the various surgical units – plastic surgery, thoracic surgery, vascular surgery and orthopaedic surgery – they were ready to take on and perform a considerable amount of work. Those involved in providing this replantation service were: Dr. E. Herndl, Dr. W. Stock, Dr. J. Heiss, Dr. K. Werber, Dr. W. Götz, Dr. K. Glas, Dr. H. Bartels, Dr. G. Ingianni, Dr. G. Meyer-Busche and Dr. H. Schmück. The outstanding photographic documentation was provided by the Department of Photography of the Surgical Unit of the T.U., Munich. The authors are grateful for the support which they have recieved from the sisters, physiotherapists, occupational therapists and from all personnel in the operating theatres. The authors also acknowledge the help and support of Springer-Verlag and especially Miss TISMER for her considerable efforts in typing the manuscript. Much of the work was supported by the firms of Ethicon – Hamburg, Thomae-Biberach, Aesculap – Tuttlingen and the authors gratefully acknowledge the financial assistance from the Volkswagen Foundation, which made much of the experimental work possible.

Munich

E. BIEMER
W. DUSPIVA

Contents

Part 1 Technique of Microvascular Surgery and Preliminary Experimental Studies 1

I. Development of Microvascular Surgery 3

II. Technical Equipment 4
1. Operating Microscope 4
2. Accessories and Documentation 7
3. Operating Seats 9
4. Instruments 9
5. Suture Material 15

III. Experimental Microvascular Surgery 16

IV. Suture Technique in Microvascular Surgery 17
1. Preliminary Remarks 17
2. End-to-End Anastomosis 18
3. End-to-Side Anastomosis 28

V. Complications of Microvascular Suture 30
1. Assessment of Microvascular Anastomosis 30
2. Patency Test 30
3. Microthrombectomies 30
4. Micro-vein Grafts 30
a) Indications for Micro-vein Grafts 33
b) Donor Sites for Micro-vein Grafts 35
c) Rules for Micro-vein Grafts 36

VI. Micromorphological Evidence at the Site of Anastomosis in Small Vessels 40

VII. Medical Prophylaxis and Treatment of Vessel Thrombosis and Spasm 47
1. Local Measures 47
2. Systemic Measures. 47

References 49

Part 2 Clinical Microvascular Surgery 53

A Replantation with Microvascular Anastomosis (microreplantation) 55

I. Definitions and Nomenclature 56

1. Replantation 56
2. Amputation 56
3. Total Amputation 56
4. Subtotal Amputation 56
5. Revascularisation 57
6. Replantation: Macro- and Micro-replantation 58

II. Classification of Amputations in the Hand 59

III. Indications for Replantation 59

IV. Guide-lines for the Primary Treatment of Amputation Injuries 62

V. Replantation Technique 63
1. Wound Debridement 64
2. Bone Shortening 64
3. Osteosynthesis 65
4. Suturing of the Flexor Tendon and Tendon Sheath 67
5. Arterial Anastomosis 67
6. Nerve Suturing 68
7. Management of the Extensor Tendon Apparatus . . . 68
8. Vein Anastomosis 68
9. Skin Closure 68
10. Dressings 69
11. Medicinal Treatment 69

VI. Considerations of Differing Levels and Mechanisms of Amputation 70
1. Levels of Amputation in the Hand 70
2. Guillotine Amputations 75
3. Crushing Injuries 75
4. Severe Crushing and Combination Injuries with Damage to the Amputated Part 76
5. Avulsion Injuries 79
6. Degloving Injuries 79

VII. Primary Replacement of Destroyed Phalangeal Joints . . 85

VIII. Primary Finger Transplantation 88

IX. Post-operative Management 89

X. Physical Management 94

XI. Secondary Operations 95

XII. Results 97

XIII. Microreplantation of Other Parts of the Body – (e.g., toes, ears, scalping injuries, and penile amputations) 99

XIV. Replantation Service 104

B Tissue Transplantation with Microvascular Anastomosis . . 105

I. Development of Tissue Transplantation Using Microvascular Anastomosis 105

II. Definitions and Nomenclature 106
III. Indications for Free Tissue Transplantation 106
IV. Preparations for Tissue Transplantation 107
V. Operating Technique 108
1. General Operative Plan 108
2. Medicinal Treatment 109
3. Post-operative Treatment and Supervision 110
4. Complications 110
VI. Free Flap Transplantation 116
1. Development 116
2. Advantages and Disadvantages of Free Flap Transplantation 116
3. Special Requirements for Free Flap Transplantation 117
4. Donor Sites 118
a) Groin Flaps (fat flap, iliac flaps) 118
b) Dorsalis Pedis Flaps (interdigital fold flap, toe pulp flap) 121
c) Delto-Pectoral Flap 123
d) Temporal Flaps 123
e) Axillary Flaps 123
f) Retro-Auricular Flaps 128
VII. Combined Skin and Muscle Flap Transplantation (musculo-cutaneous flaps) 129
VIII. Combined Skin Flap with Bone Transplantation (osteo-cutaneous flaps) 130
IX. Bone Transplantation 131
X. Muscle Transplantation 133
XI. Transplantation of the Omentum 134
XII. Toe Transplantation 134
References 143
Subject Index 147

Part 1

Technique of Microvascular Surgery and Preliminary Experimental Studies

I. Development of Microvascular Surgery

The well proven technique of continuous vessel suture which gives excellent results in larger vessels under the naked eye, unfortunately proves difficult when dealing with vessels with an outer diameter of less than 2 mm: under the naked eye the vessel lumen can no longer be safely identified. It is easy with such suturing techniques to suture the back wall of the vessel or, by inverting the suture, create a stenosis at the suture site. The problem of uniting smaller vessels with an outer diameter of 0.3–2 mm has largely been solved in the last two decades with the development of microsurgical operative techniques. The advantage of these techniques lies in the optical enlargement, which permits much better identification of the lumen of these thin vessels than can be achieved with the naked eye. The vessel stumps are easily identified and, using fine suture material and instruments, can be repaired exactly, so that no constriction or distortion occurs at the site of anastomosis. Magnification on a small scale is possible using loupe-spectacles (up to times 6, see Fig. 1), and larger scale magnification is possible using the operating microscope. There are certain disadvantages using the operating microscope: these must be taken into consideration, especially the reduction in the field of vision.
A wide variety of techniques for joining small vessels has been attempted in the last few years, e.g. pure sticking plaster, sticking plaster in conjunction with holding sutures, rings, small capillary tubes, clips and various suture devices (Johns 1947; Swenson and Gross 1947; Bikfalvi et al. 1953; Samuels 1955; Androsov 1956; Inokuchi 1958; Carter and Roth 1958; Nathan 1960; Urschel and Roth 1961; Nakayama et al. 1962; Hafner et al. 1963; Mozes et al. 1963; Ballinger et al. 1963; Gonzales and Nathan 1963; Sigel and Acevedo 1963; Williams and Takaro 1963; Chase and Schwartz 1963; Stirling 1964; Takaro 1964; Padula et al. 1965; Smith 1966; Blümel and Gottlob 1968; Kalkowski et al. 1970; Östrup 1976; Matras et al. 1977; Pearl et al. 1977). The majority of these techniques which have been used in animal trials rely on cannulisation of the vessel lumen and for the most part can be performed with the naked eye. Many of these methods, however, have common disadvantages e.g. media necrosis caused by the sticking of the foreign material, reduced tensile strength, lumen constriction, the presence of a permanent foreign body in the lumen and, in particular, the restriction of the techniques because of the size of the materials used. Nevertheless, new methods are constantly being developed and it is possible that many of these techniques e.g. sticking with "Fibringlue"[1] may gain acceptance, when used in conjunction with the operating microscope techniques in the future, similar to the techniques used in microsurgery of nerves (Matras et al. 1973; Duspiva and Biemer 1976; Kuderna 1976).
Very good results can be achieved in suturing of nerves with an outer diameter of 0.3–2 mm, using simple sutures of fine nylon under operating microscope control. The greatest variation in technique is in the suturing of arteries, veins, and vein transplants by end-to-end and end-to-side anastomosis. Equilibrium can be achieved up to a certain degree and even vessels of an outer diameter of only 0.3 mm can still be anastomosed with comparative safety (O'Brien 1977).
Microsurgical suture techniques in small vessel surgery have greatly developed in the last two decades since the work of Jacobson et al. in 1960. Buncke 1965 and 1966 reported the first series of replantations of amputated parts in experimental animals. The first successful replantation in a human was performed in Japan (Komatsu and Tamai 1968) where microsurgical techniques were used to replant a totally amputated thumb. About the same time, there appeared in the literature the first reports concerning free tissue transplantation using microvascular anastomosis in animal

1 Fa. Immuno, Vienna, Heidelberg

trials (Krizek 1965). The first clinical cases were reported by Daniel and Taylor (1973) and O'Brien et al. (1973b).
There has been continuous development and improvement of operating microscopes, instruments and surgical techniques, and new clinical applications for microsurgery have followed. As in the German-speaking nations, there are presently many centres throughout the world where replantation and free tissue transplantation using microvascular techniques are routinely performed.

II. Technical Equipment

1. Operating Microscope

Much of the preparatory work in microvascular surgery can best be performed using loupe-spectacles (see Fig. 1). The magnification varies from 2 to 6 times and allows a greater view of the operative field than can be achieved under the microscope. For the actual microvascular suturing, it is necessary to employ greater magnification, which is supplied by the operating microscope (see Fig. 2). At the present time, there are a variety of models of operating microscopes, which are suitable for microvascular surgery. The authors' experience lies mainly with microscopes manufactured by Zeiss. For experimental work, the OPMI 6 (see Fig. 5) and the wall-mounted OPMI 9 with appropriate attachments are generally used. In the clinical situation, stereoscopic double microscopes with fibre-optic illumination, such as the OPMI 2 and the OPMI 7 D are used. Such microscopes enable the assistant to perform his duties accurately. For practical courses in microsurgery, the OPMI 1 U7 (see Figs. 3 and 4) on a table

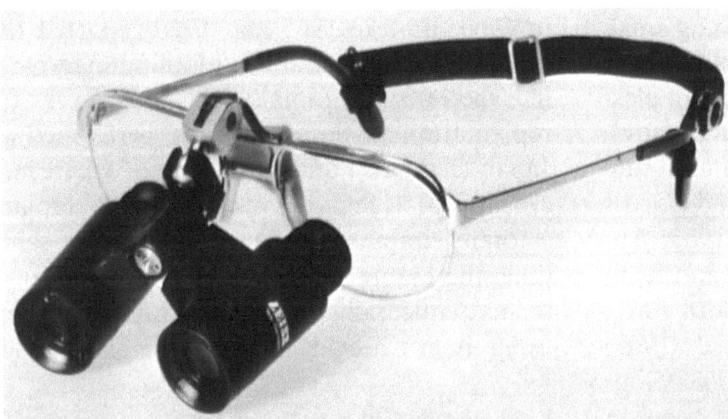

Fig. 1. Loupes (Zeiss)

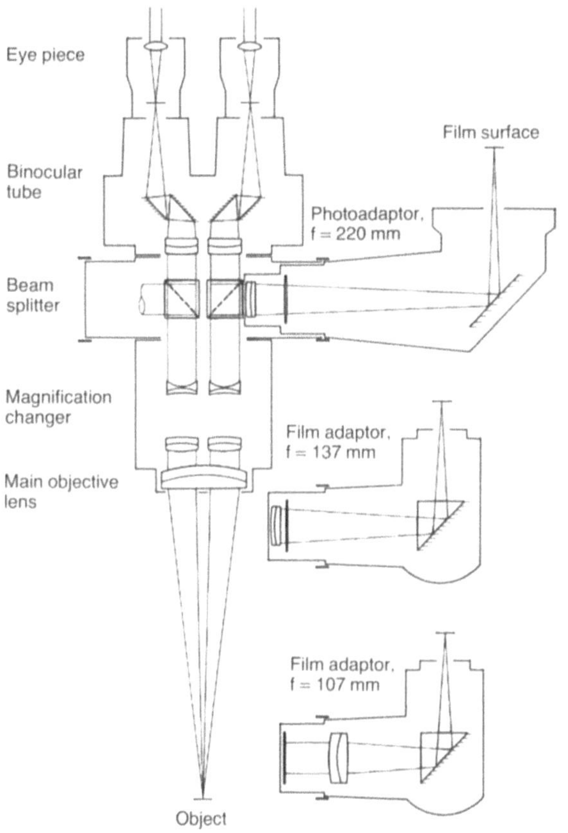

Fig. 2. Schematic diagram of an operating microscope (courtesy of Zeiss)

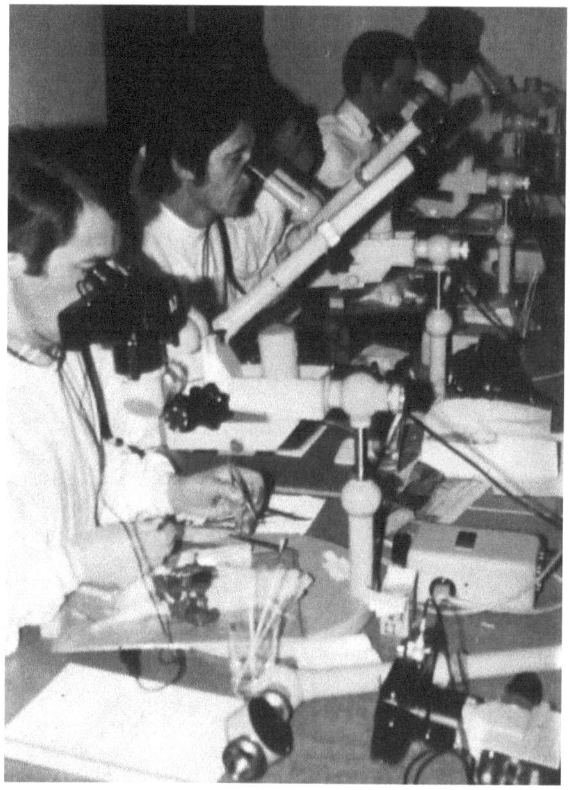

Fig. 3. Table microscope in use during an instructional operating course

stand has proved reliable and allows a large number of participants to operate independently.

The technical details, the mounting and control mechanisms of the many operating microscopes that are available on the market can be found in the appropriate instruction manuals produced by the manufacturers. In this Chapter several of the operating microscopes produced by Zeiss are illustrated and described in detail.

Particularly important when using the operating microscope, is to obtain precise focusing at the highest level of magnification, since only then can an exceedingly long operation be performed without fatigue. Great care should be taken with the operating microscope and, when not in use, it should be carefully covered.

In our experience, the foot-pedal switches can cease to function if they should become encrusted with blood during an operation. Our current practice is to protect the foot-pedal switch during use by placing it in a plastic

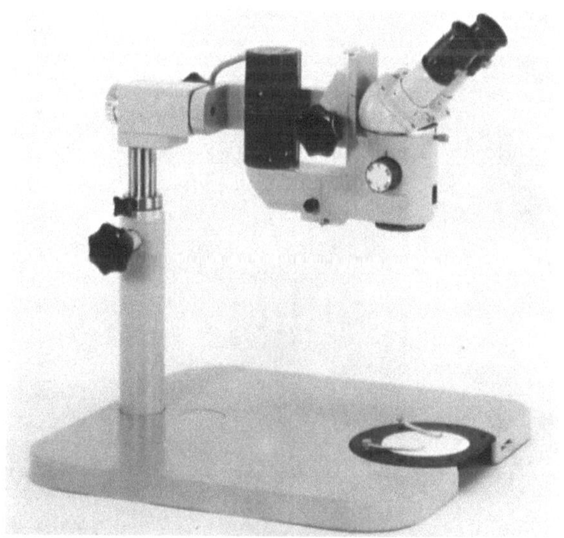

Fig. 4. The OPMI 1 U7 type of microscope on a table stand, for use in an instructional operating course. An f = 175 mm interchangeable objective is used and the instrument has complete sterilizable attachments for manipulating the microscope. There is a built-in Galilei alternator with 5 levels of magnification and attachments for a variety of adaptors. 3 lighting variants are possible: standard lighting with 6 V lamps, high performance lighting using halogen lamps 12 V (OPMI 1/H) or fibre-optic lighting (OPMI 1/F)

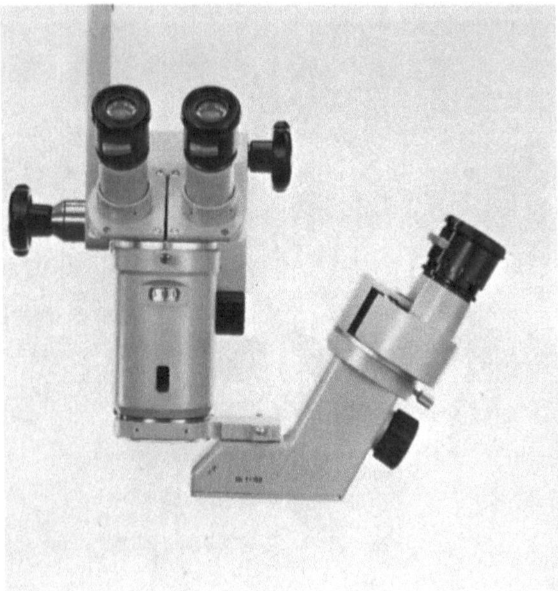

Fig. 5. Zoom microscope OPMI 6 with assistant microscope at 8°. For plastic and reconstructive microsurgery, the microscope and accessories are frequently installed on a portable floor support or a ceiling-mount (not shown in the picture). The most commonly used microscope is at present a zoom microscope which the operator controls by a foot control switch, thus being able to chose the most suitable magnification for each case. The zoom system extends from 1:4 and if required, can be adjusted manually. Co-axial illumination (6 V, 30 w) is used to light the operating field. For the assistant, a co-observer microscope can be mounted on a support ring which rotates around the main microscope. The angle of vision between the assistant microscope and the main microscope amounts to only 8°. In practice this means that the assistant maintains a stereo-optic picture with almost the same field of view as the operator. When needed, a 3-step Galilei change (not shown in the picture) can be fitted between the body of the assistant's microscope and the binocular tube. The main microscope is focused by an electric motor controlled by the foot switch, whereas the assistant's microscope is focused manually by means of a push-button

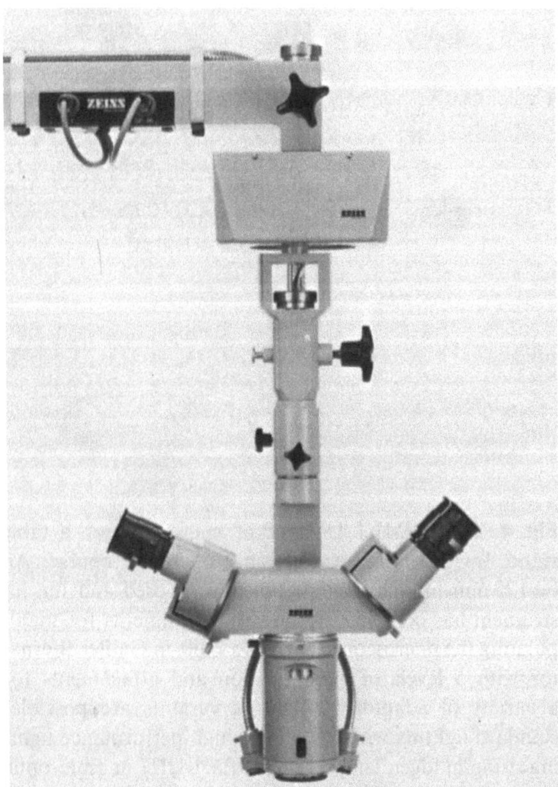

Fig. 6. OPMI 7D, with coordinated coupling. The coordinated coupling, sometimes referred to as the XY coupling is useful for fine adjustment of the microscope. It is controlled by an electric motor and allows displacement in a horizontal direction of about 50 mm, with an adjustment speed of 3.5 mm per second. This is so calculated to allow prompt positioning of the microscope, even at relatively high magnification. The main microscope is a zoom microscope, permitting continuous magnification change within a range of 1:5. There is a stereo beam splitter on which two straight binocular tubes with appropriate eye-pieces are mounted. This arrangement enables both the operator and the assistant to have exactly the same angle of view and the same stereo optic advantages with regard to the operating field

bag. Damage to the cables, by kinking or running over while transporting the microscope, can lead to the loss of individual functions and great care should be taken when transporting the microscope within the hospital.

2. Accessories and Documentation

Different attachments for the microscope are important in building up a comprehensive system (see Figs. 8 and 9): fibre-optic lighting, electronic flash-gun, co-observer tubes (Fig. 7), dual microscope, beam-splitter with possibility for photography (Super 8 mm and 16 mm) and colour T.V. adaptor. The assistant microscope – 8° – acts as an independent microscope, being secured on a carrying ring which allows rotation round its own and the main microscope's axis. In the middle of the carrying ring, an operating field magnifier × 2, can be mounted and it can be used simultaneously with the assistant's microscope. Beam-splitters, 50 and 70, permit accessories for co-observation and documentation to be simply and quickly mounted. Beam-splitter 50 is particularly suited for co-observer tubes, supplying the same amount of light to the tube and to the main microscope. Beam-splitter 70 directs more light to the attachments and is more advantageous for the recording accessories. With co-observer tubes, the assistant can see the operating field at the same angle as the surgeon. The monocular as well as the stereo co-observer tubes can be used

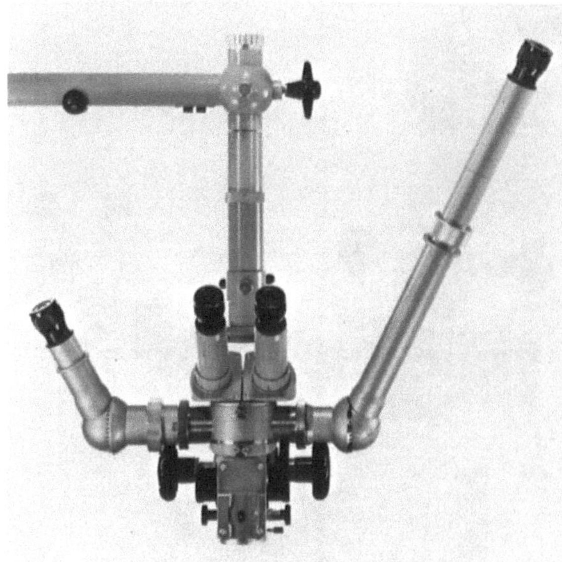

Fig. 7. Short and long co-observer tubes mounted on the microscope

in differing directions and, with the extended observer tube, the operating field can be observed without disturbing the operating team.

The photo-adaptor, f = 220 mm, fits on one of the beam-splitters and can be used with all objectives on the main microscope. With Galilei exchange and a × 2 lens attachment, a × 10 magnification can be obtained for each lens. The photographic attachment is used with the microscope lenses f = 125 mm and f = 200 mm. In addition, three photographic lenses (125/1, 125/2, 200/1.25) can be used with this attachment or combined with × 2

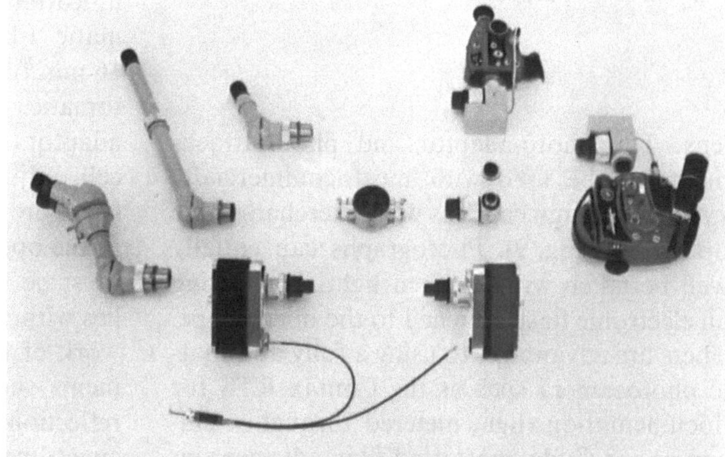

Fig. 8. Accessories for co-observation and documentation: cine, photo and TV cameras, co-observer tubes and adaptors

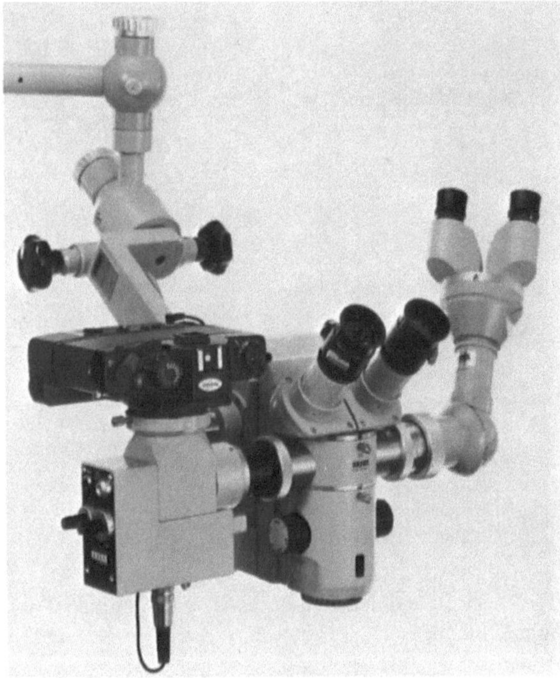

Fig. 9. Zoom microscope, with co-observation and equipment for documentation. Although only one observation beam with the main microscope can be used for the stereo co-observer tube, it is still possible using binocular eye pieces to obtain a stereo optic view of the operating field. Nevertheless, this stereo view is inevitably less good than that obtained in the main microscope. Two different mechanically controlled focusing positions allow the assistant to position the co-observer binocular tube in the appropriate place. By using a reversion prism, the picture of the microscope operating field can be orientated in the correct way. In addition to the stereo co-observer tube, there are also monocular co-observer tubes in two differing lengths (these latter tubes do not, of course, give a stereo optic view of the operating field). For documentation, an automatic photoadaptor with a 35 mm camera, as illustrated, is available. Instead of a 35 mm camera, a cine camera or TV camera can be attached as required, provided that the proportion and weight of these cameras is sufficiently small. Such cameras necessitate appropriate cine film or TV adaptors

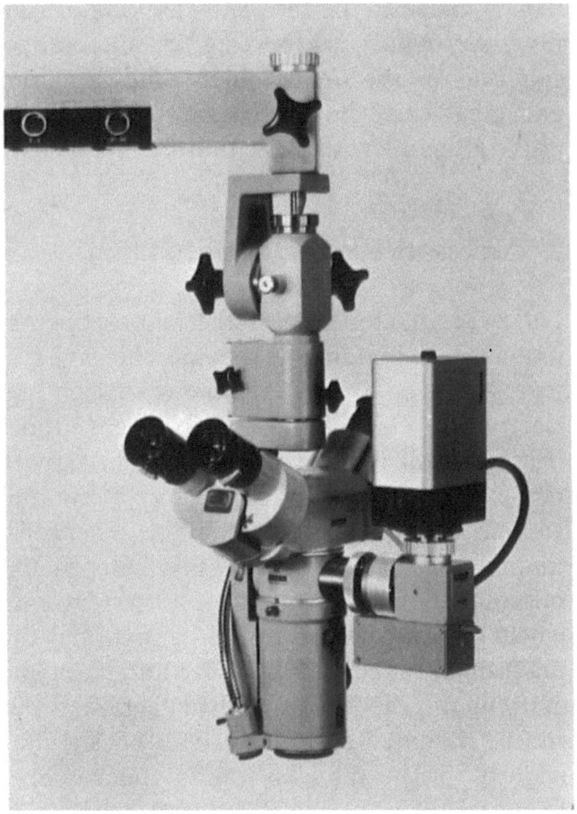

Fig. 10. Colour TV camera mounted directly onto the microscope

lens. The photo-adaptor and photo-attachment can be used with most commercially available 35 mm cameras with interchangeable optics (see Fig. 9). Photographs can equally well be taken with halogen lighting or using an electronic flash attached to the microscope. There are advantages to using a fully automatic photocamera such as the Contax RTS for documentation (light metered through a silicon photo diode, motorised film, advance single frame infra-red distance release, selective in-reflection of the data, etc.).

The beam splitter also accepts any of the three cine adaptors available (f = 74 mm for Super 8 film; f = 107 mm and f = 137 mm for 16 mm film). The adaptors for a 16 mm film differ in the degree of magnification and field of vision; the f = 107 mm adaptor has lower magnification but a larger field of vision. Automatic film adaptors for Super 8 mm and 16 mm film cameras were developed with automatic diaphragm and automatic photo adaptor (see Fig. 10). With the help of a photo cell, adjustments of diaphragm and shutter speed are at one's disposal and documentation of the operation is very much facilitated. Care must be taken that the part to be illustrated lies within the right angle of the ocular framework of the field view obtained. Dull instruments should be used to avoid troublesome reflection in the photography, particularly in cine films.

Colour T.V. transmission, because of the high light requirements of the cameras, suffered initial difficulties (Littmann et al. 1975). Despite these difficulties, T.V. cameras for use on the operating microscope are available. It is also possible to mount a small, lightweight 35 mm camera directly on to the operating microscope or, by using an optical link system (viz. picture transmission extension by Wittmoser and optical system by Hopkins), to transmit the image to a separately mounted camera. Other surgical specialties have already had experience of such optical extensions (Mauermayer 1976).
Colour T.V. transmission is particularly useful as a teaching-aid in courses dealing with microsurgical operating techniques. It is thus possible for a large number of observers to follow the operation (Biemer et al. 1978b) and the authors have been pleased with their results using the mobile "Telemed-System" made by Lemcke.

3. Operating Seats

Special operating seats with detachable, sterilizable arm-rests have proved very reliable, particularly in these, often protracted, operations (see Figs. 11 and 12). These seats are easily adjustable, the seat height being controlled by the foot control, so that the surgeon and assistant can always maintain optimal seat positions appropriate to their heights. Such comforts enable the operation to be performed smoothly and without fatigue. The adjustable arm-rests largely eliminate hand and arm tremor.
Alternatively, a satisfactory seat position can be achieved with swivel stools, using as a substitute for arm-rests, layers of hospital linen under the arms for support, or by using appropriately cut-out operating tables.

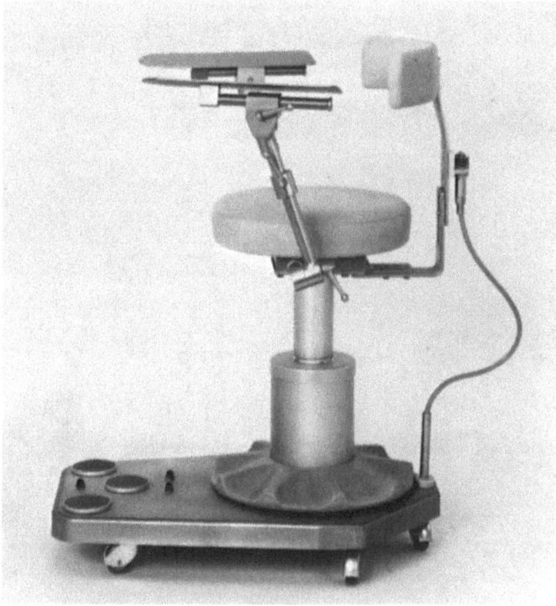
11

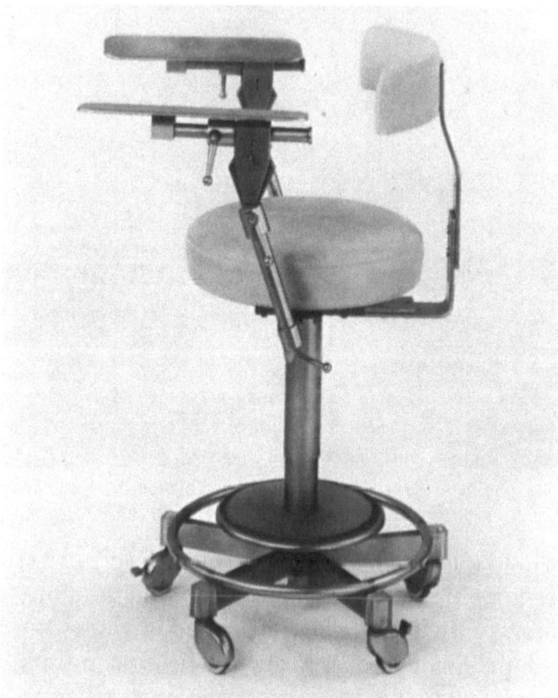
12

Figs. 11, 12. Operating seat – above with control pedals – below without control switches. Both illustrations show removable, sterilizable and fully adjustable arm-rests (Zeiss)

4. Instruments

The number of instruments necessary for microvascular surgery is small: forceps, knot forceps, scissors, and vessel clips (see Fig. 13). The fine forceps originated from the watchmaker, jewellers forceps, whereas the remaining instruments developed from microsurgical research and the operative techniques in related surgical fields.
Microinstruments must be treated very carefully: the instruments are kept together for

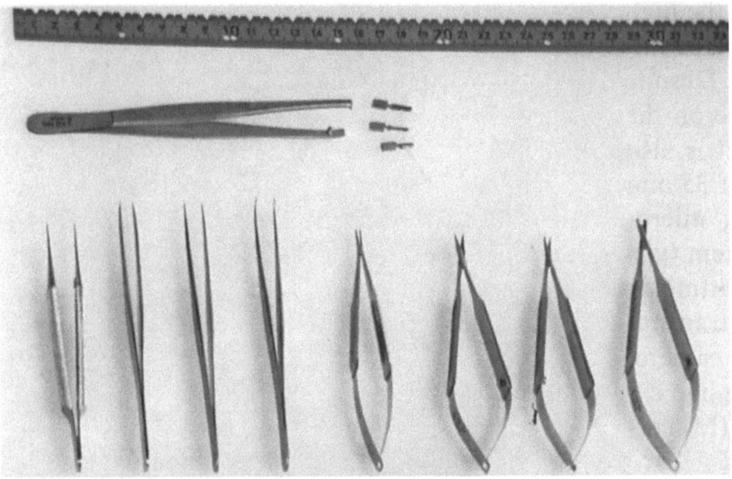

Fig. 13. Basic microsurgical instrumentation

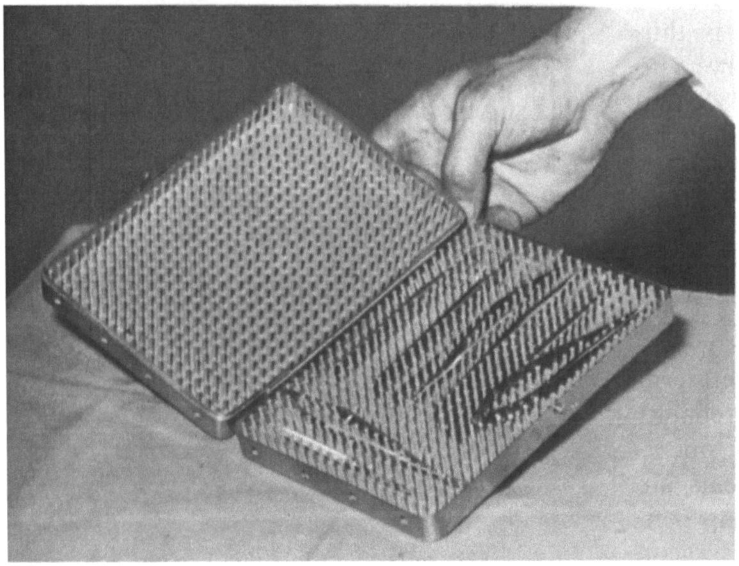

Fig. 14. Microsurgical metal case, containing instruments secured in rubber studs. This offers completely safe and secure storage and the possibility of sterilization (Aesculap)

safe-keeping and sterilization in metal containers with specifically designed dividers to hold the instruments secure. The fine points are protected by inserting them into silicone tubing.

Cleaning is best performed in an ultrasonic cleaner. Instruments with a ratchet are not suitable for microsurgery since the jerkiness of the ratchet action makes the finest work impossible.

Instruments may have flat or rounded barrels. Instruments with half rounded grips have the advantage that rotation of the instrument around a longitudinal axis is feasible using only the fingers, while the mid-hand can remain at rest and fully supported. In flat barrelled instruments, rotation requires movement of the whole hand, and to this end the grip is somewhat firmer. In the main, the half rounded design with gripping handle appears to dominate.

Instruments with a length of 11–12 cm are most suitable for microsurgical operations for both animal experiments and for re- and transplantation surgery. Longer instruments can inadvertently touch the microscope or cable, thus endangering the sterility of the operation. It is essential to clean the instruments during the operation to prevent encrusted blood and adherent tissue interfering with the precise function of the instruments. Another problem worth some attention is magnetisation of the

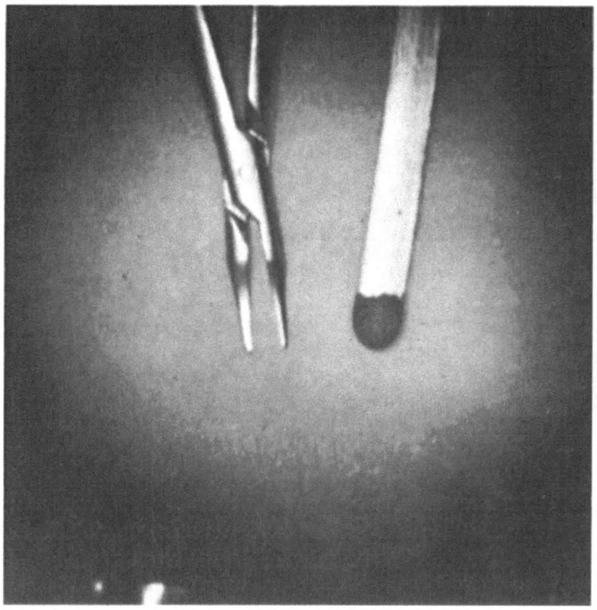

Fig. 15. Needle holder (Detail)

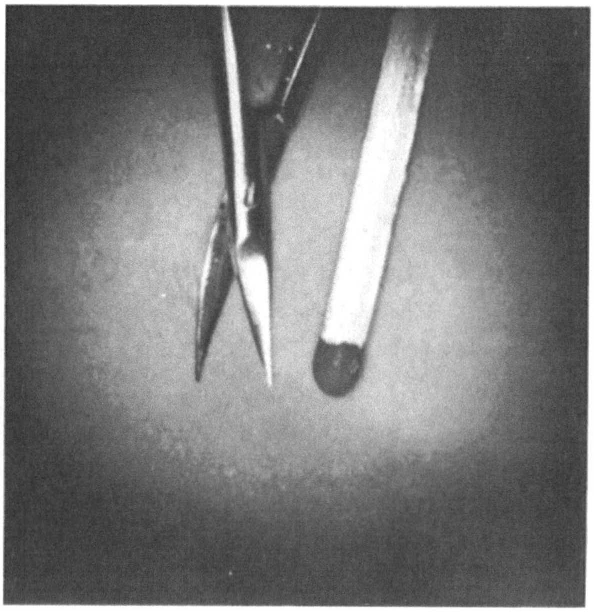

Fig. 16. Fine spring scissors (Detail)

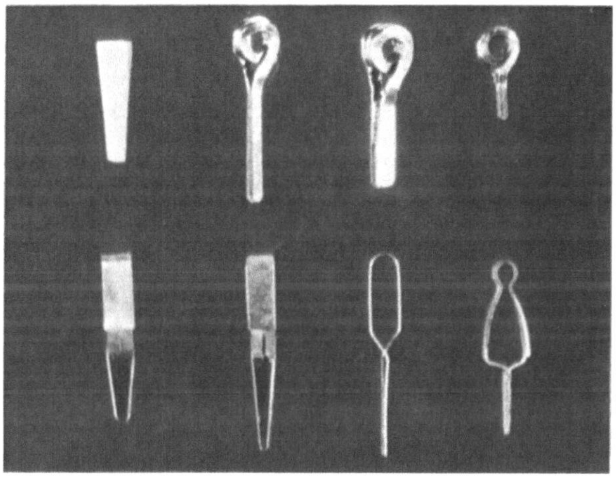

Fig. 17. Differing types of microvascular clamps. *Upper row,* from left to right (Acland, Scoville-Lewis). *Lower row,* from left to right (Biemer, Chinese Model)

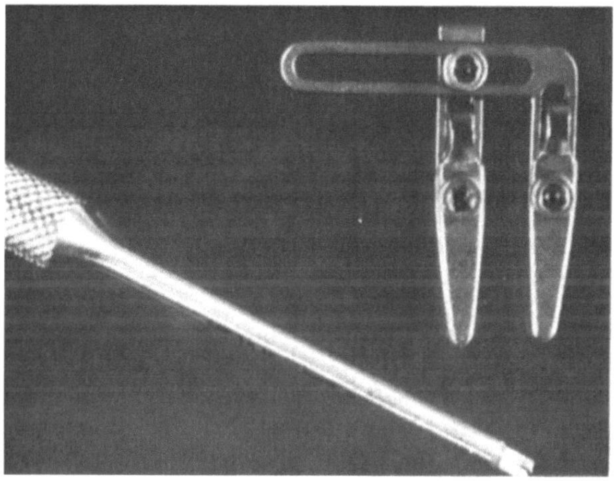

Fig. 18. Approximator clamp with adjustable closing pressure (Aesculap)

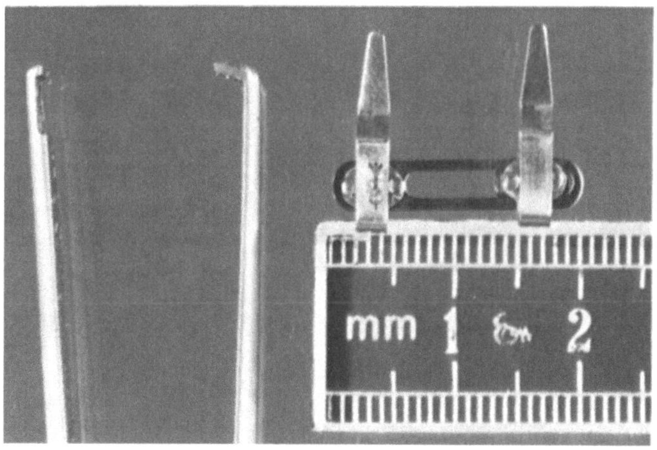

Fig. 19. Approximator clamp with fixed, nonadjustable closing pressure (Aesculap)

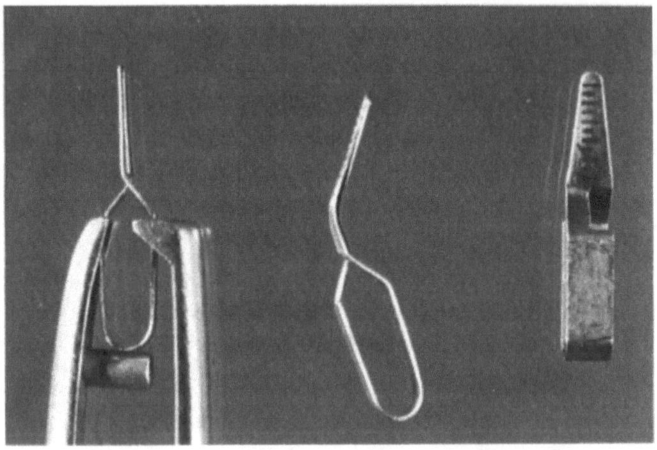

Fig. 20. Vessel clamps designed by Biemer (Aesculap), with calibrated area of compression (18, 20, 21 g per mm^2) and printed measure. Also shown are the specially designed application forceps

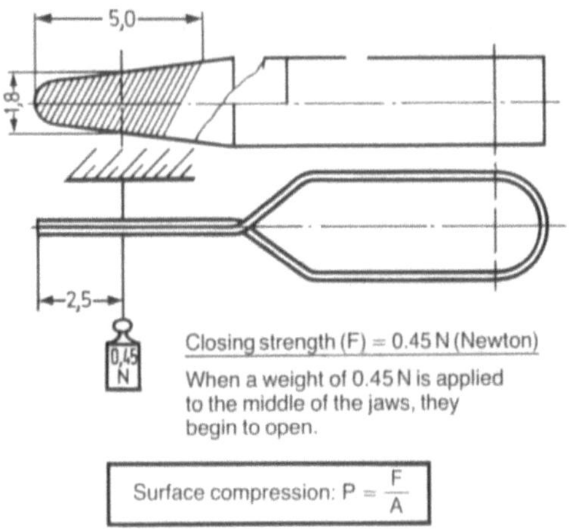

Example of calculation

Artery ∅ 0.80 mm

Breadth of clamp at the measuring point 1.80 mm

Surface (A) = ½ length × breadth of clamp $= \frac{2.51\,\text{mm}}{2} \times 1.8\,\text{mm} = 2.26\,\text{mm}^2$

Surface compression $P = \frac{F}{A} = \frac{0.45\,\text{N}}{2.26\,\text{mm}^2} = 0.20\,\text{N/mm}^2$

Fig. 21. Calculation of the closing strength and surface compression of vessel clamps (reproduced by kind permission of Aesculap)

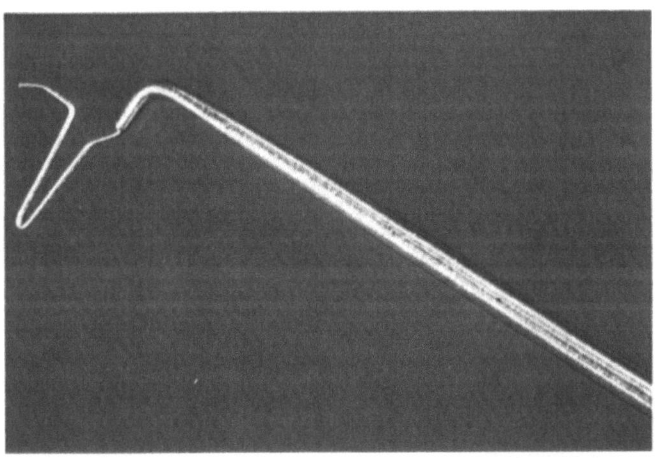

Fig. 22. Vein spreader designed by Biemer (Aesculap)

instruments, since it is very troublesome if the needle becomes pulled from the needle-holder and forceps by magnetic forces.

The basic instrumentation (see Fig. 13) comprises straight jeweller's forceps (nos. 2–5) and curved jeweller's forceps (no. 7), with fine or coarse points; the latter allows the curved jeweller's forceps to be used as a needle-holder (Acland 1975).

An early development was a forcep with a small plateau at the point, thus enabling more secure handling of the suture in a larger area of the forcep. It is most useful to be able to perform small repairs oneself, such as regrinding the points of forceps, and to this end a grindstone is included in the equipment (e.g., Degussit, fine, no. 90203, – Degussa). Also included in the microsurgical instrumentarium are suture-tying forceps with straight and gently curved jaws (Barraquer, Castroviejo) and straight and gently curved spring scissors (Wescott, Castroviejo).

Vessel-clamps or clips (see Fig. 17), are necessary, not only to interrupt blood flow during vessel anastomosis, but also to prevent retraction of the vessel stumps in the surrounding soft tissue and hold the vessel ends in a favourable position for suturing.

Various types of approximating clamps (Acland, Piza-Katzer, Biemer, among others), are used only in animal experiments or for training and instruction in microsurgical techniques (see Figs. 18 and 19). The authors have found that, in the clinical situation, single small clips are most versatile and practicable; they take up less room and are more considerate to the vessel wall. The forcible approximation of the vessel ends for suturing, using approximator clamps, endangers the vessel wall and leads to subsequent stretching of the anastomosis. The body of any vessel clamp should be as smooth and as compact as possible so that suture material does not become entangled. Among the many clamps in current use are those of Mayfield, Heifetz, Scoville-Lewis, Acland and Biemer. Important in any clip is the pressure exerted over a given area and this is partly derived from the closing strength (see Fig. 21). Too great a closing pressure gives rise to pressure damage of the vessel intima (Acland 1974), but on the other hand, too little closing strength allows the vessel clamps to slip easily to the side. Small plastic syringes, with blunt, polished fine cannulae are used to irrigate the operating area and, in addition, to flush out the vessel ends. The authors use heparinised Ringer's lactate (10 E/ml) at room or body temperature, for irrigation. Careful dilatation and flushing of clamped vessel stumps can readily be achieved with a drip of heparinised Ringer's lactate administered via the syringe and cannula, and controlled by jeweller's forceps. Complementary to the aforementioned instrumentation are some special instruments which have been developed for microvascular surgery. A "counterloop" which allows the vessel wall to be supported while the needle is inserted, thus avoiding the necessity to pick up the vessel wall and hold it with forceps (Acland 1972b). 2 cm long pieces of measuring tape, with millimetre divisions is most useful for experimental examination and for recording and documenting details of operations. Coloured background material made in plastic or metal (yellow, green or blue), has also proved most useful for vessel anastomosis (Terzis et al. 1974; Daniel and Terzis 1977). A vein strut (see Fig. 22), which allows careful stretching of the lumen, and special vein scissors (see Figs. 25 and 26), which act like a guillotine and thus avoid flushing of fine vessels during cutting.

Further specialised instruments should also be mentioned: Pneumatic needle-holders (Salmon and Assimacopoulos 1964) and irrigators

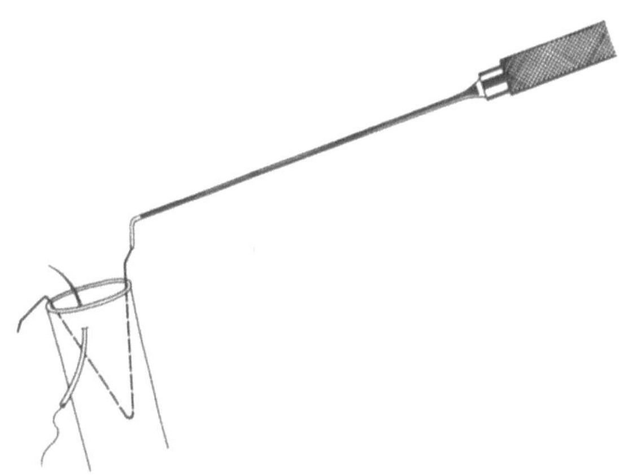

Fig. 23. Diagramatic representation of the microvascular spreader

24 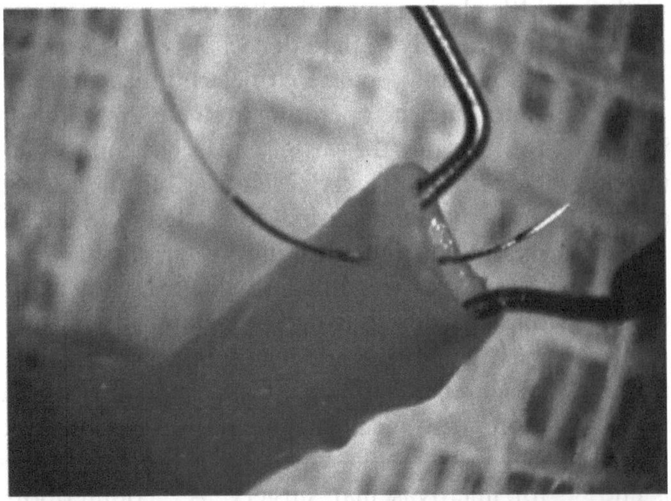

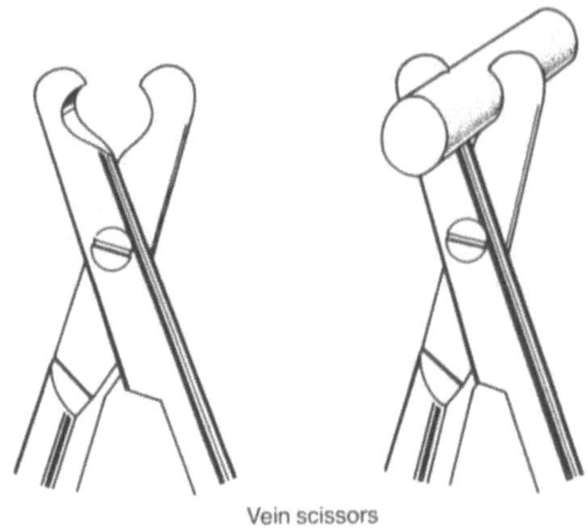

Fig. 26. Diagramatic representation of the vein scissors

25 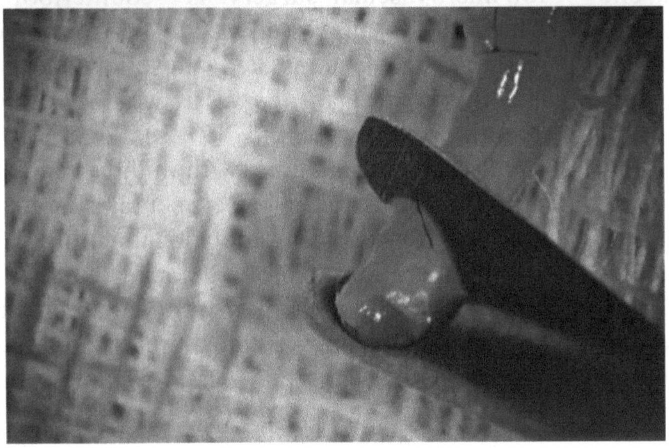

Fig. 24. Vein spreader designed by Biemer (Aesculap)

Fig. 25. Vein scissors designed by Biemer (Aesculap)

(Rigg 1975b). Pedal-operated microsurgical instruments: low-pressure hydraulics (Buncke and Schulz 1966): compressed air (Salmon et al. 1964): electricity (Parel et al. 1970): "Bowden"-pullers (Acland 1972b). Equally noteworthy is the "Saran-Wrap Cuff" technique, used to seal microvascular anastomosis (McLean and Bunke 1973).

Other equipment which is generally used in plastic surgery has taken on a new significance; for example, the bipolar-coagulator. Similarly, Doppler equipment (see Fig. 27), which is used to seek out subcutaneous vessels and monitor blood flow through microvascular anastomosis (Karkowsky and Buncke 1975; Aoyagi et al. 1975).

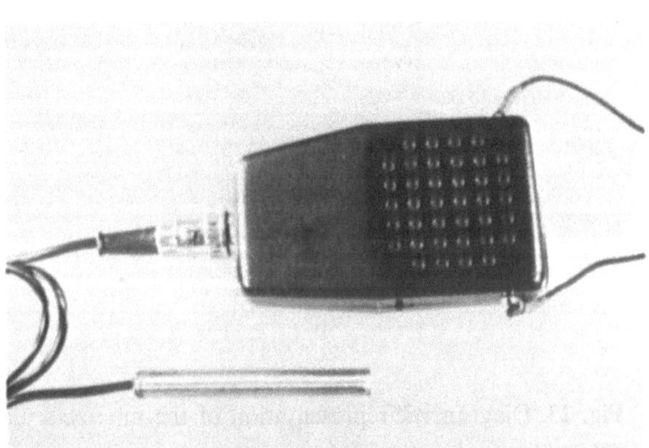

Fig. 27. Portable Doppler instrument (Sonicaid, Kranzbühler & Son)

5. Suture Material

The most commonly used suture material is nylon of strength 10/0 and 11/0, with diameters of 25 μ and 15 μ respectively – e.g., EP1 (0.2) or alternatively EP1 (0.1) by Ethicon (see Fig. 29). The authors mostly favour 10/0 nylon (25 μ), because of the advantage of the higher tensile strength. For microsurgical purposes these sutures are armed with $^{3}/_{8}$ round body needles of types BV2, BV4 and BV6 (needle diameter 0.14, 0.10 and 0.07 mm respectively). Previously, the 10/0 nylon thread was also available with the more curved TF10 needle.

Cutting needles are not suitable for vascular surgery. The length of suture material should be trimmed to 5–7 cm by the surgeon or the operating nurse, thus allowing both the needle and the end of the thread to be maintained within the field of vision.

Sutures with metalised points (O'Brien and Hayhurst 1973) and fine resorbable suture material (10/0 Vicryl from Ethicon) should also be mentioned. Round bodied needles can be held more readily in the jaws of needle holders if they are partially flattened at the end. A further suture material which is extensively used is that developed by Acland and termed "vascular" by the Company Spingler and Tritt, with 18 μ nylon thread and a 70 μ, 4 mm long, $^{3}/_{8}$ round bodied needle.

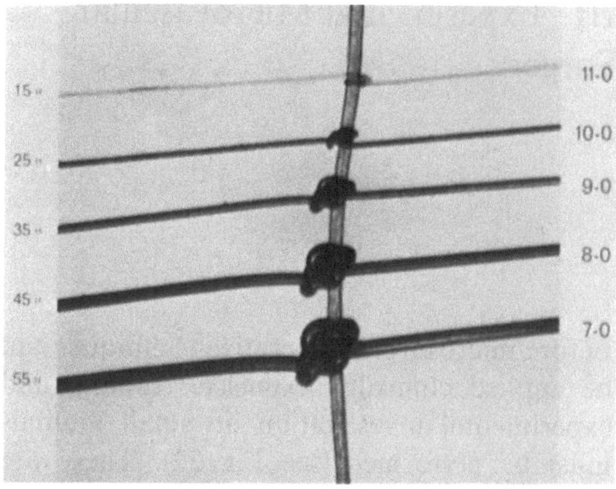

Fig. 28. Nylon suture varying from 7/0 to 11/0. For comparison, the sutures have been knotted around a woman's hair (reproduced by kind permission of Ethicon)

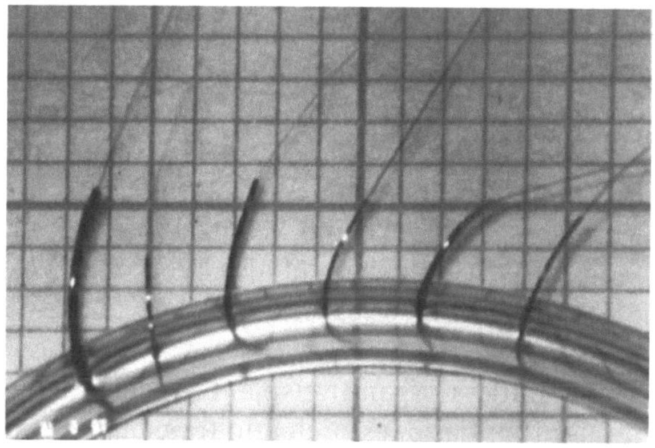

Fig. 29. Microsurgical suture material armed with differing needles for use in microvascular surgery

III. Experimental Microvascular Surgery

Before microsurgical operative techniques can be applied clinically, extensive training and experimental investigation on small animals must be performed (see Fig. 32). There are countless training and trial models on different animal types described in the literature:

Rats	(Salyer and Kyger 1973; Strauch and Murray 1967; Piza-Katzer 1974; Duspiva and Biemer 1976; Rigg 1975b, among others)
Rabbits	(Piza-Katzer 1974; Buncke and Schulz 1966; O'Brien and Shanmugen 1973)
Pigs	(Daniel and Williams 1973)
Monkeys	(Buncke and Schulz 1965)
Dogs	(Goldwyn et al. 1963; Krizek et al. 1965)

The countless organ-transplant models in the rat used for basic research into transplantation immunology will not be dealt with in detail. Such operations were performed mainly with loupe spectacles and continuous suture techniques. A useful survey is published by Medrano-Heredia et al. (1976).

Portions of rubber glove are useful as an initial suture exercise. Thereafter, the abdominal aorta of the rat, with an outer diameter of 1–1.5 mm is suitable for mastering the techniques of microvascular suture. The more advanced surgeon can operate on the femoral artery, the common carotid artery, the inferior epigastric artery of rats and may even perform free tissue transplantation of skin and subcutaneous tissue and other organs. Similar techniques can be employed in the rabbit where there are somewhat larger anatomical proportions. Especially in larger animals, all variety of free tissue transplantation utilising microvascular anastomosis can be learned and investigated.

Anaesthesia for Experimental Animals

In addition to well known ether anaesthesia, certain narcotics are suitable: Rompun (Bayer, Leverkusen) (16 mg = 0.8 ml/kg body weight) and Ketanest (Parke Davies & Co., Munich) (100 mg = 2 ml/kg body weight), given intramuscularly. The effective narcosis is in the order of 90–120 min and there follows a long after-sleep. Subsequent injections of $^1/_4$ of the initial dose can be administered every 90 min. Good anaesthesia can also be achieved with Thalamonal (Janssen Ltd., Düsseldorf) (2 ml/kg body weight) i.m. Here there is possible respiratory depression and it is important to ensure that the nostrils of the animal are freely held and observed. The duration of anaesthesia is again in the region of 90–120 min. In the rabbit, anaesthesia is achieved using 0.1 mg = 0.2 ml/kg body weight, i.m; Rompun 4 mg = 0.2 ml/kg body weight i.m; Ketanest 50–70 mg = 1.0–1.4 ml/kg body weight, i.m. The duration of anaesthesia is in the region of 30–45 min and subsequent injections of Rompun and Ketanest may be given, or alternatively Natrium Pentobarbital 30 mg/kg body weight may be given slowly intravenously. The duration of anaesthesia amounts to around 30 min and subsequent injections can be given.

The appropriate anatomical region of the anaesthetised animal is shaved and loose hairs are carefully removed. It may even be worthwhile using a desinfectant solution for careful

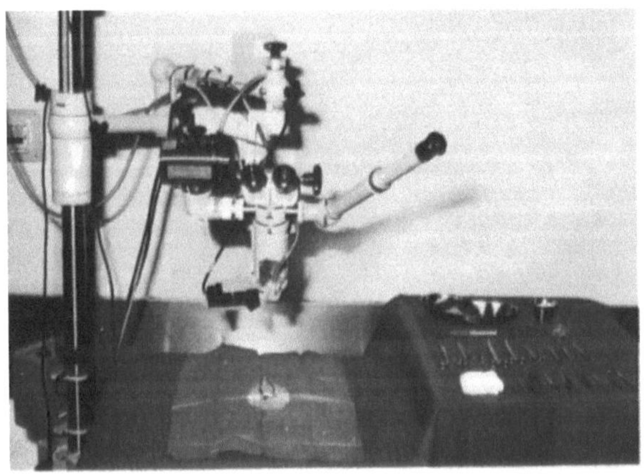

Fig. 30. Laboratory for practising microsurgical suturing techniques

cleaning of the area, since hairs in the operating field are very troublesome. The experimental animal is fixed to a cork board or a small animal operating table. The operation commences with the appropriate skin incision and presentation and exposure of the desired operating field. The soft tissue is retracted with wound-props or can be held to the side by spearing with cannulae. The operating microscope is then swung into position and a comfortable sitting position with appropriate seat height is adopted, with the forearm and hands supported on a broad surface. The preparation of individual vessels can be accomplished effortlessly, using a mixture of blunt and sharp dissection. The simplest exposure is the approach to the femoral artery. Preparation of the aorta is more difficult, since too vigorous dissection can easily tear the neighbouring vena cava which is easily damaged, resulting in profuse and often fatal bleeding. The vessels, particularly the veins of the experimental animals, are distinctly more delicate than comparable human vessels and therefore demand especially careful preparation.

IV. Suture Technique in Microvascular Surgery

1. Preliminary Remarks

Microvascular suturing has now become routine, being performed in countless centres for microvascular surgery throughout the entire world with individual modifications to certain details. The following section deals with the authors' particular technique for microvascular suture in the rat aorta; modifications and their sources will be mentioned.

Firstly, there are a few important rules which are pre-requisites for the success of a patent microvascular anastomosis:

1. A comfortable seat position and precise focussing.
2. Good exposure and visualisation with retraction of the soft tissue using holding threads. Assessment of the vessel ends and the placing of the sutures is carried out at 20–30 times magnification and the sutures knotted under 4–10 times magnification.
3. Meticulous atraumatic preparation of the vessel stumps.
4. Vessels are sufficiently exposed and only healthy, non-traumatised tissue is anastomosed.
5. Vessels of approximately the same diameter are anastomosed as for as is possible.
6. Tension at the anastomosis should be avoided.
7. Kinking and twisting of the vessel ends should be avoided, since the resulting turbulence is known to lead to thrombosis (Smith et al. 1972).
8. End-to-end anastomoses are technically simpler than end-to-side anastomoses.
9. The anastomoses should not lie in immediate proximity to bifurcations, since the resultant turbulence encourages thrombus formation (O'Brien 1977).

10. The anastomosis of a small vessel into a larger vessel should be avoided because of the resultant turbulence. By contrast, the anastomosis of a larger vessel into a smaller one does not suffer this problem (O'Brien 1977).
11. Always remove cut pieces of suture material in order to avoid confusion when tying knots.
12. Avoid crushing the vessel and damaging the intima by applying forceps only to the adventitia.

2. End-to-End Anastomosis

(see Fig. 31a–l)

The vessel is first divided or, if previously sectioned, the vessel stumps are trimmed. This can be performed in a straight or oblique fashion (Buncke and Schulz 1966; Jacobson and Katsumura 1965; Harii 1975; Nishikawa and Yonekawa 1976; O'Brien 1977).

A cutting plane at right angles to the axis of the vessel is the one most commonly used in microvascular surgery. It is usually necessary to clamp the vessel stumps, since suturing in a bloodless field without clamps can seldom be achieved.

Adventitia and periadventitial tissue, which hang into the vessel lumen and sometimes conceal the lumen are everted or removed. Sometimes a portion of adventitia is excised from the vessel stump, or the adventitia may be pulled in the direction of the vessel and then cut off level with the vessel amputation. Adventitia which is introduced into the vessel lumen by suturing leads to thrombosis at the anastomosis site (Seidenberg et al. 1958). The question of whether the adventitia should be stripped from the vessel ends, and how far distant from the site of the anastomosis this should be performed, is still not clear. Seidenberg et al. (1958), removed the adventitia totally for up to 3 mm from the proposed anastomosis. Hedberg (1962), Chase and Schwartz (1963), and Smith (1966) removed the adventitia. Acland (1973) found no evidence of thrombosis developing in small vessels after preparation of the adventitia. O'Brien (1977) nevertheless advises only the removal of the peri-adventitial tissue.

Following this preparation, the vessel ends are dilated and stretched, particularly when collapsed or constricted by spasm. In this way, one may compensate for small callibre differences. It must be stressed, however, that the intima must not be injured by this technique (Hedberg 1962). The lumen is then flushed out with heparinised Ringer lactate solution (10 E/ml). This completes the dilatation of the lumen and removes retained blood and existing blood clot. The vessel ends can now be advanced towards one another. In the experimental situation or training model, this can be achieved using a vessel approximator. In the clinical situation, the vessel ends should be sutured as they lie, without instrumental help. The anastomosis is performed using interrupted sutures tied instrumentally, since a continuous suture easily leads to a stricture. The needle holder is held in a pen-holder grip with the needle in the middle or, alternatively, in the rear half of the jaws. The needle should thereby point in the appropriate direction. This facilitates an easy tangential insertion from outside to in, through all layers of the wall. O'Brien (1977) favours a perpendicular insertion through the vessel wall since the resultant trauma is less. However, with this technique the back wall is more easily transfixed. The distance of the insertion point of the needle from the end of the vessel stump should be approximately twice the thickness of the vessel wall. The gentle curve of the needle leads the suture through the vessel wall and the needle must not be pushed deeply into the vessel lumen for fear of injuring or transfixing the back wall of the vessel.

The initial sutures should always be inserted in two steps and not in one pull through both stumps, since, by regaining the needle in the middle, it is easier to choose the site to puncture on the other stump. The opposite vessel stump can be held by micro-forceps applied to the adventitia, and the needle passed from inside to outside. The suture is carefully pulled in the direction of the vessel axis and knotted with one double throw and two counter-rotating single throws, thus securing the knot. Suturing with short threads (ca. 5 cm long) has repeatedly proved reliable, and enables the needle to be held throughout the knotting process. With the needle thus held, the suture-carrying end points medially to the knot instrument. The needle is then led upwards in a direction vertical to the microscope and back into the operating field, thus forming a favourable sling suitable for instrumental knotting. When using a long thread, the needle must be laid aside and the suture advanced through the tissue bit by bit; for the next suture, the needle must be found and retrieved.

The former technique is thus quicker and avoids possible damage to the thread. In addition, if the suture is applied with too great tension, the needle is wrenched from the suture and in fact this acts as a sign that the anastomosis is under excessive tension. The suture is tied in a lengthwise direction of the vessel in order to avoid lateral distortion of the anastomosis. The suture must not be tied too tightly, otherwise extensive media necrosis can occur at the site of the anastomosis. Judgement here, relies more on sight rather than feel. Following completion of the suture, the short end is trimmed while the other end can be left long to act as a holding thread.

The second suture is inserted into the front wall of the vessel at an angle of 120° to the first suture. This allows the back wall of the vessel to fall gently backwards when the holding sutures are distracted and prevents this wall from being easily transfixed during suturing of the front wall (asymmetric biangulation, Cobbett 1967a, b). The front wall is completed using interrupted sutures, either commencing at one end or subdividing into segments to ensure good adaptation progressively and eversion. The ends of the sutures are cut short and throughout the procedure the area is regularly flushed with heparinised Ringer's solution.

The back wall of the vessel can be prepared for suturing by turning over the vessel clips. Sometimes it is not possible to turn over the clips, due to lack of space, and then the back wall can be exposed by pulling through the holding sutures, thus turning the back wall to the front (Fig. 32u).

On occasions the back wall can be completed from both sides, using a kind of "climbing thread technique" (similar to the technique described by Fujino and Aoyagi 1975). This way, one end of the last suture is kept long and acts as a new holding thread to pull the vessel forward.

Arteries and veins are handled in a similar fashion, the only difference being the number of sutures required. Arteries with an outer diameter of 1 mm require about 8–10 sutures, whereas veins of similar diameter require only 4–6 sutures. In all cases, as few sutures as possible should be used in order to limit the degree of trauma to the vessel wall. Very fine veins with an outer diameter of under 0.5 mm are sometimes best sutured under a flowing blood stream without clamps. Although visualisation is poorer, this is compensated by the expanded lumen.

The vessel clips are removed after completion of the anastomosis, first removing the distal clamp and then the proximal one. Initially there is bleeding between the interrupted sutures and this is readily controlled by laying on, or gently pressing on a compress. In a few minutes, the anastomosis is sealed by a layer of thrombus and fibrin – this process lasts about 10 min (Acland 1973). Using the "cuffing" technique, a faster sealing of the anastomosis in arteries can be achieved, thus avoiding blood loss: a narrow strip of film is laid round the anastomosis, fastened with a clip and left "in situ" for about 3 min (McLean and Buncke 1973). This technique also reduces the number of sutures required, but is not suitable for vein anastomosis, since these anastomoses easily collapse (O'Brien 1977).

The application of fibrin plasters, which, with thrombin, bring about coagulation, can save suture material and achieve a fast sealing of the suture site (Matras 1977).

The individual steps in microvascular suturing technique are again portrayed in the following series of illustrations, showing anastomosis of the abdominal aorta in the rat, a vessel with an outer diameter of 1.5 mm.

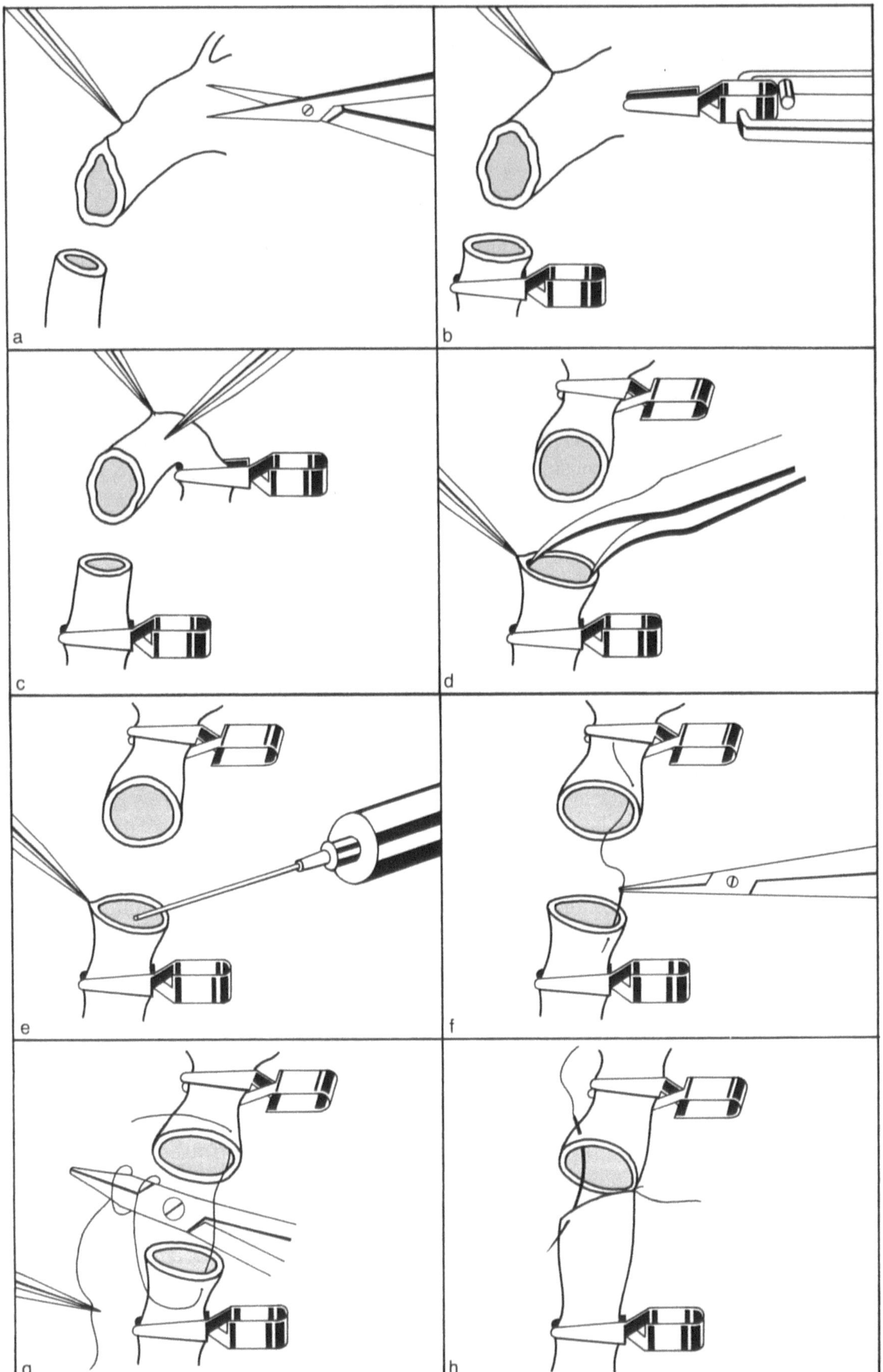
a
b
c
d
e
f
g
h

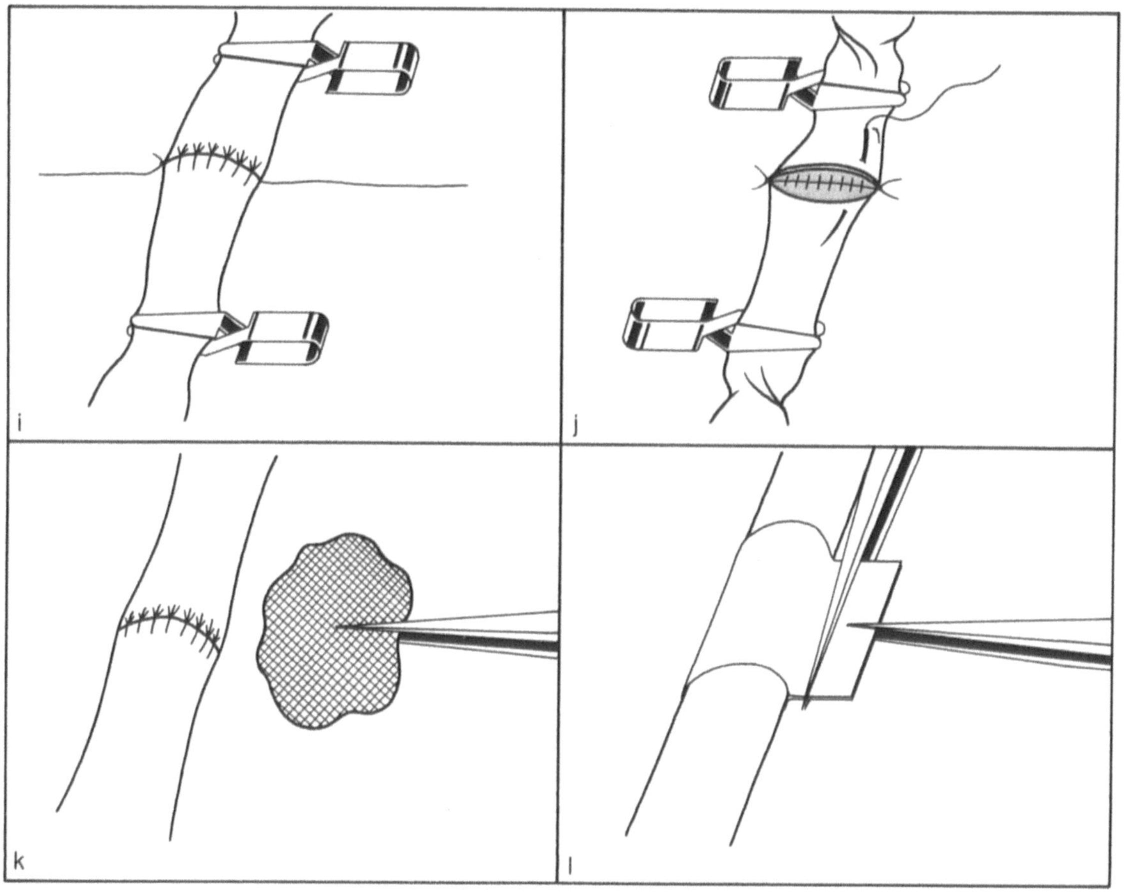

Fig. 31a–l. End-to-end anastomosis. **a** Identification and exposure of the vessel stumps. When necessary the ends are trimmed to healthy tissue. **b** Clamping of the vessel stumps as necessary. **c** Stripping of periadventitial tissue and excision of portions of adventitia, so that no adventitia hangs into the lumen. **d** Careful opening and dilating of the vessel lumen. This can be used to equilibrate small differences in calibre. **e** Removal of small blood clots by irrigating the lumen with heparinised Ringer's solution. **f** Interrupted sutures passing through all layers of the vessel wall. The sutures are inserted at a distance from the edge of the vessel stump, approximating that of the thickness of the vessel wall. **g** Instrumental tying of the suture material with 2–3 counter-rotating knots. **h** Insertion of the second suture at an angle of 120° on the anterior wall of the vessel. Where necessary, these sutures are left long as holding sutures. **i** Completion of the anterior wall with interrupted sutures. **j** Suturing of the posterior wall once the clamps and holding sutures have been turned over. **k** Removal of the clamps following completion of the anastomosis. Light pressure with a swab or a compress aids the sealing of the anastomosis. **l** Some authors sheath the anastomosis by covering it with a layer of film (McLean & Buncke 1973)

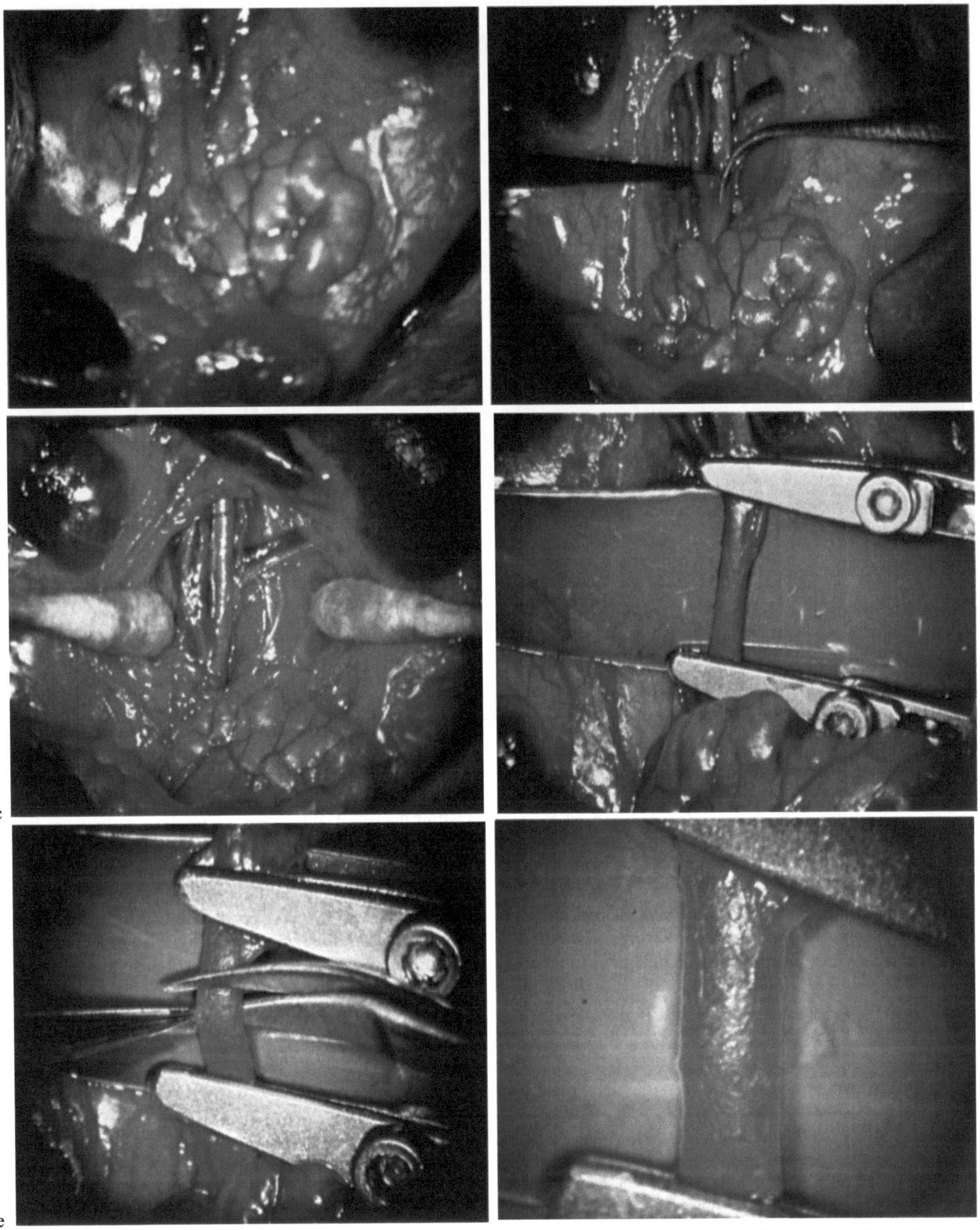

a b c d e f

Fig. 32 a–c. Low power view of the retroperitoneal structures in the rat. The loops of intenstine are held away to the right by a swab and the preparation of the aorta is performed partly using sharp, but predominantly blunt dissection using two cotton buds or swabs or forceps

Fig. 32 d–f. The aorta is carefully separated from the inferior vena cava and is held with an approximator clamp. A coloured plastic strip placed under the vessel will improve the contrast for photography. Under medium magnification, the further preparation of the vessel can be performed and the vessel divided

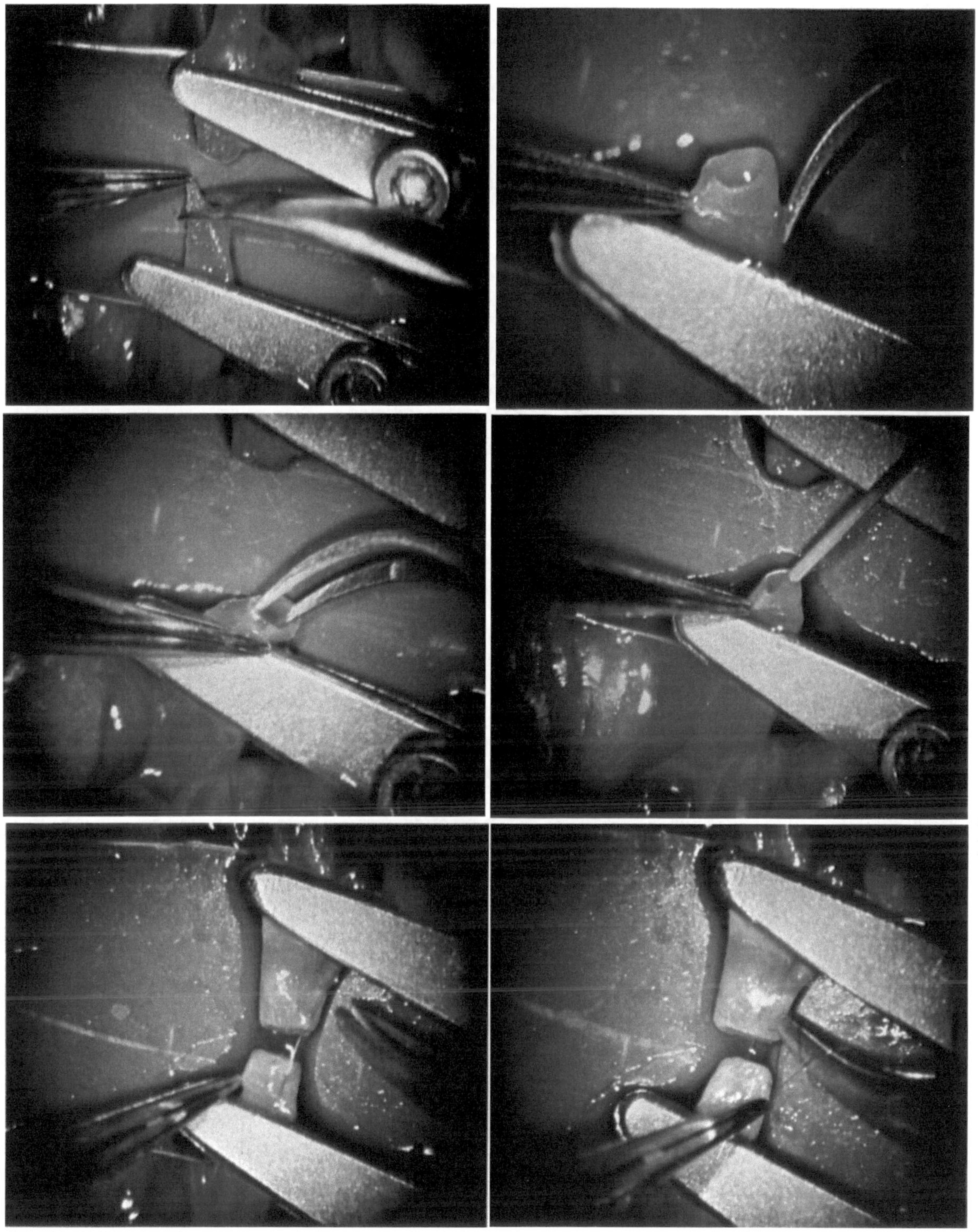

g h i j k l

Fig. 32 g–i. The vessel stumps are prepared for suturing. The adventitia is trimmed or stripped back and the collapsed lumen gently dilated

Fig. 32 j–l. The lumen is flushed out with heparinised Ringer's solution and the first suture inserted and tied, using instruments

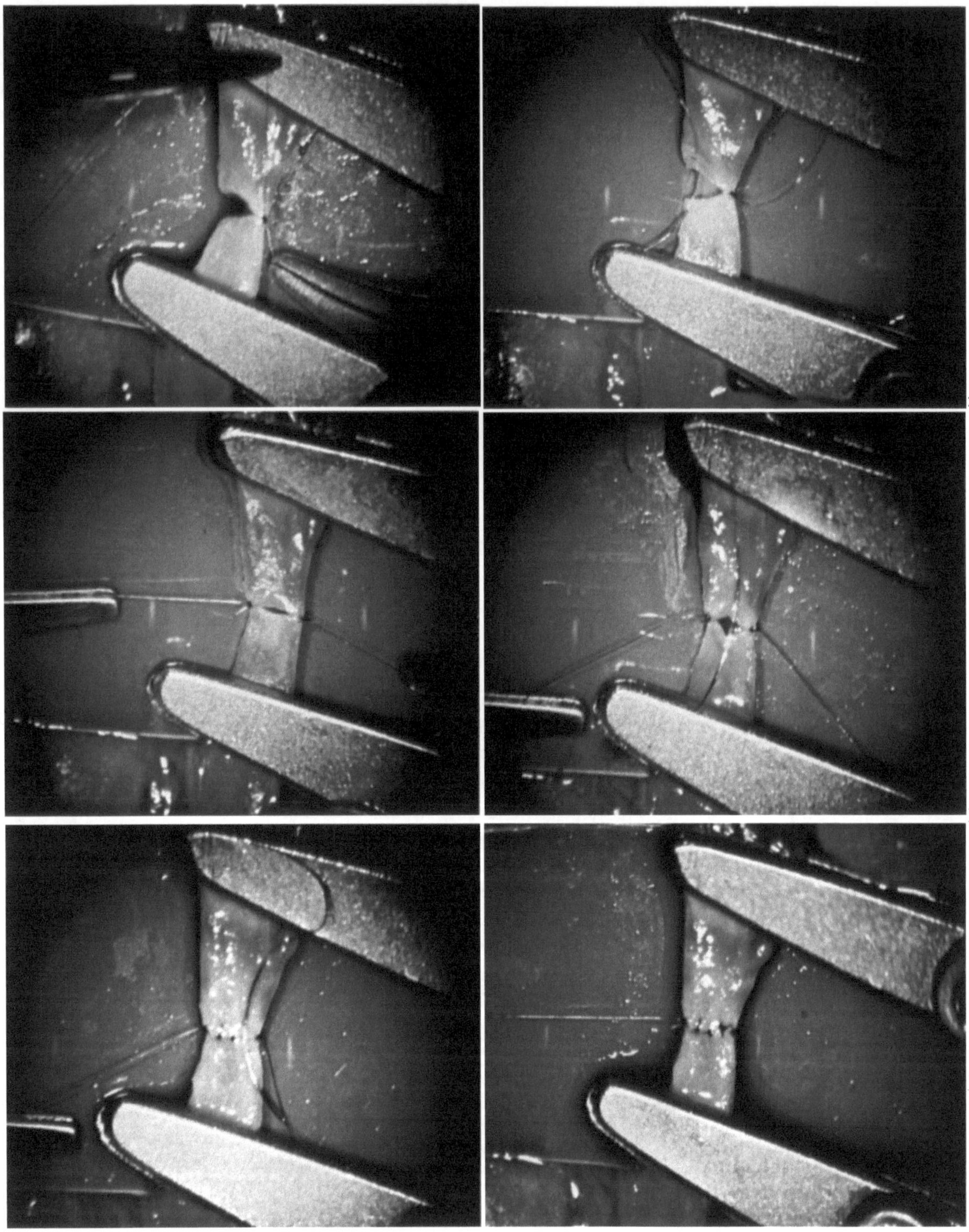

m n o p q r

Fig. 32 m–o. When tying the suture, the pull on the thread is made in a lengthwise direction of the vessel so as to avoid distortion of the anastomosis. The second suture is inserted into the anterior wall of the vessel at an angle of 120° to the first. These first two sutures can be left long and used as holding sutures, allowing easy manipulation of the anastomosis

Fig. 32 p–r. The anterior wall of the anastomosis is completed with interrupted sutures

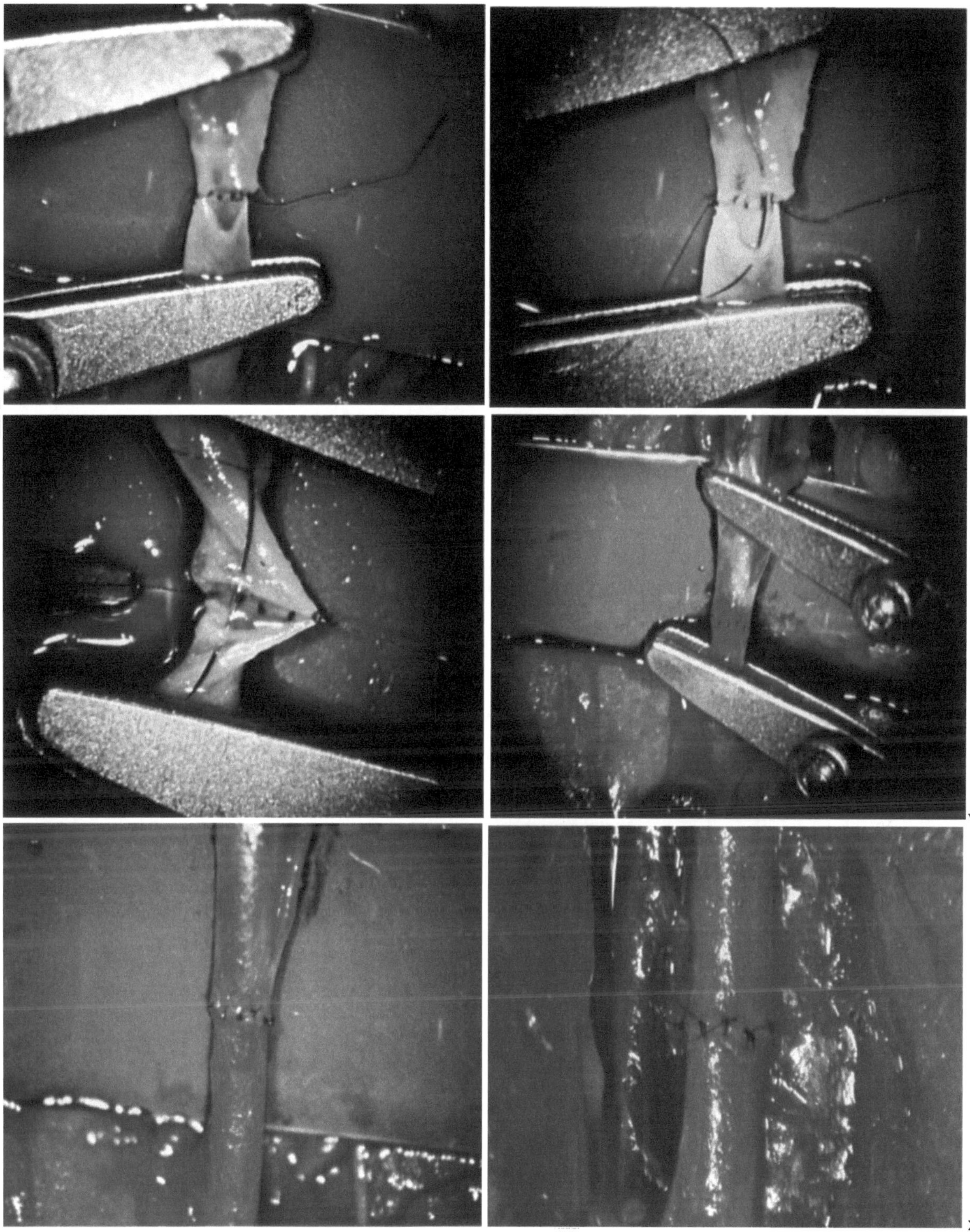

s t u v w x

Fig. 32 s–u. Following completion of the anterior suture line the entire vessel, together with the approximating clamp, is turned over so that the posterior wall can now be sutured under good vision. Sometimes the vessel clamps or approximating clamps cannot be flapped over because of the lack of space. In such cases, the anastomosis must be turned over using the holding sutures. Suturing is thus technically more difficult and it is easier to make mistakes such as distorting the anastomosis or transfixing the back wall of the vessel with a suture

Fig. 32 v–x. Following completion of the posterior suture line, the distal vessel clamp is opened first. The anastomosis is swiftly sealed by a permanent adherent thrombus and then the proximal vessel clamp can be removed to allow free blood flow

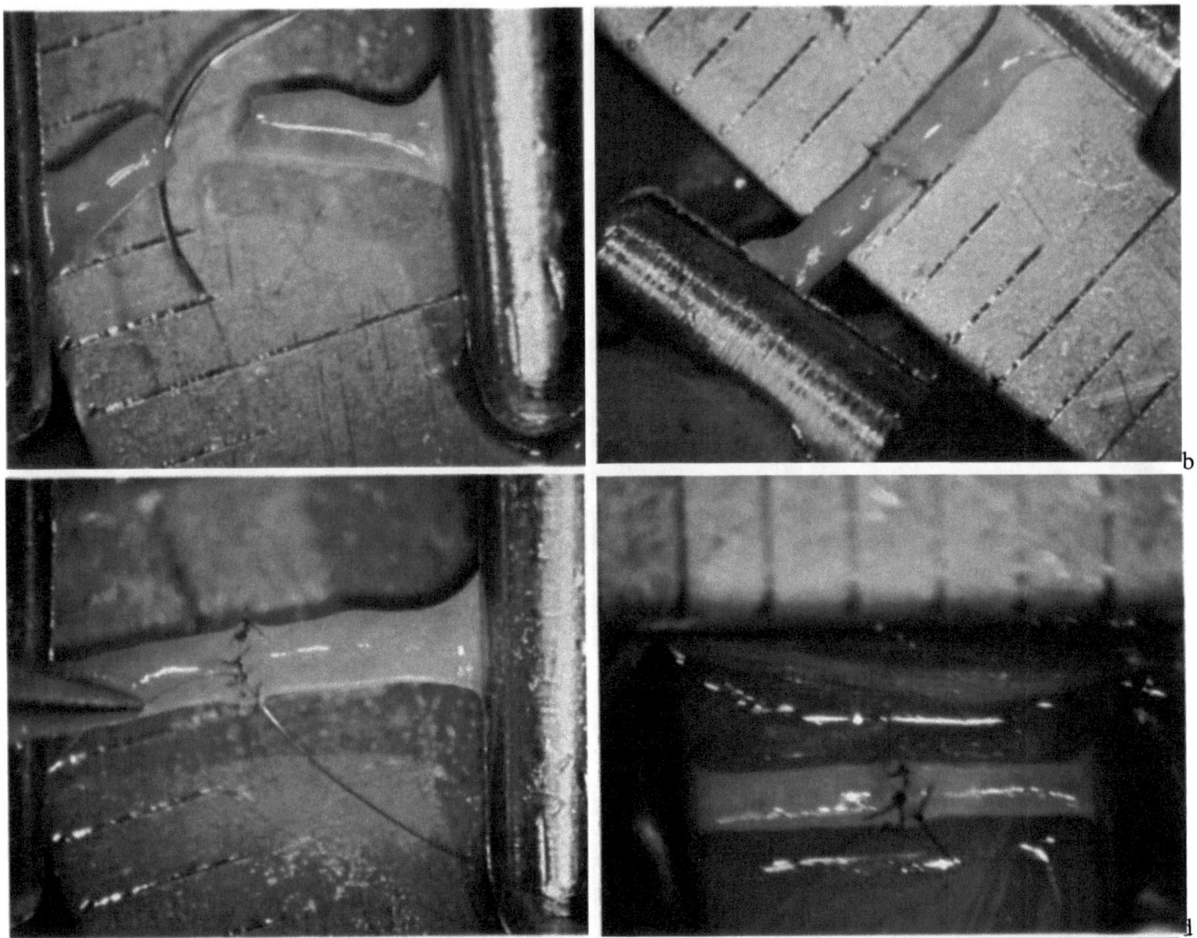

33a b c d

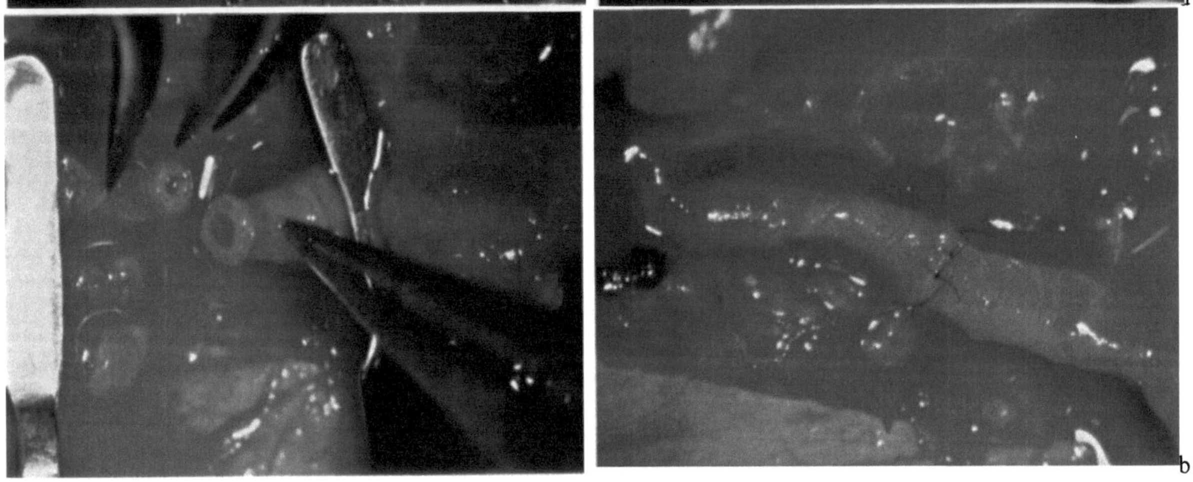

34a b

Fig. 33 a–d. Suturing of the femoral artery in the rat – an outer diameter of 0.8 mm

Fig. 34 a, b. Anastomosis of a small human artery: in contrast to the vessels in the rat, the more developed vessel wall in the human is clearly visible

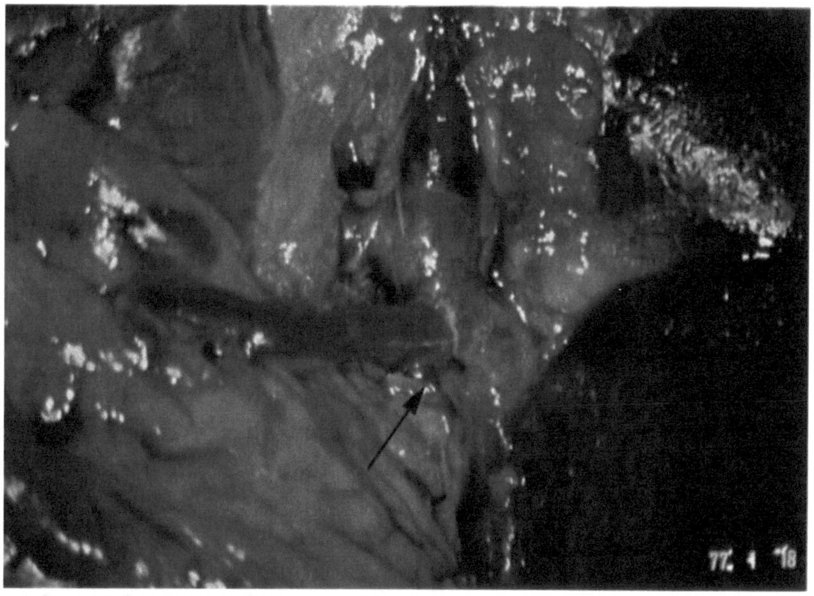

Fig. 35. Model for an end-to-side anastomosis using the carotid artery of the rat. A by-pass using a transplanted piece of femoral artery is used. Clamping of the carotid artery permits an easy check for patency of the by-pass

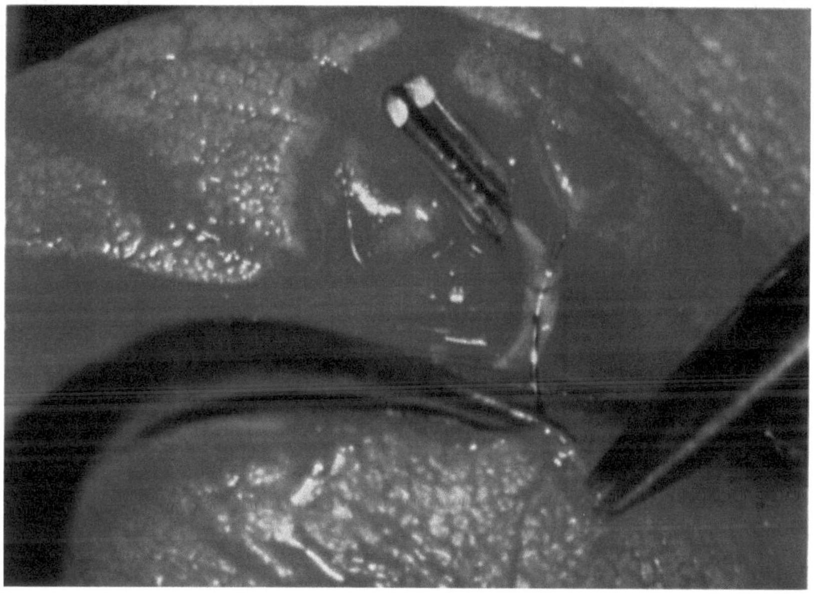

Fig. 36. End-to-side porto-caval shunt in the rat

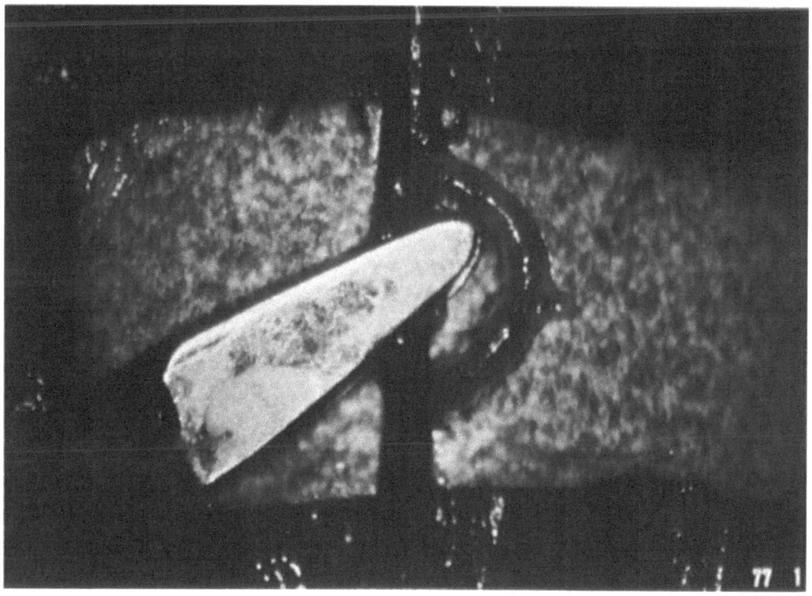

Fig. 37. Anastomosis of a digital artery in a child

3. End-to-Side Anastomosis
(see Fig. 38a–f)

In many cases the donor vessel cannot be sacrificed and the somewhat more difficult end-to-side anastomosis must be chosen. The angle of junction does not appear to influence thrombus formation (Acland 1977). To obtain a side opening in the vessel wall, which is as near as possible to the lumen of the proposed recipient vessel, the following technique has proved most useful: the needle is inserted into the wall of the donor vessel and this wall is then raised and an appropriate oval hole cut out with scissors. Popov et al. (1977) recommend a simple transverse incision which, thanks to the inherent stretching capability of the vessel, can be converted to a round hole; the anastomosis is performed using interrupted sutures. Often the entire flap can be rotated round the vessel hilum, thus turning the anastomosis so that suturing can be performed under good exposure. If this is not possible, then the back wall can be sutured with the knots on the outside and subsequently the front wall in the usual manner. To assess the patency of the lumen, it is occasionally most useful to leave the last 2 or 3 sutures untied. Similar techniques have been described by Rigg (1975a) and Nathan (1976). A beautiful practice model for end-to-side anastomosis technique is the carotid artery bypass in the rat (see Fig. 35): the femoral artery of the rat can be used as a graft. A practice model for an end-to-side vein anastomosis is the porta-caval shunt in the rat and here, because of the size of the vessel, a continuous suture may be useful.

The technique of end-to-side microvascular anastomosis is illustrated in Fig. 38a–f.

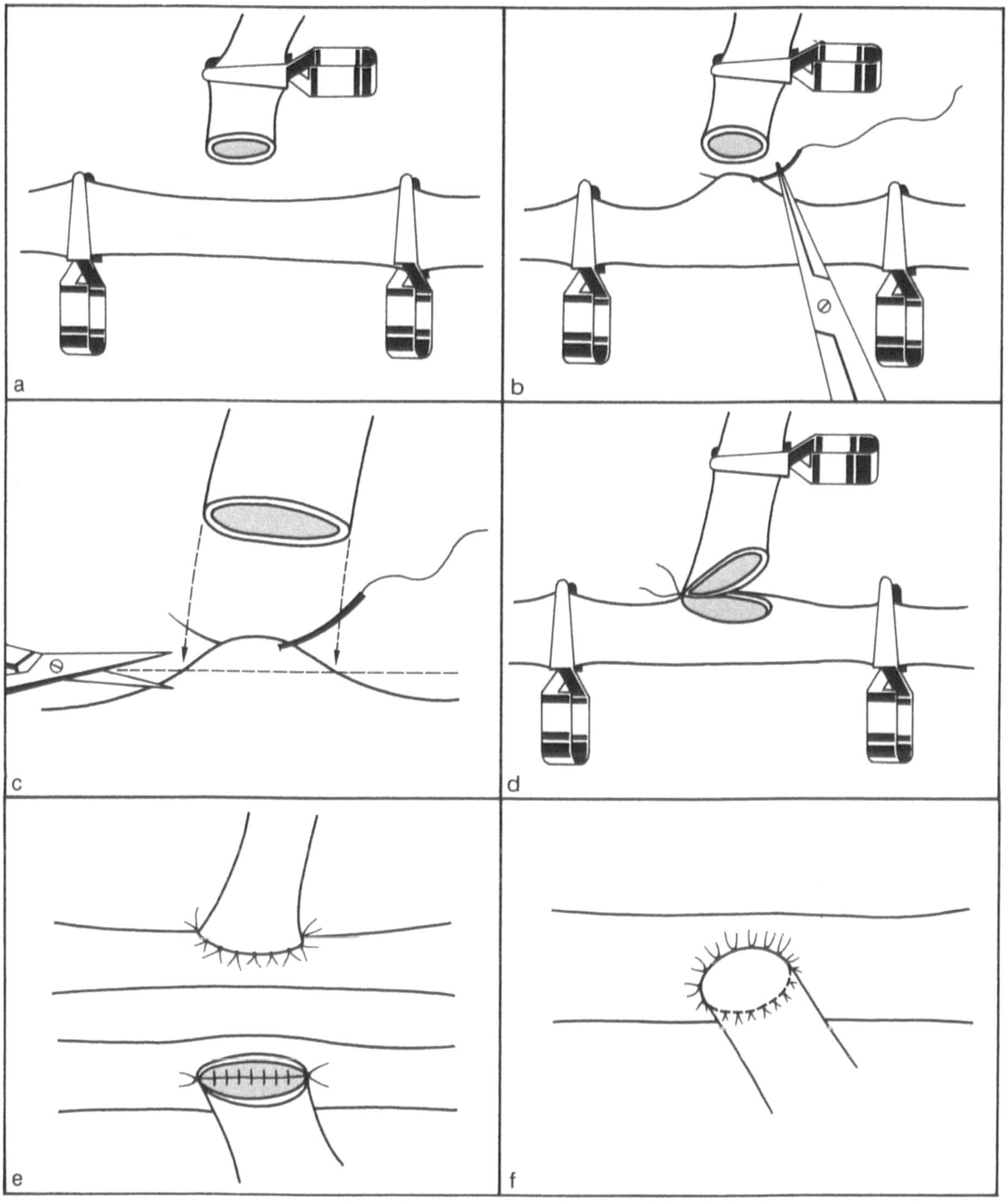

Fig. 38. a Preparation and clamping of vessels. **b** Lifting of the vessel wall by inserting the needle. **c** A segment of vessel wall is cut out with fine scissors. Either – **d** anastomosis commencing at one corner and continuing in a circular fashion using interrupted sutures or – **e** suturing the posterior wall following turning over the entire pedicle and clamps. **f** By this means the anastomosis can be completed under good vision

V. Complications of Microvascular Suture

Since, as a general rule, the entire operation depends on impeccable vessel anastomosis, when there is questionable patency, one or two sutures can be removed and the lumen inspected directly. At the site of the thrombosed suture site, a micro-thrombectomy can be performed.

1. Assessment of Microvascular Anastomosis

As previously mentioned, following the release of blood flow, a permanent thrombosis forms at the site of the anastomosis, and should be fully developed after around 10 min. Thereafter, the question is whether or not the anastomosis is patent. The blue, shiny appearance of a thrombus, the pale flaccid vessel segment and lack of bleeding from the tissue distal to the anastomosis, all point to a complete blockage of the anastomosis. A reddish coloured dilated distal vessel segment with pulsating arteries and fresh bleeding distal to the suture sites is indicative of a patent anastomosis. A thrombus can sometimes be felt by quite gentle palpation and stretching of the anastomosis with micro-forceps. Occasionally, fully unfolding the lumen may indicate patency of the anastomosis. However, successive massaging or even crushing of the suture site must be guarded against, since further trauma will lead to certain occlusion by thrombus.

2. Patency Test

O'Brien (1977) described a patency test for end-to-end anastomosis which can be modified for end-to-side anastomosis: the blood flow is occluded distal to the anastomosis by gently applying jeweller's forceps and squeezing the vessel wall. A second pair of forceps applied at this point empties the contents of the vessel in a distal direction. The vessel is then occluded distally by applying pressure to the micro-forceps and the proximal occlusive forcep is released. If the anastomosis is patent, the previously emptied segment of vessel will fill swiftly from a proximal direction.

3. Microthrombectomies

The 'milking' of thrombus material which has formed at the site of the anastomosis in a distal direction, is largely unsuccessful. Also, the opening of the thrombosed anastomosis by dividing individual sutures and expressing the thrombus almost never leads to success, since the reason for the thrombosis at the suture site lies frequently in damage to the vessel wall, especially the intima in the region of the anastomosis. This may be caused by crushing, over-dilatation or by excessive tension between the sutured vessel ends. Further causes are splitting and twisting at the suture site or inadequate microvascular suturing technique with excessive trauma or transfixation of the back wall or evertion of the adventitia with resulting constriction. In some cases, a segmental thrombosis arises in an area of vessel wall damage at some distance from the anastomosis, causing occlusion of the vessel. In such cases, if the local vessel damage is minimal, an attempt can be made to remove the thrombus via a side-branch, by means of micro-forceps or using the smallest Fogarty catheter. In nearly every occasion following a thrombectomy, the area of the anastomosis where the thrombus occurred, must be resected (Fig. 52a–c). Prior to re-anastomosis, the vessel ends should be carefully inspected.

4. Micro-vein Grafts

Frequently in microsurgery, as in vascular surgery, there is a necessity to bridge vessel defects and here, small calibre autologous vein grafts are required. Fujikawa and O'Brien (1975) investigated autologous micro-vein grafts to bridge arterial and venous vessel defects in rabbits. They found a similar throm-

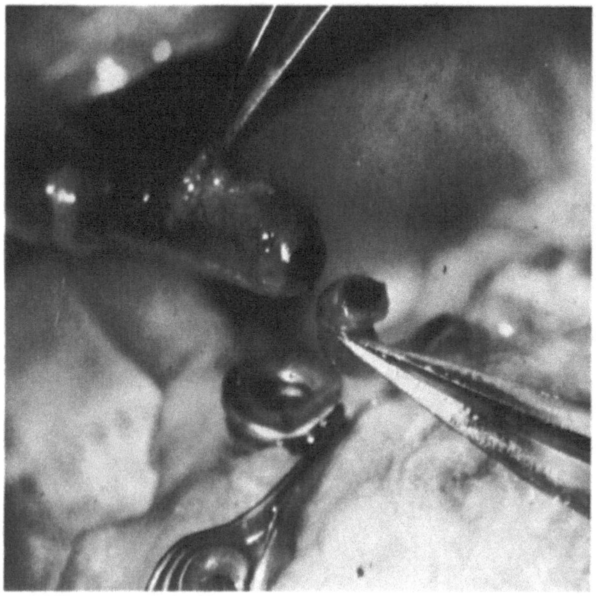

Fig. 39. Thrombosis at the site of microvascular anastomosis in a human vessel

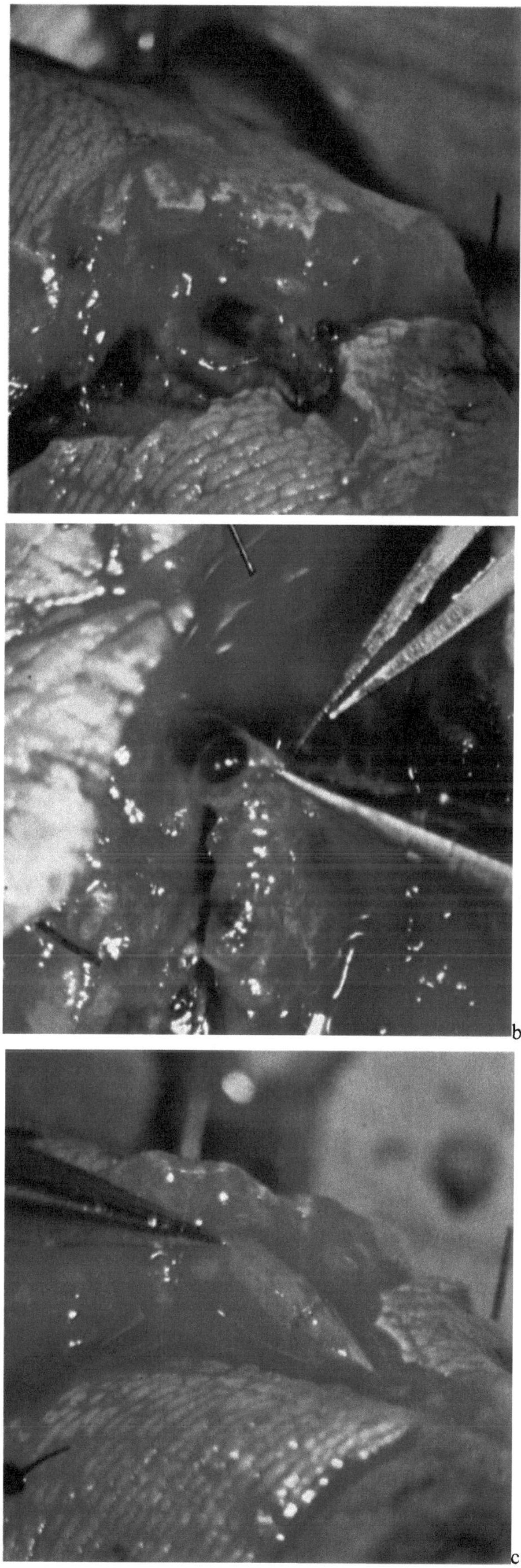

40a

b

c

Fig. 40 a–c. Thrombosis of a dorsal digital vein. The thrombus is expressed using straight micro-forceps. The vessel is then reanastomosed following resection of the previous anastomosis

41
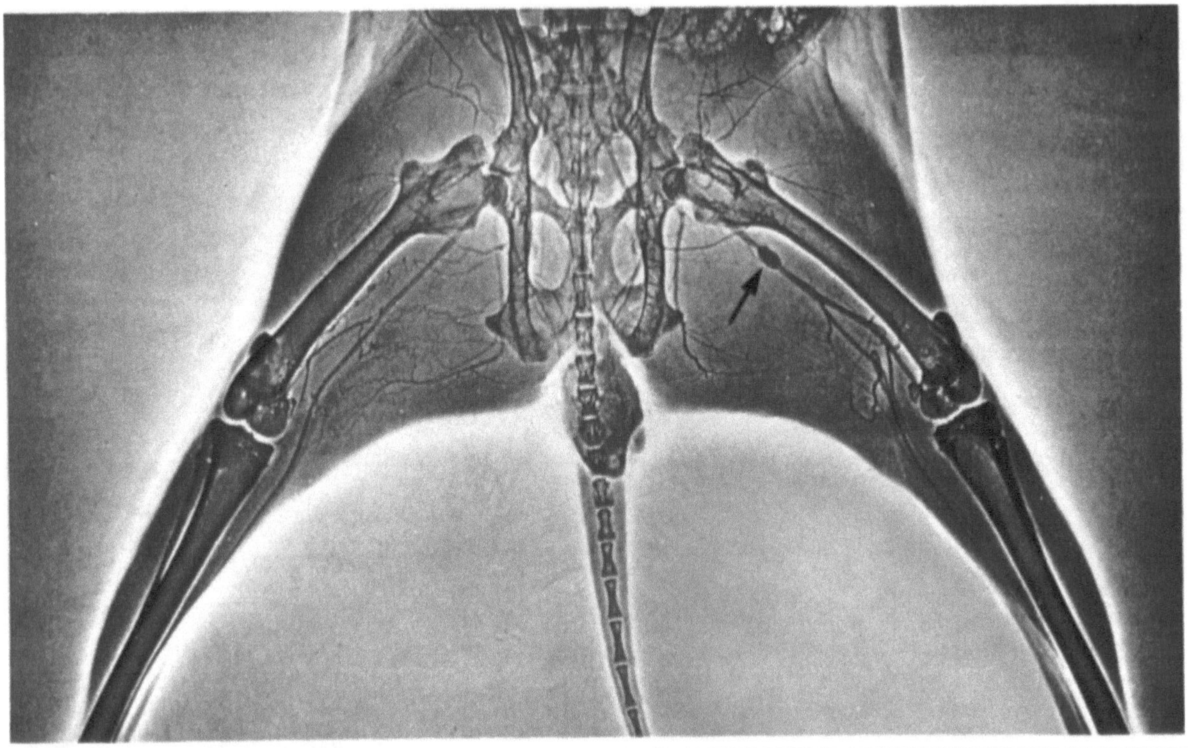

42
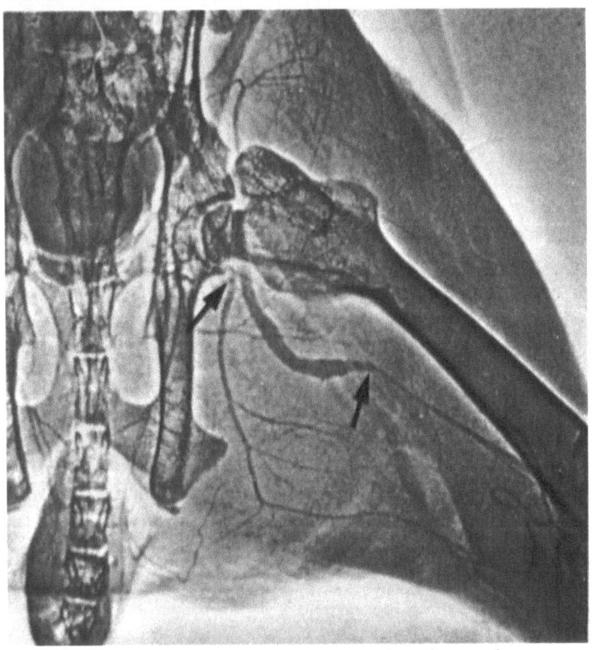

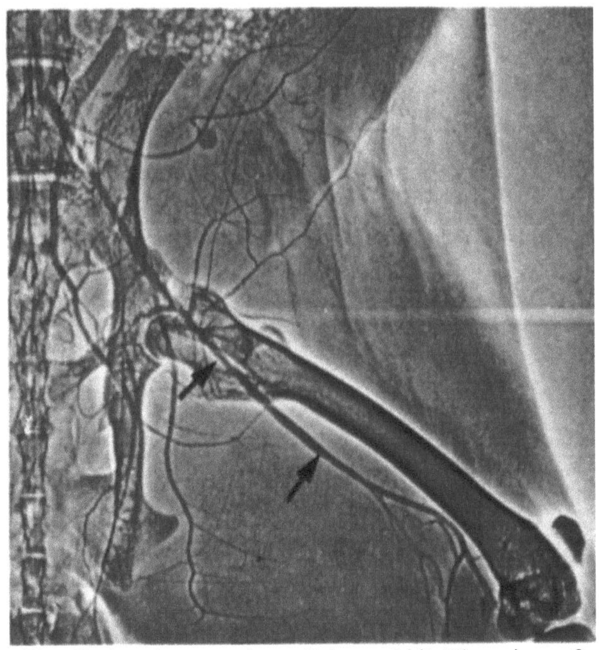
43

Fig. 41. Autologous vein graft in the left femoral artery in a rabbit. Vein graft of too large a calibre has been chosen (see arrow). (Intravenous xero-arteriography)

Fig. 42. Autologous vein graft in a rabbit. Too long a graft has been chosen (see arrow) (intravenous xero-arteriography)

Fig. 43. Autologous vein graft in a rabbit. The vein graft is of the correct length and correct calibre. The anastomoses (see arrows), are scarcely recognisable (intravenous xero-arteriography). The x-ray pictures were performed at the Institute for X-ray Diagnosis at the Clinic "Rechts der Isar" of the TU Munich (Director Prof. A. Anacker) by Dr. B. Kramann bosis rate in both groups of 10–20%, independent of the graft length. The authors' experimental investigations using autologous vein grafts in the femoral artery in rabbits, yielded the following results (Table 1).

Table 1. Results of differing lengths of vein graft in the rabbit. Grafts of femoral vein inserted into the femoral artery

	Length of graft	Patency	Thrombosis
Group A no. = 16	0.9–1.5 cm	15	1
Group B no. = 13	2.2–2.7 cm	12	1
Group C no. = 12	3.0–3.7 cm	12	0

This research was performed in collaboration with the Institute for Experimental Surgery and with the Institute for X-ray Diagnosis at the TU Munich (T.H. Holzmann, I. Wriedt-Lübbe, B. Kramann, E. Biemer, and G. Blümel 1978)

Histological examination 3 weeks after grafting showed a new interior lining, comprising a single layer of endothelial cells. There was evidence of thickening of the wall with deposition of collagen and layering of elastic threads in a longitudinal fashion. Simultaneously, there was thickening of the adventitia by the formation of new collagen. This thickening of the vessel wall after 6–8 weeks frequently totalled 10 times that of a normal wall. In about one-quarter of the grafts, calcification of the sub-endothelial layer occurred. After 8 weeks, the thickening of the wall regressed, little by little, and after 4 months totalled only 1.5 to 2 times (see Figs. 44–46). These changes in the vessel wall were independent of both the suture technique and the length of the graft: furthermore, they did not appear to influence patency.

a) Indications for Micro-vein Grafts

1. Vessel defects (arterial or venous).
2. Difficult anastomoses with short vessel stumps.
3. To by-pass bifurcations and tributaries.
4. Tension at the site of anastomosis.
5. Differing vessel calibre.

In replantation, the loss of length at the vessel ends can be accommodated mostly by shortening of the bone. This is more difficult in subtotal amputations where shortening must be limited because of retained structures. In crushing and especially in avulsion injuries, there are always vessel defects to be bridged in order to achieve re-anastomosis. In all these instances, both the arterial and venous anastomoses can be achieved using a graft. It is often necessary to perform an anastomosis using a very short vessel stump. In such cases, turning of the vessel to enable suturing of the back wall is not possible, and this produces considerable technical difficulties in managing the back wall adequately. These difficulties can be avoided by the use of a small graft, and by simply folding, not turning, the graft, the back wall of the anastomosis can be presented and completed with fewer problems. Particularly in the dorsum of the hand, there may be no opposing vein stump, due to soft tissue loss or wound debridement.

Using micro-vein grafts, it is possible to anastomose displaced vessels, or those at a distance from the vessel end. This greater variability of possible anastomosis allows the functionally most competent vessels to be anastomosed and increases the certainty of the operative procedure.

A principal rule in microsurgery is to avoid tension at the anastomosis. Such tension can appear frequently in the clinical situation, even when there is no actual loss of vessel length. It can arise where the anastomosed vessels do not lie in opposition, or where one vessel stump is held retracted by a side branch. In such situations, a short vein graft facilitates suturing and increases anastomotic patency. In addition, by avoiding tapering of the vessel, which occurs when it is pulled in a length-wise direction under too much tension, the tendency to thrombosis is reduced.

Where the segment of a vessel is destroyed by an amputation injury (e.g. tangential amputations, crushing and avulsion injuries), then vessels of differing size require to be joined. This is particularly frequent in free tissue transplantation with end-to-end anastomosis to larger vessels. The use of an oblique cut on the smaller calibre vessel rarely leads

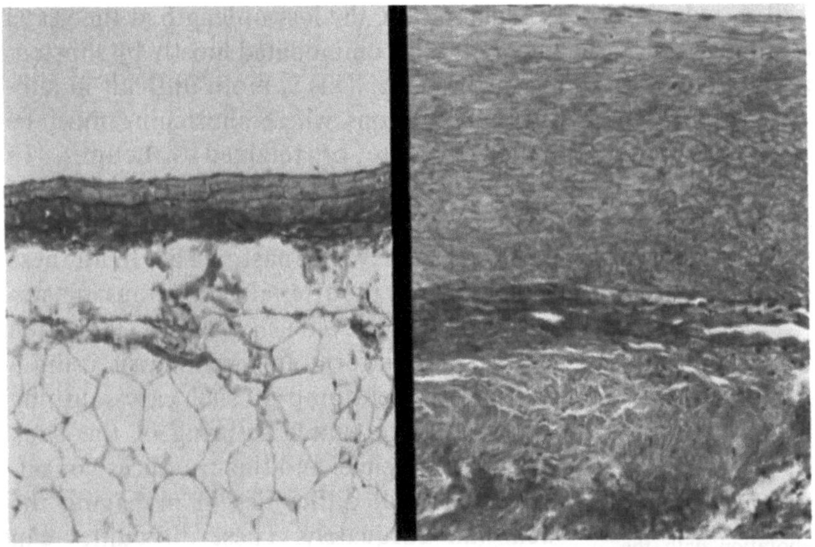

Fig. 44. Histological section of the femoral vein of the rabbit: v. – Gieson elastic stain ×47 magnification: left – normal vessel; right – 6 weeks following implantation into the femoral artery of the same animal. Increase in thickness of the vessel wall, predominantly the result of sub-endothelial thickening[2] ×10

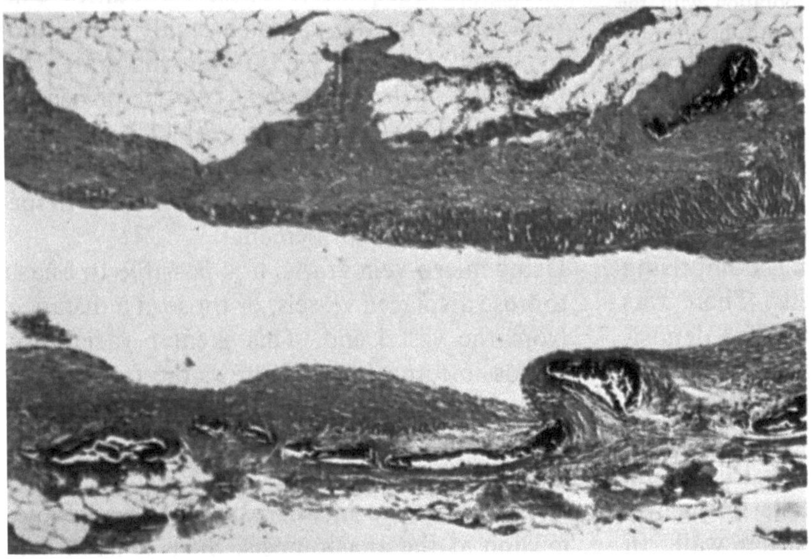

Fig. 45. Histological section through the wall of the femoral vein in the rabbit $2^1/_2$ months following implantation into the femoral artery; Kossa stain, ×18.9 magnification. Areas of calcification are clearly visible[2]

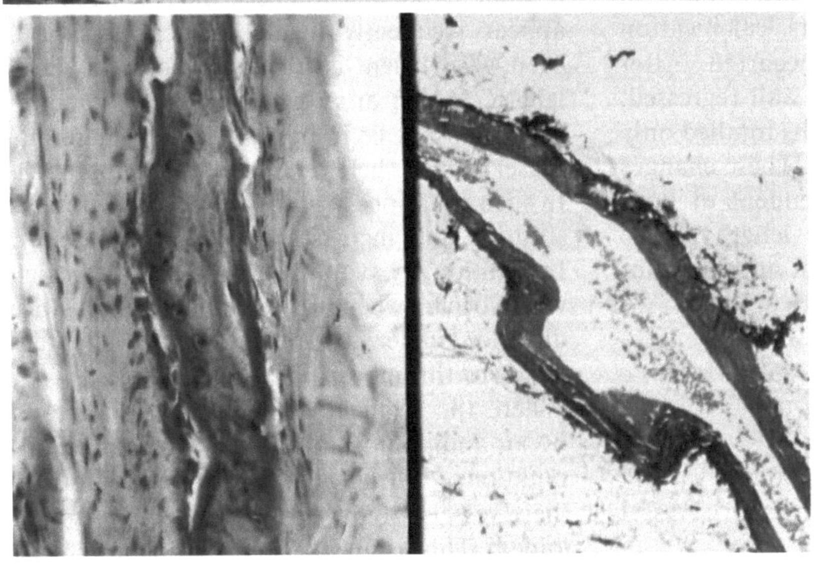

Fig. 46. Histological section through the wall of the femoral artery in the rabbit, 4 months following implantation into the femoral artery. Left – elastic stain; right – toluidin blue stain. The build-up of fibrous tissue is clearly visible[2]

2 The histological investigations were performed in the Institute for Experimental Surgery at the Clinic "Rechts der Isar" of the TU Munich (Director Prof. G. Blümel) by Dr. I. Wriedt-Lübbe

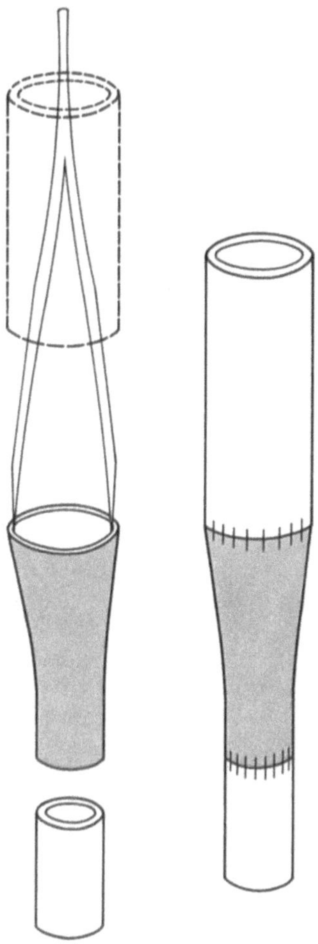

47

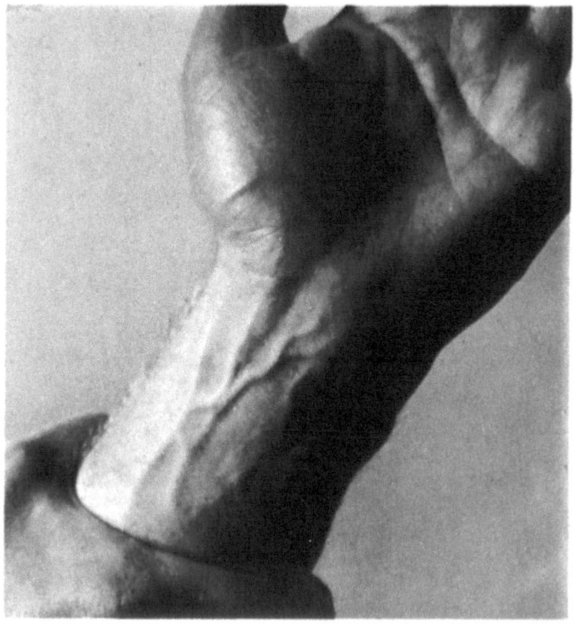

48

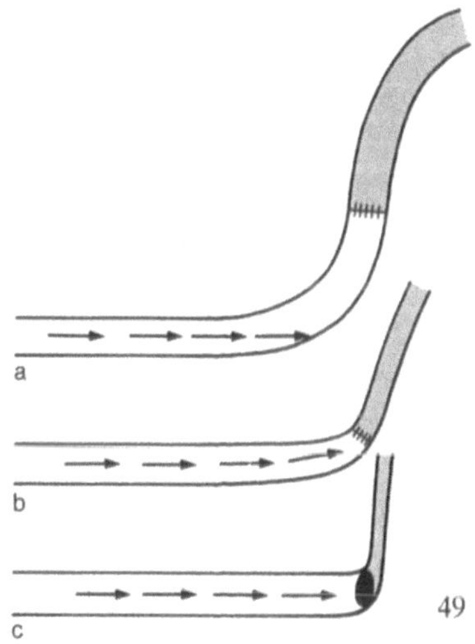

49

Fig. 47. The calibre difference between the two vessel ends can be accommodated gradually by differential dilatation of the vein graft

Fig. 48. The most suitable donor site for micro vein grafts is the volar surface of the wrist

Fig. 49 a–c. When a vein graft is used to bridge an arterial defect and is sutured at an angle, the pulse waves tend to attempt to straighten the artery, particularly when a short graft is used. This leads – **a** to a reduction in the tension in the vein graft; **b** to a reduction of the angle of junction, and **c** to thrombosis finally

to an appropriate enlargement of the vessel cross-section, and the anastomosis is more difficult to perform when compared to an end-to-end anastomosis of equal diameter vessels. In addition, the oblique cut gives rise to bending and kinking, which are unfavourable for good blood flow. Insertion of a vein graft allows more favourable conditions with an uninterrupted passage for blood flow (see Fig. 47). The greater elasticity of veins permits the gradual transition from the differing dilatation performed at both ends of the graft.

b) Donor Sites for Micro-vein Grafts

The most suitable donor site for micro-vein grafts, particularly in replantation in the hand region, is the volar side of the wrist and forearm. In this region, clearly visible and easily presented veins of the appropriate length, i.e. about 1–3 mm in diameter, can be obtained (see Fig. 48). In addition, even in obese patients, these veins lie relatively superficially and, by applying gentle pressure to the forearm, can be made to dilate and bulge out.

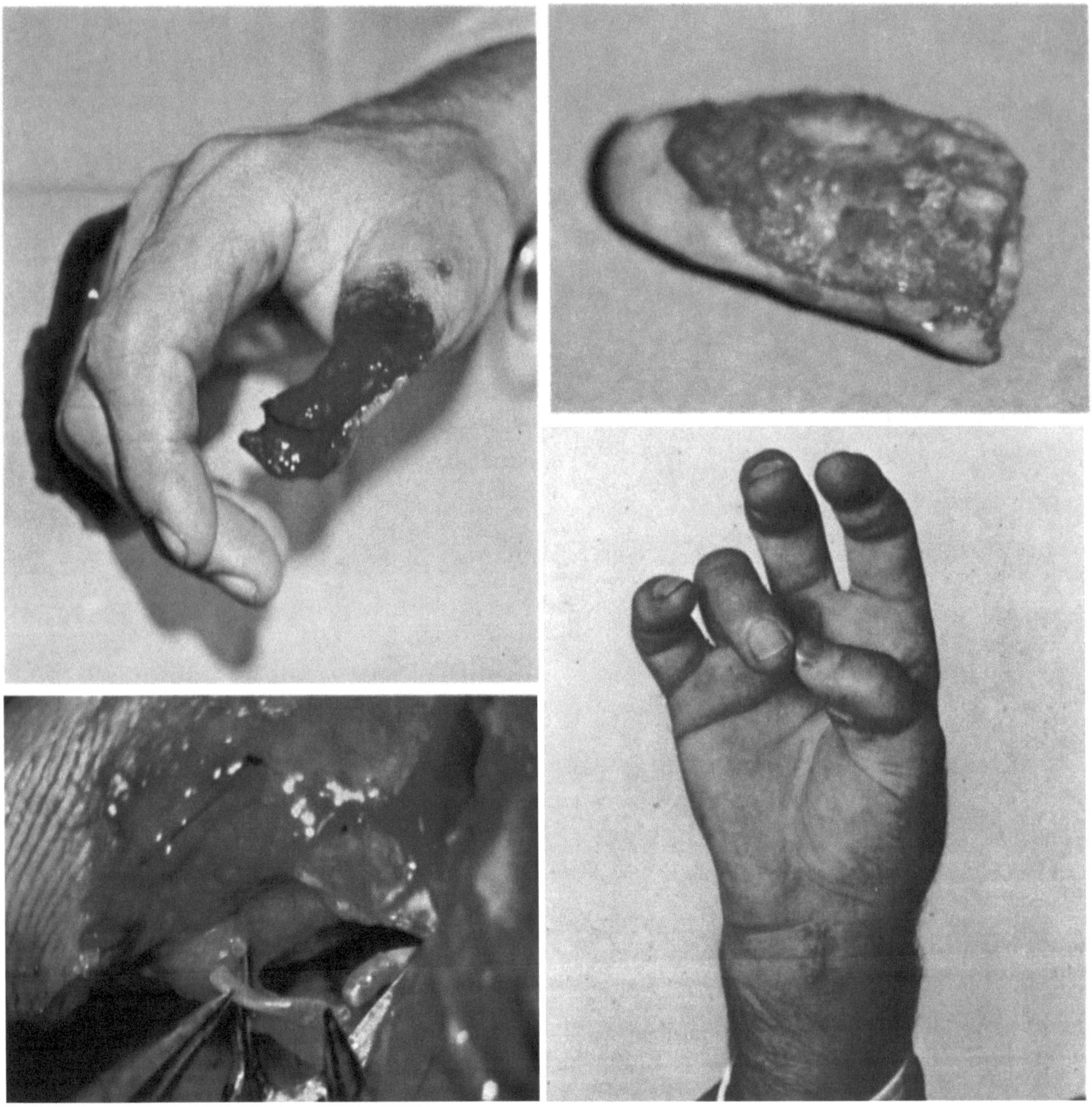

a b c d

Fig. 50a–d. Oblique total amputation of the thumb with destruction of the volar arteries. To avoid further shortening of the thumb, the vessel loss is replaced using vein grafts

Their removal does not disturb the venous drainage of the replant, which primarily proceeds via the dorsum of the hand. It is important to exactly ligate all side branches before using the vein graft, otherwise thrombosis may develop at these sites. This ligation is best performed using the microscope and 10/0 nylon suture material. The vein graft must not be traumatised and should be cleared of all surrounding tissue, otherwise subsequent atrophy of this tissue can lead to occlusion following transplantation. The graft should be kept moist with Ringer's solution, to prevent drying out.

c) Rules for Micro-vein Grafts

1. Equivalent diameter of graft.
2. Correct length of graft.
3. Removal of all surrounding tissue.
4. Precise ligation of side branches at their source.
5. Avoid right angled arterial-venous junctions (Fig. 44).

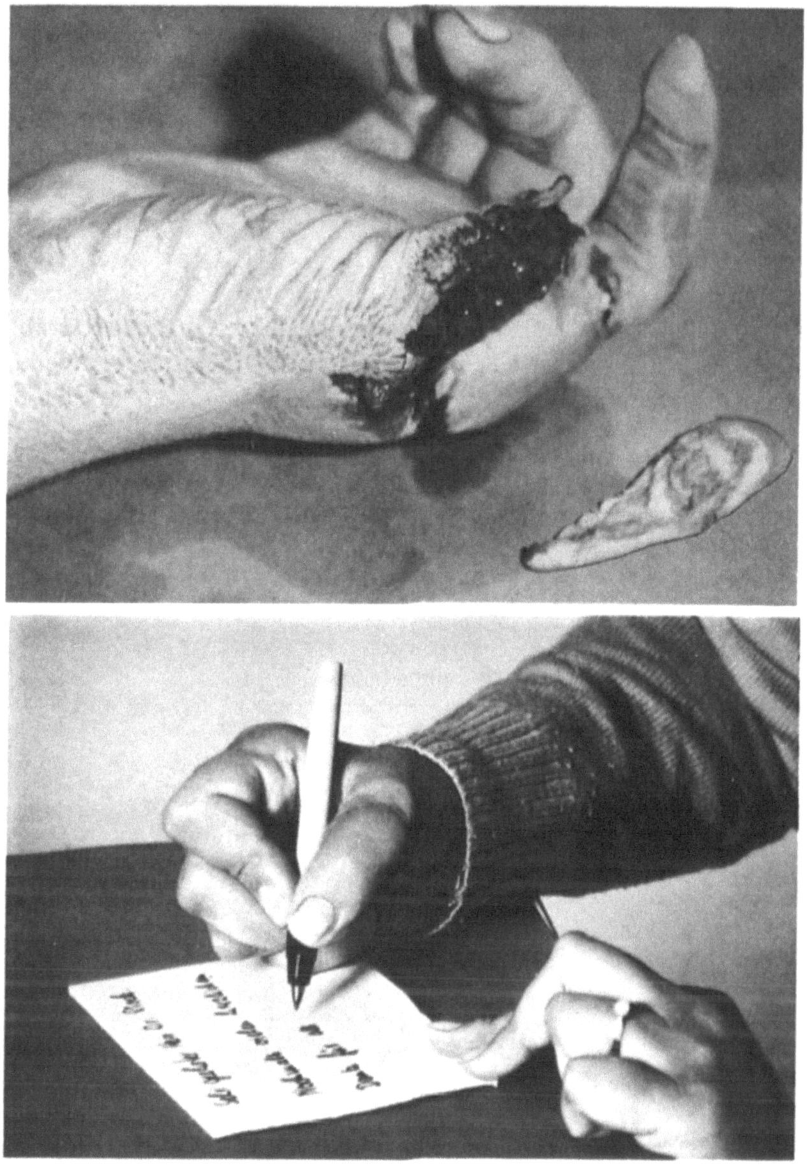

Fig. 51 a, b. Similar case to Fig. 50

a

b

It is important to estimate the dimensions of the vein in its normal position, so that a graft of the appropriate diameter can be taken, since the graft frequently collapses into a spastic state. Following relief of the spasm, a graft of too great a calibre may be "in situ", giving rise to a pseudo-aneurysmal dilatation. Twisting of the arterial stump, which can arise from the previously mentioned oblique arterial venous anastomosis, should be avoided. The aim should be to obtain a tapering vein graft which, under the pulsating pressure of blood flow, aligns itself in a straight line with the artery. The more sharp angled anastomosis gives rise to thrombus formation (see Fig. 49). The authors have been able to deal with avulsion injuries, which have the worst prognosis in replantation surgery, by the frequent use of micro-vein grafts, and thus obtain healing (O'Brien et al. 1973a; American Replantation Mission to China 1973).

In addition, because vein grafts allow the possibility of further shortening the vessel ends up to absolutely healthy tissue, early thrombosis over a fairly large area can be avoided. Certainly, the technique offers prophylaxis against later vessel occlusion. In the authors' experience, there is no necessity to use arterial grafts. Such grafts are difficult to obtain and lack distensibility and adaptability to deal with differing vessel diameters.

Follow-up examination of 38 microvascular

operations, in which one or more vein grafts were used, yielded the following results (Biemer 1977).

Successful Clinical Use of Micro-vein Grafts in 38 Cases. The most frequent clinical use for vein grafts is found in replantation surgery (see Figs. 50a–d and 51a, b).
In the microsurgical replantation service of the clinic "Rechts der Isar", one or more microvein grafts were used in approximately every fifth replantation.

Table 2

Replantations	32
Vein graft to vein (length 4–35 mm)	22 (2 thromboses)
Vein graft to artery (length 10–70 mm)	10 (0 thromboses)
Transplantations	6
Vein graft to vein (length 20–40 mm)	4 (2 thromboses)
Vein graft to artery (length 25–30 mm)	2 (1 thrombosis)

Other Types of Vessel Grafts in Microvascular Surgery

1. Dacron prostheses.
2. Lyophilised, homologous vein grafts.

The initial experimental analysis of the dacron prostheses shows a relatively high thrombosis rate after the 3rd day[3].
Lyophilised homologous vessel grafts yield more favourable results, but a definite conclusion cannot be made at this time.

3 This research was performed in collaboration with the Institute for Experimental Surgery of the Clinic "Rechts der Isar", Munich

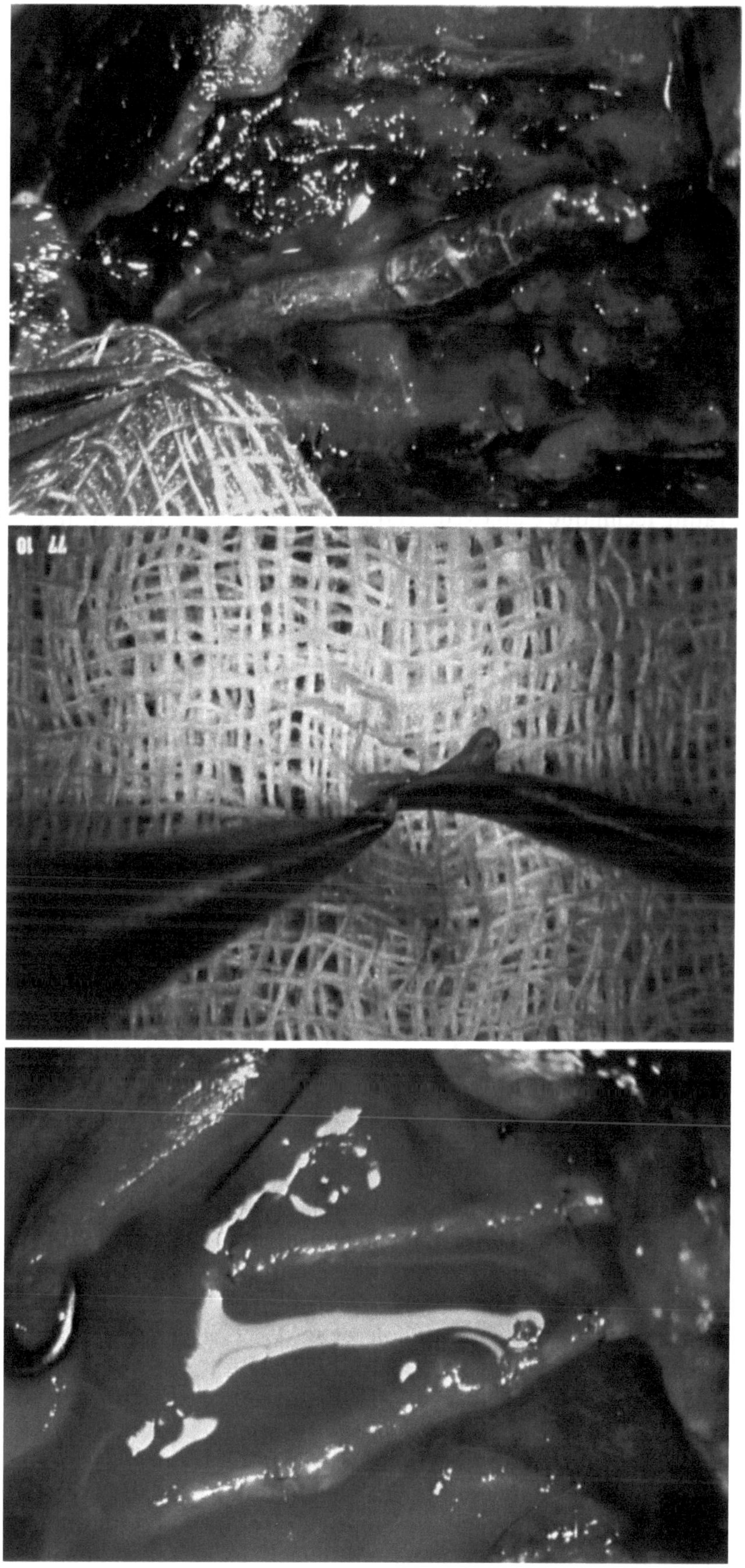

a

b

c

Fig. 52. a Thrombosed dorsal digital veins. **b** Preparation of a micro vein graft. The periadventitia is removed and side branches ligated exactly under the microscope. **c** Micro vein graft sutured in position

VI. Micromorphological Evidence at the Site of Anastomosis in Small Vessels

Following the re-establishment of blood flow, the anastomosis becomes sealed by a layer of thrombus which adheres to the vessel wall and on which fibrin accumulates. This thrombus does not enlarge if healthy vessel wall is anastomosed, and a careful atraumatic operating technique employed, so that the lumen is not narrowed or occluded significantly. Despite a careful stuture technique, vessels with an outer diameter of below 0.5 mm, particularly the very fine vein, frequently undergo occlusion by thrombus in the area of the anastomosis. O'Brien (1977), has compiled the patency rates obtained in animal experiments by different authors.

Investigation of the micromorphological appearance at the suture site at different times post-operatively, indicates the changes that occur in the tissue leading to re-endothelialisation (Baxter et al. 1972; O'Brien 1977; Murray et al. 1966; Poole et al. 1958; Buck 1961; Harashina et al. 1976).

The time required for full endothelialisation appears to vary between 1 and 4 weeks. Veins appear to require more time than arteries (O'Brien 1977; Bos 1977). The authors have found that anastomosis of the rat aorta and femoral artery have, in individual cases, shown small intima defects at 3 weeks post-operatively, whereas after 4 weeks post-operatively, the re-endothelialisation was complete (see Figs. 53–55). The origin of this "neo-intima" is not fully clear (Poole et al. 1959; Zweifach 1959; Ghani and Tibbs 1962; Nomura 1970). Harashina et al. (1976) investigated the rôle of differing sizes of sutures used in the anastomosis on the rate of patency but a correlation was not established. In addition, the suture projecting into the lumen did not have such a strong thrombogenic effect, as had been previously suggested. Nishikawa and Yonekawa (1976) investigating the healing of microveinous anastomosis, drew attention to the importance of time scale in such investigations. They showed that a recanalisation of a thrombosed anastomosis first of all occurred at 2 weeks post-operatively and that the possibility of recanalisation was more marked in veins than in arteries. O'Brien (1977), on the other hand, found no evidence of recanalisation at 2 weeks post-operatively in either arteries or veins.

Media necrosis and subintimal hyperplasia (see Figs. 53 and 56), are characteristic findings at the site of microvascular anastomoses and are evidently dependent on the degree of trauma to the vessel wall (Björkerud 1969; Lendvay and Owen 1970; O'Brien 1977; Bos 1977).

Subintimal hyperplasia is particularly pronounced in vessels of replanted digits, and here possibly the length of time of cooling of the digit may play a rôle (see Fig. 56). Scanning electron-microscopy of small vessels and microvascular anastomoses (Thurston et al. 1976; Servant et al. 1976; Duspiva and Biemer 1976; Frost and Hess 1969; O'Brien 1977; Szabo 1977), gives information on the morphological appearance of the inner surface of small vessels (see Figs. 57–61). Changes and defects caused by suturing, clamping, instruments, suture material and technical mistakes, such as bad adaptation, tears of the intima projecting into the lumen, tension of the anastomosis and stretching at the anastomosis, can all be clearly demonstrated. Also, the process of sealing of the anastomosis by adherent thrombus up to full re-endothelialisation, can be observed. Scanning electron-microscopic technique is particularly good for detecting threads of neo-intima which could project into the vessel lumen.

Fibrinolysis – Autographic Investigation of Microvascular Anastomoses (see Figs. 62–65)

Fibrin deposition and the resultant fibrin dissolution is, to a great extent, dependent on local factors and the fibrinolytic system lies at the heart of the matter, particularly localised plasminogen activator in the endothelial cells (Todd 1959, 1961, 1964; Warren 1964; Büttner and Schmidt 1972).

Fig. 53. Media necrosis in the aorta of the rat four weeks following end-to-end anastomosis (H & E × 90)

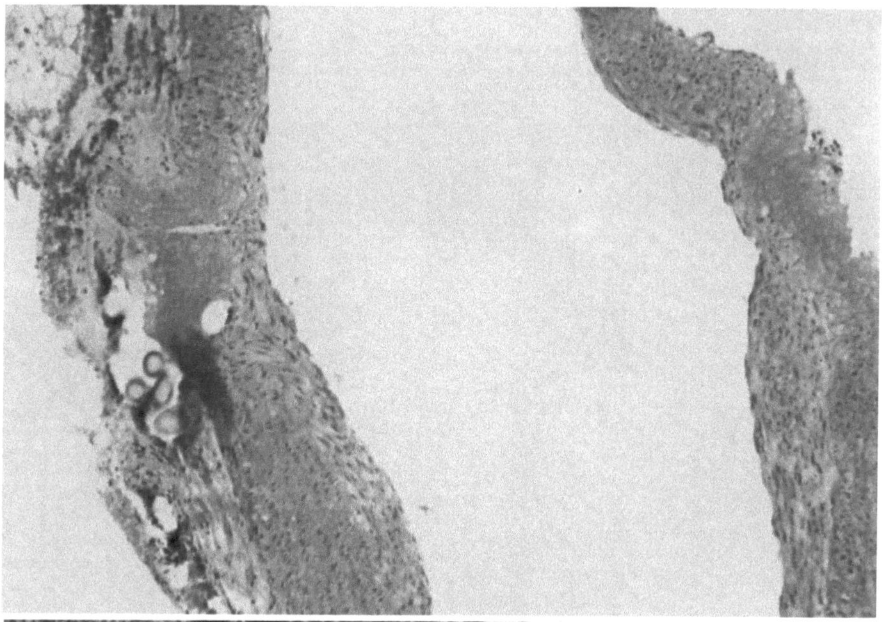

Fig. 54. Femoral artery of the rat three weeks following end-to-end anastomosis (Ladewig × 150). A small intimal defect is still present at the suture site

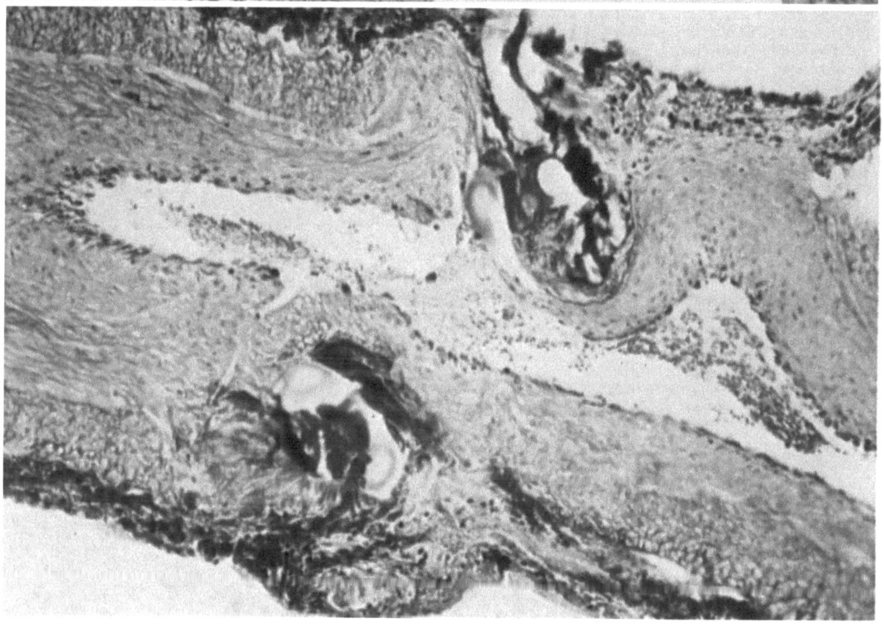

Fibrinolysis-autographs following the method of Todd (1958) were performed in 17 microvascular anastomoses in the aorta and femoral artery of the rat over a period of 1–74 days post-operatively.[4]

The quantity of plasminogen activator can be detected in the following way: – 10 μ thick cryostat slices of the tissue to be investigated are laid on slides coated with a plasminogen-holding fibrin film and incubated at 37° C for 180 minutes. During this time, the tissue plasminogen activator converts the plasminogen in the fibrin film to plasmin so that the fibrin is topographically lysed. The areas of lysis show up with H and E stain under the microscope as bright halos and can be evaluated quantitatively, according to the method of Pandolfi (1972). In the normal rat aorta, the plasminogen activator activity is predominantly in the adventitia and is relatively weak in the intima. In order to exclude a non-specif-

4 These investigations were performed in collaboration with Frau Dr. Ingrid Wriedt-Lübbe and Prof. Dr. G. Blümel at the Institute for Experimental Surgery of the TU in Munich

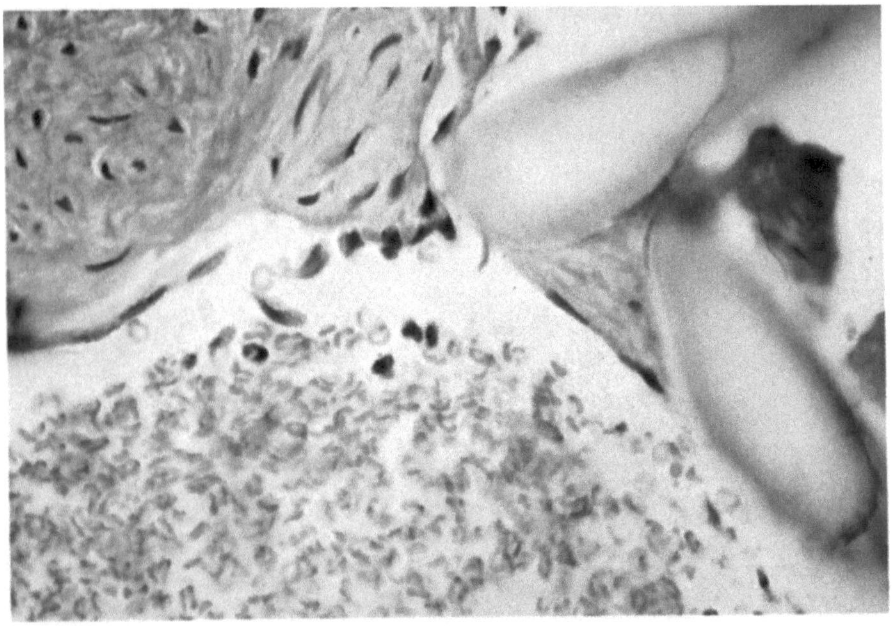

Fig. 55. Section showing subintimal hyperplasia and neointima in the femoral artery of the rat eight weeks following end-to-end anastomosis (E.V.G. × 500)

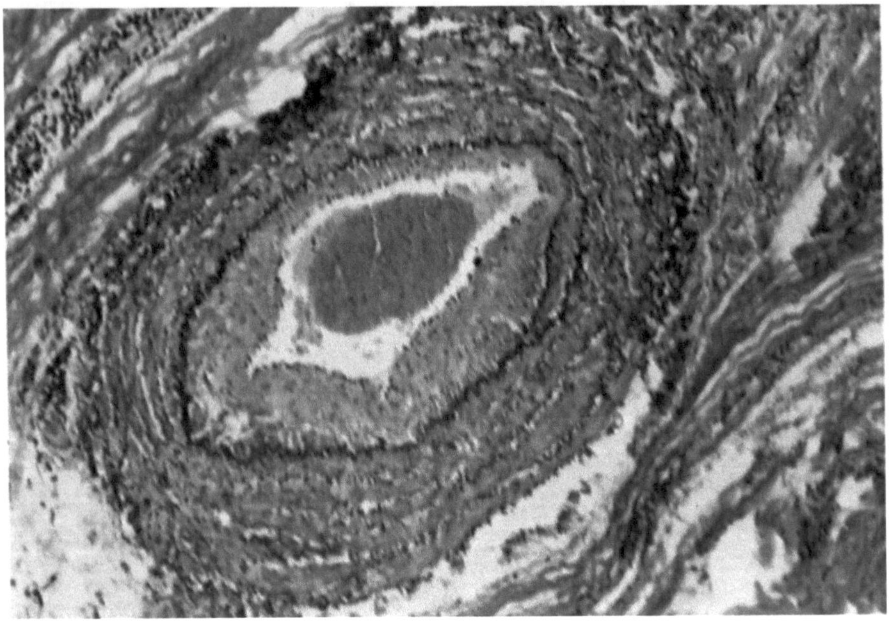

Fig. 56. Digital artery twelve weeks following replantation in a case in which amputation was performed on functional grounds. Notice the strongly developed subintimal hyperplasia. The digit was cooled for 12 h prior to arterial anastomosis (E.V.G. × 120). The authors thank Prof. W. Gossner and Priv. Doz. Dr. L. Ratkow (Institute for Pathology at the TU Munich) for this photograph

Fig. 57. Scanning electron-microscope picture of the anastomosis site in the rat aorta at the end of the operation. The anastomosis is sealed by small platelet thrombus and fibrin (× 450)

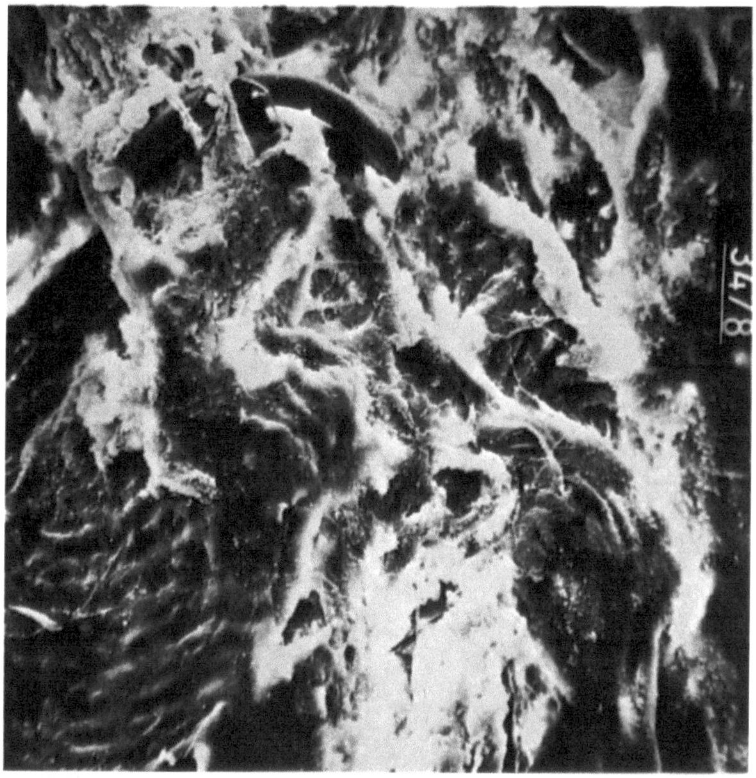

Fig. 58. The appearance of the anastomosis site in the rat aorta two days post-operatively. The anastomosis is securely sealed by permanent thrombus adherent to the vessel wall. The 10/0 nylon suture material projects into the lumen (× 450)

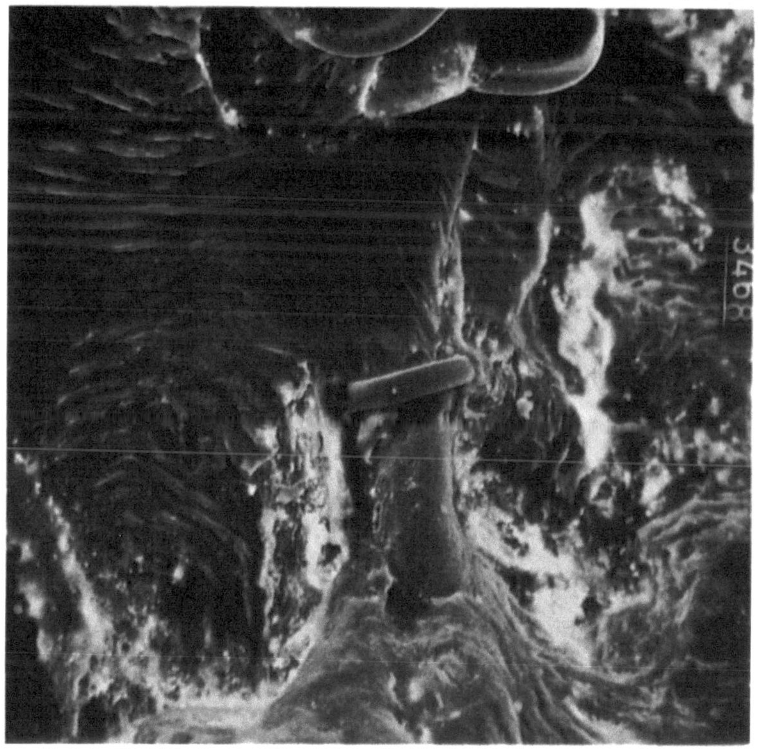

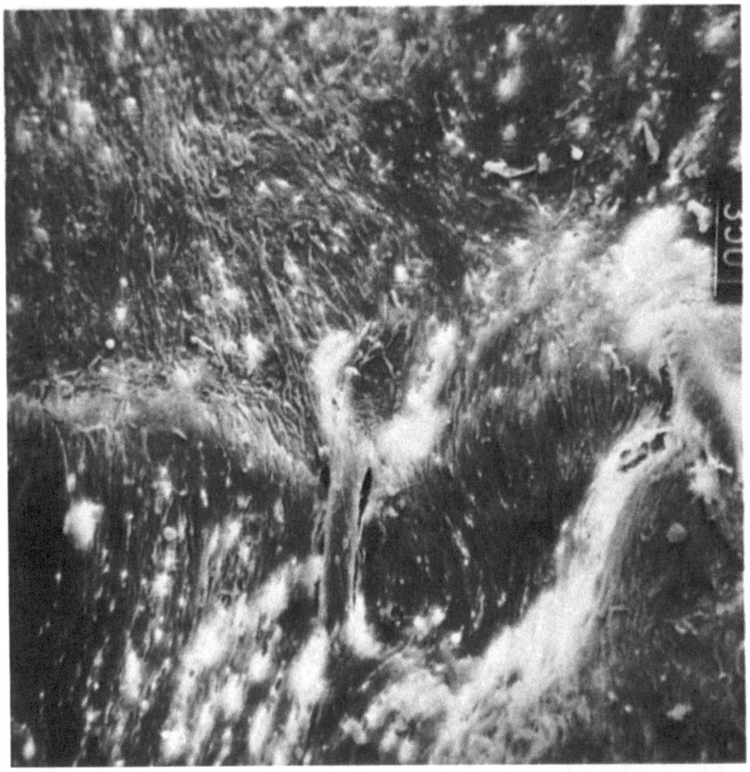

Fig. 59. Re-endothelialisation beginning at the anastomosis site in the rat aorta at two weeks post-operatively (×450)

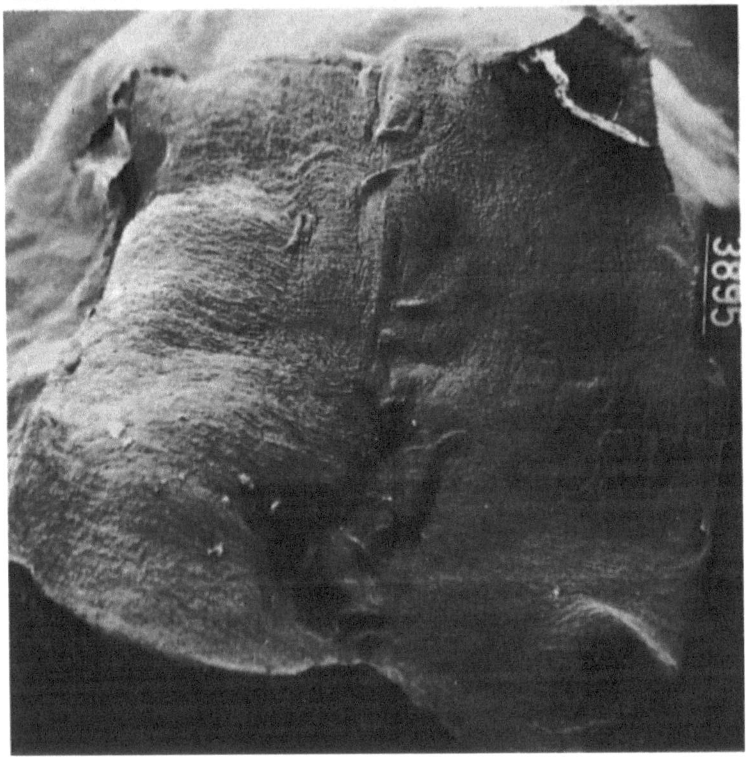

Fig. 60. Re-endothelialisation is completed at the suture site in the rat aorta at eight weeks post-operatively (×90)

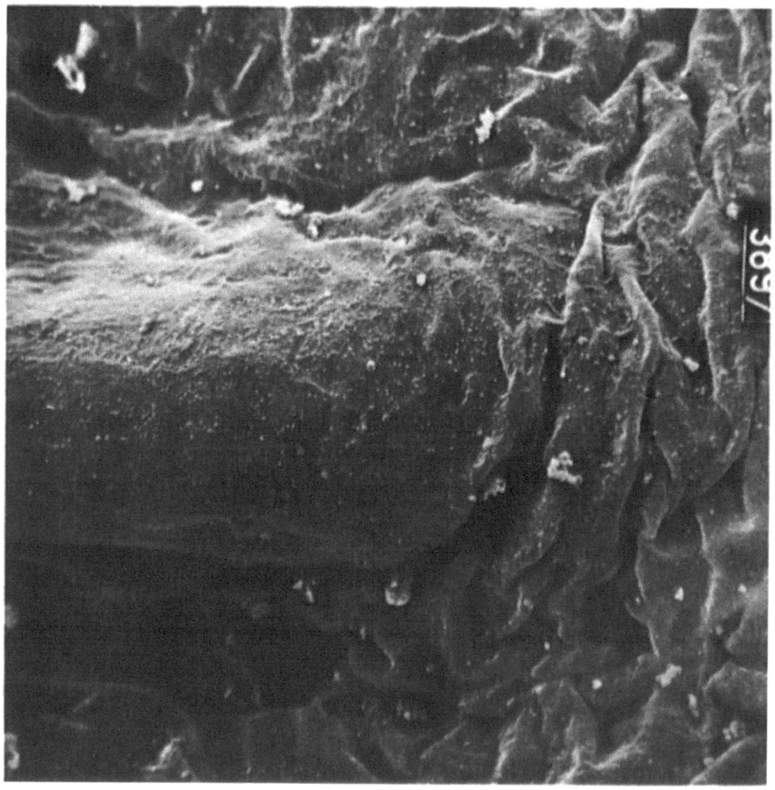

Fig. 61. Endothelium covering the 10/0 nylon suture material (section from Fig. 60)

ic proteolyse, a slice of each tissue sample was placed on a plasminogen-free fibrin film and in no case was lysis demonstrated.

At 24 hours post-operatively, plasminogen activator activity was not demonstrated in either the aorta or the femoral artery. In the initial post-operative period, thrombus on the vessel walls in the area of the anastomosis, could be demonstrated. Also, at 8 days post-operatively no fibrinolytic activity was demonstrated in the intima, although there was thrombus in the lumen. Proceeding from the adventitia, in the immediate vicinity of the suture line, a strong fibrinolytic activity was detected. The highest level of lysis was achieved at 14 days post-operatively (see Fig. 64). The great increase in activity of the plasminogen activator was restricted to the immediate vicinity of the anastomosis and was localised in both the intima and the adventitia. Sections from the remaining vessel wall and from control vessels showed analogous behaviour. After 1–$2^1/_2$ months, a raised plasminogen activity could still be demonstrated around the site of the anastomosis and the intensity of the "lysis" was only slightly reduced when compared to the results obtained after 14 days. The remaining sections from the vessel wall, with completely patent lumen, showed a normal fibrinolytic activity.

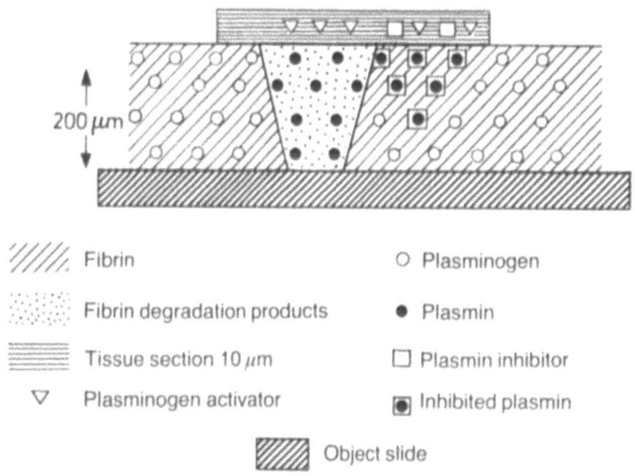

Fig. 62. Diagram of fibrinolysis autography

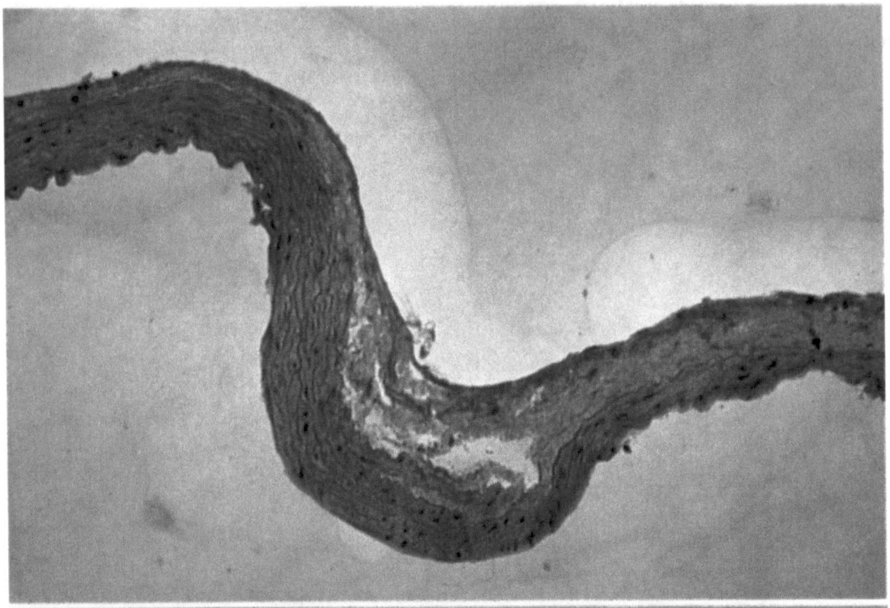

Fig. 63. Fibrinolysis autograph of the normal rat aorta. Plasminogen activator activity is found at the adventitia and it is relatively weak in the area of the intima (180 × 30)

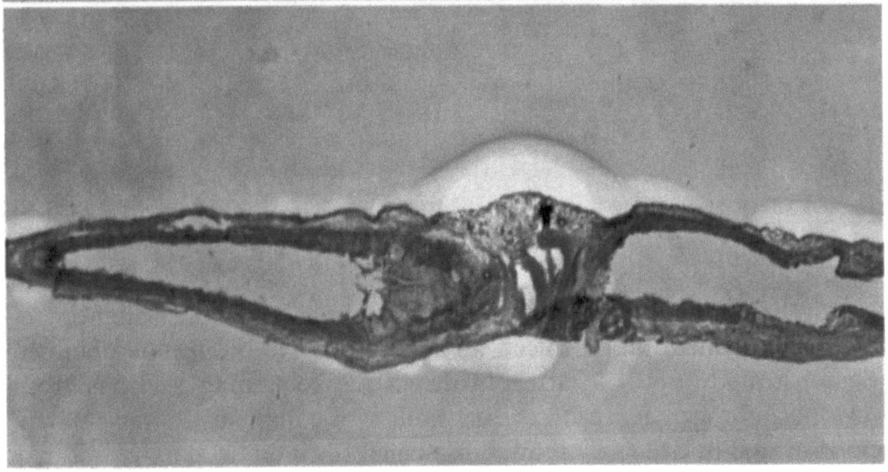

Fig. 64. Fibrinolysis autograph of the aorta of the rat ten days following microvascular suturing (180 × 25)

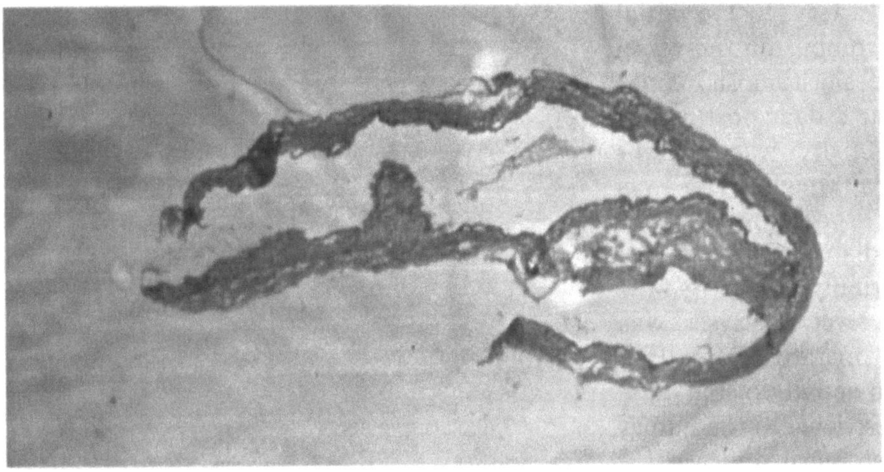

Fig. 65. Fibrinolysis autograph of the aorta of the rat $2^1/_2$ months after microvascular suturing. The increased plasminogen activator activity is clearly recognised at the suture site (180 × 25)

VII. Medical Prophylaxis and Treatment of Vessel Thrombosis and Spasm

Impeccable operating technique in the performance of a microvascular anastomosis is the best guarantee for a lasting patency of the anastomosis without using anticoagulants (O'Brien et al. 1973; Hayhurst et al. 1975; Horton et al. 1975; Duspiva et al. 1976). Attempts are made to avoid thrombosis in the vessels by the prophylactic and therapeutic doses of differing medicaments, particularly in high risk cases such as very thin vessels, vessel disproportion, traumatic or degenerative changes in the vessel wall (which have not been avoided by resection and graft interposition) as well as other complications which may arise. Such measures may be applied in a systemic or local fashion.

1. Local Measures

Acland (1972a) described the use of isotonic magnesium sulphate solution applied locally to obtain vessel dilatation and prevent thrombosis. Fujimaki et al. (1977) however, could show no improvement in the patency rate of microvascular anastomosis using this method. Elcock and Fredrickson (1972) could show no improvement in the patency rate by flushing the vessel stumps with heparinised sodium chloride solution when compared with physiological saline controls. Nevertheless, most authors use heparinised solutions in microvascular suturing since, by reducing local coagulation in the operating field, the overall view is improved. Local vessel spasm can be relieved by direct application of 1% procain, 4% papaverin (Nishikawa and Yonekawa 1976) or dipyridamol (O'Brien 1977).
Favourable results can be achieved in relieving vessel spasm by using warm physiological solutions (sodium chloride or Ringer solutions) and therefore no cold flushing liquids should be used on the vessels.
In the majority of cases, however, the relief of spasm depends mainly on the passage of time. An example of this was supported by Anderl (1977) where an operation had to be stopped because of severe vessel spasm and was subsequently completed with success the following day. The ideal uniformly successful medical treatment for the elimination of vessel spasm has not yet been developed.

2. Systemic Measures

Systemic medical treatment in microvascular surgery has 3 aims.

1. To prevent blood coagulation.
2. To inhibit the associated platelet aggregation.
3. To improve blood flow and thereby the microcirculation.

Several authors have reported increased patency rates in the experimental situation following the use of anticoagulants (Elcock and Fredrickson 1972; Kolar et al. 1973; Ketchum et al. 1974).
In replantation surgery, many authors perform heparinisation using different dosages and varying durations of treatment (O'Brien 1973; Lendvay 1973; Hayhurst et al. 1974; Duspiva and Biemer 1976; Biemer and Duspiva 1976a and b; Schmidt-Tintemann et al. 1976, Mandl et al. 1977, Ikuta 1977, Biemer et al. 1977). In contrast, in free tissue transplantation, the majority of authors do not use heparin (Harii et al. 1974; O'Brien et al. 1974; Hayhurst et al. 1975; Biemer et al. 1976; Mandl et al. 1977; Duspiva et al. 1977).
An undesirable and often serious complication is bleeding, which can even occur at a distance from the operating site (Poole and Bowen 1977). The countless experimental and clinical works on the effects of heparin on arterial and venous blood flow, will not be dealt with in greater detail here. A wide variety of dosages have been used, but a work worth reference is that of Kakkar et al. (1971).
Cumarine as an anticoagulant agent has been employed very rarely in microvascular sur-

gery. Dipyridamol[5] acts as a platelet aggregation inhibitor (Harker and Slichter 1970; Emmons et al. 1965) and thus inhibits thrombus formation (Hirsch 1965; Mayer 1973).
Scharrer (1969) and Reuter (1970) showed in their investigations that acetyl-salicylic acid[6] likewise inhibited small platelet aggregation and served as a prophylaxis against thrombosis. Acetyl-salicylic acid was released onto the market in injection form[7] and can thus be given pre- and intra-operatively by intravenous injection (Vinazzer et al. 1975; Schricker et al. 1977).
Low molecular weight dextran activates the fibrinolytic system, reduces the adhesiveness of platelets and promotes the micro-circulation (Fischer and Wimmer 1965). In animal experiments an increased survival rate of pedicle skin flaps has been shown (Olivari 1975). Close attention must be paid to the dosage instructions, since one of the side effects that has been described is that of anaphylactic reaction (Michelson 1968).
Pluronic F 68, which is a surface tension agent, lowers the blood viscosity, improves the micro-circulation and reduces the adhesiveness of platelets (Ketchum et al. 1974).
Davies (1976) described a method of sympathetic blockade to combat vessel spasm in replantation surgery. Following occlusion of the circulation with a bandage, 20 mg of guanethidine in sodium chloride solution, together with 500 units of heparin is injected into the extremity, prior to replantation of the amputated part. The individual medical measures used by the authors in their microsurgical operations, will be detailed in the following clinical section.

5 Persantin, Thomae & Co
6 Colfarit, Bayer & Co
7 Aspisol, Bayer & Co

References

Acland R (1972a) Prevention of thrombus in microvascular surgery by the use of magnesium sulphate. Br J Plast Surg 25:292

Acland R (1972b) New instruments for microsurgery. Br J Surg 59:181

Acland R (1972c) A new needle for microvascular Surgery. Surgery 71:130

Acland R (1973) Thrombus formation in microvascular surgery: an experimental study of the effects of surgical trauma. Surgery 73:766

Acland R (1974) Microvascular anastomosis: a device for holding stay sutures and a new vascular clamp. Surgery 75:185

Acland R (1975) Notes on the handling of ultrafine suture material. Surgery 77:507

Acland R (1977) Personal communication

Anderl H (1977) Diskussionsbemerkung. 8. Tagung der Vereinigung der Deutschen Plastischen Chirurgen, Erlangen. In: Geldmacher J (Hrsg) Mikrovaskuläre Chirurgie, Plastische Chirurgie, Handchirurgie. Verlag für Lehrmittel, Wissenschaft und Forschung, S 56

Androsov PJ (1956) New method of surgical treatment of blood vessel lesions. AMA Arch Surg 73:902

Aoyagi F, Fujino T, Ohshiro T (1975) Detection of small vessels for microsurgery by a doppler flow meter. Plast Reconstr Surg 55:373

Ballinger WF, Fineberg C, Giglio D (1963) Repair of small blood vessels with minimal interruption of flow. J Surg Res 3:475

Baxter TJ, O'Brien BMcC, Henderson PN, Bennet PC (1972) The histopathology of small vessels following microvascular repair. Br J Surg 59:617

Biemer E (1977) Microvenous grafts in microvascular surgery. Br J Plast Surg 30:197

Biemer E, Duspiva W (1976a) Erfolgreiche Replantation eines völlig abgetrennten Daumens. Münch Med Wochenschr 118:711

Biemer E, Duspiva W (1976b) Erfolgreiche Replantation der Mittelhand. Münch Med Wochenschr 118:473

Biemer E, Duspiva W (1976c) Free microvascular transfer of a groin flap to the scull after scalp avulsion. Chir Plast 3:277

Biemer E, Duspiva W, Hebeler W (1978a) Demonstrationsbeispiele für die Ausbildung in der Mikrochirurgie der Gefäße und Nerven. Visodata 78, München (16.–20. Jan 78), Symposion Av-Medien in der Medizin

Biemer E, Holzmann Th, Schöneich H, Wriedt-Lübbe I, Kramann B, Blümel G (1978) Gefäßersatz in der Mikrochirurgie. Wissenschaftliche Ausstellung. 95. Tagung der Deutschen Gesellschaft für Chirurgie. Langenbecks Arch Chir 347:697

Bikfalvi A, Dubecz S (1953) Observations in animal experiments with mechanised vessel suture. J Int Chir 5:481

Björkerud S (1969) Reaction of the aortic wall of the rabbit after superficial, longitudinal mechanical trauma. Virch Arch [Path Anat] 347:197

Blümel G, Gottlob R (1968) Histologische Untersuchungen an mit Alkylcyanoacrylaten behandelten Gefäßen. In: Klebstoffe in der Chirurgie. Symposium, Wien 1967. Gottlob R, Blümel G (Hrsg). Verlag der Wiener Med. Akademie, Wien, S 181

Bos KE (1977) Histopathology of microvascular anastomoses. Postgraduate course of microsurgical techniques, Maastricht (19.–21. 5. 1977)

Buck RC (1961) Intimal thickening after ligature of arteries. An electron-microscopic study. Circ Res 9:418

Buncke HJ, Schulz WP (1965) Experimental digital amputation and reimplantation. Plast Reconstr Surg 36:62

Buncke HJ, Schulz WP (1966) Total ear replantation in the rabbit utilizing micro-miniature vascular anastomoses. Br J Plast Surg 19:15

Büttner D, Schmidt FC (1972) Über die fibrinolytische Aktivität der Venenwand. VASA 1:24

Carter EL, Roth EJ (1958) Direct nonsuture coronary artery anastomosis in the dog. Ann Surg 148:212

Castroviejo R (1952) Improved needle holders. Trans Am Acad Ophthalmol Otolaryngol 56:929

Chase MD, Schwartz SI (1962) Consistent patency of 1,5 millimeter arterial anastomoses. Surg Forum 13:220

Chase MD, Schwartz SI (1963) Suture anastomosis of small arteries. Surg Gynecol Obstet 117:44

Cobbett JR (1976a) Small vessel anastomosis. Br J Plast Surg 20:16

Cobbett JR (1976) Microvascular surgery. Surg Clin North Am 47:521

Daniel RK, Taylor GI (1973) Distant transfer of an island flap by microvascular anastomosis. Plast Reconstr Surg 52:111

Daniel RK, Williams BC (1973) The free transfer of skin flaps by microvascular anastomoses. Plast Reconstr Surg 52:16

Daniel RK, Terzis JK (1977) Reconstructive microsurgery. Little Brown and Co, Boston

Davies KH (1976) Guanethidine sympathetic blockade: its value in reimplantation surgery. Br Med J I:876

Duspiva W, Biemer E (1976) Technik der Mikrogefäßchirurgie. Med Welt 27:852

Duspiva W, Biemer E (1977) Komplikationen bei der freien Gewebeübertragung mit mikrovasculären Anastomosen. Handchirurgie 9:71

Duspiva W, Blümel G, Haas S, Wriedt-Lübbe I (1977) Eine neue Methode der Anastomosierung durchtrennter peripherer Nerven. Langenbecks Arch Chir [Forum Suppl] 77:100

Elcock HW, Fredrickson JM (1972) The effect of heparine on thrombosis at microvenous anastomotic sites. Arch Otolaryngol 95:68

Emmons P, Harrisson MJG, Honour AJ, Mitchei IRH (1965) Effect of pyrimidopyrimidine-derivate and thrombusformation in the rabbit. Nature 208:255

Fischer M, Wimmer H (1965) Aktivierung des fibrinolytischen Systems durch niedermolekulares Dextran. Bibl Haematol 23:1278

Frost H, Hess H (1969) Untersuchungen zur Pathogenese der arteriellen Verschlußkrankheiten. Klin Wochenschr 47:245

Fujikawa S, O'Brien BMcC (1975) An experimental evaluation of microvenous grafts. Br J Plast Surg 28:244

Fujimaki A, O'Brien BMcC, Kurata T, Threlfall GN (1977) Microsurgical repair of 0,5 mm vessels. Zitiert nach O'Brien (1977)

Fujino T, Aoyagi F (1975) A method of successive interrupted suturing in microvascular anastomoses. Plast Reconstr Surg 55:240

Ghani AR, Tibbs DJ (1962) Role of blood borne cells in organisation of mural thrombi. Br Med J 1:1244

Goldwyn RM, Lamb DL, White WL (1963) An experimental study of large island flaps in dogs. Plast Reconstr Surg 31:528

Gonzalez EE, Nathan P (1963) A new method for anastomosing blood vessels by manual applied clips. Angiology 14:178

Hafner CD, Gogarty TJ, Cranley JJ (1963) Nonsuture anastomosis of small arteries using a tissue adhesive. Surg Gynecol Obstet 116:417

Harashina T, Fujino T, Watanabe S (1976) The intimal healing of microvascular anastomoses. Plast Reconstr Surg 58:608

Harii K, Ohmori J, Ohmori S (1974) Free deltopectoral skin flaps. Br J Plast Surg 27:231

Harii K (1975) Fundamental technique of microvascular surgery. Neurol Surg 3:889

Harker LA, Slichter SJ (1970) Studies of platelet and fibrinogen kinetics in patients with prosthetic heart valves. N Engl J Med 283:1302

Hayhurst JW, O'Brien BMcC, Ishida H, Baxter TJ (1974) Experimental digital replantation after prolonged cooling. Hand 6:134

Hayhurst JW, O'Brien BMcC (1975) An experimental study of microvascular technique, patency rates and related factors. Br J Plast Surg 28:128

Healy JE, Clark RL, Gallager HS, O'Neill P, Sheena KS (1962) Nonsuture repair of blood vessels. Ann Surg 155:817

Hedberg SE (1962) Suture anastomosis of small vessels following relief of spasm by hydrostatic pressure dilation. Ann Surg 155:51

Hirsch Y (1965) Increased platelets adhesiveness in recurrent venous thrombosis and pulmonary embolism. Br Med J II:797

Holzmann TH, Wriedt-Lübbe I, Kramann B, Biemer E, Blümel G: An experimental study of venous grafts in microvascular surgery – a functional and micromorphological investigation. Paper at 13 Congress of European Society for Surgical Research, Helsinki, May 21–24 1978

Inokuchi K (1958) A new type of vessel suturing apparatus. AMA Arch Surg 77:954

Ikuta Y (1977) Replantation surgery in the upper extremity. Handchirurgie 9:51

Jacobson JH, Suarez EI (1960) Microsurgery in small vessel anastomosis. Surg Forum 11:243

Jacobson JH, Suarez EI (1962) Microvascular surgery. Prog Cardiovasc Surg 41:220

Jacobson JH, Katsumura T (1965) Small vein reconstruction. J Cardiovasc Surg 6:157

Johns TNP (1947) A comparison of suture and nonsuture methods for the anastomosis of veins. Surg Gynecol Obstet 84:939

Kakkar VV, Field ES, Nicolaides AN, Flute PT (1971) Low doses of heparin in prevention of deep-vein thrombosis. Lancet II:669

Kalkowski H, Urbaszek W, Günther K, Splith G (1970) Experimentelle Untersuchungen mit einer nahtlosen Gefäßanastomose nach Payr. Z Exp Chir 3:16

Karkowsky J, Buncke HJ (1975) Plast Reconstr Surg 55:682

Ketchum LD, Wennen WW, Masters FW, Robinson DW (1974) Experimental use of pluronic F 68 in microvascular surgery. Plast Reconstr Surg 53:288

Kleinert HE, Kutz JE, Atasoy E, Neale HW, Serafin D (1974) Replantation of non-viable digits; 10 years experience. J Bone Joint Surg 56:1092

Kolar L, Wieberdink J, Reneman RS (1973) Anticoagulation in microvascular surgery. Europ Surg Res 5:52

Komatsu S, Tamai S (1968) Successful replantation of a completely cut-off thumb. Case Report. Plast Reconstr Surg 42:374

Krizek TJ, Tani R, Desprez JD, Kiehn CL (1965) Experimental transplantation of composite grafts by microsurgical vascular techniques. Plast Reconstr Surg 36:538

Kuderna H (1976) Klinische Anwendung der Klebung von Nervenanastomosen mit Fibrinogen. Fortschr Kiefer Gesichtschir 21:135

Lendvay PG, Owen ER (1970) Microvascular repair of completely severed digit: fate of digital vessels after six months. Med J Aust 2:818

Lendvay PG (1973) Replacement of the amputated digit. Br J Plast Surg 26:398

Littmann G, Riedel H, Jakubowski H (1975) Mitarbeitertubus und Film-(Fernseh-)Adapter für Zeiss-Operationsmikroskope. Zeiss-Informationen 75

Mandl H, Freilinger G, Holle J (1977) Mißerfolge und Komplikationen in der Mikrogefäßchirurgie. Handchirurgie 9:63

Matras H (1977) Diskussionsbemerkung. Bayer.-Niederösterreichisches Arbeitstreffen Krems (8. 10. 1977)

Matras H, Dinges HP, Lassmann H, Mammoli B (1973) Non-sutured nerve transplantation. J Maxillofac Surg 1:37

Matras H, Chiari FM, Kletter G, Dinges HP (1977) Zur Klebung kleinster Gefäße im Tierversuch. Dtsch Z Mund-Kiefer-Gesichts-Chir 1:19

Mauermayer W (1976) Die Gliederoptik in der urologischen Diagnostik und im Lehrbetrieb. Verhandlungsbericht der Deutschen Gesellschaft für Urologie 1975. Springer, Heidelberg, S 149
Mayer JE (1973) Dipyridamol and aspirine tested against an experimental model of thrombosis. Ann Surg 178:108
McLean DH, Buncke HJ (1973) Use of the saran wrap cuff in microsurgical arterial repairs. Plast Reconstr Surg 51:624
Medrano-Heredia J, Dostal G, Löbermann H (1976) Mikrogefäßchirurgie an der Ratte. Im Dienste der Chirurgie 28, Ethicon Serie
Michelson E (1968) Anaphylactic reaction to dextrans. N Engl J Med 278:552
Mozes M, Man B, Agmon M, Adar R (1963) Small vessel anastomoses. Surgery 54:609
Murray M, Schrodt GR, Berg HG (1966) Role of smooth muscles cells in healing of injured arteries. Arch Path 82:138

Nakayama K, Tamiya T, Yamanoto K, Akimoto S (1962) A simple new apparatus for small vessel anastomosis (free autograft of the sigmoid included). Surgery 52:918
Nathan HS (1976) An alternative technique for microvascular suture. Plast Reconstr Surg 58:635
Nathan HS, Nachlas MM, Salomon RD, Halpern BD, Seligman AM (1960) Non-suture closure of arterial incisions using a rapidly polymerising adhesive. Ann Surg 152:648
Nishikawa M, Yonekawa Y (1976) Microvenous anastomosis. Chir Plast 3:263
Nomura Y (1970) The ultrastructure of the pseudo-intima lining synthetic arterial grafts in the canine aorta with special reference to the origin of the endothelial cell. J Cardiovasc Surg 11:282

O'Brien BMcC (1977) Microvascular reconstructive surgery. Churchill Livingstone, Edinburgh London New York
O'Brien BMcC, Hayhurst JW (1973) Metallized microsutures and a new microneedle holder. Plast Reconstr Surg 52:673
O'Brien BMcC, Shanmugan M (1973) Experimental transfer of composite free flaps with microvascular anastomoses. Aust NZ J Surg 43:285
O'Brien BMcC, McLeod AM, Miller GDH, Newing RK, Hayhurst JW, Morrison WA (1973a) Clinical replantation of digits. Plast Reconstr Surg 52:490
O'Brien BMcC, McLeod AM, Hayhurst JW, Morrison WA (1973b) Successful transfer of a large island flap from the groin to the foot by microvascular anastomoses. Plast Reconstr Surg 52:271
O'Brien BMcC, Morrison WA, Ishida H, McLeod AM, Gilbert A (1974) Free flap transfers with microvascular anastomoses Brit J Plast Surg 27:220
O'Brien JR, Butterfield WV (1973) Aspirin in the prevention of thrombosis. Am Heart J 86:711
Olivari N (1975) Beeinflussung der Lappendurchblutung und Nekroserate nach Verschiebeschwenkplastiken durch Pentoxiphyllin und Dextran 40. Med Welt 26:1973
Östrup LT (1976) Anastomosis of small veins with suture of Nakayama's apparatus. Scand J Plast Reconstr Surg 10:9

Padula RT, Ballinger WF (1965) A new clamp for rapid vascular anastomosis. Surgery 57:819
Pandolfi M, Bjernstad A, Nilsson IM (1972) Technical remarks on the microscopical demonstration of tissue plasminogen-activator. Thrombos Diathes Hemorrh 27:88
Parel JM, O'Brien BMcC, Crock GW, Henderson PN, Galbraith, JEK (1970) Prototypal electro-microsurgical instruments. Med J Aust 1:709
Pearl RM, Wustrack KO, Harbury Ch, Rubenstein E, Kaplan EN (1977) Microvascular anastomosis using a blood product sealant adhesive. Surg Gynecol Obstet 144:227
Phelan JT, Young WP, Gale JW (1958) The effect of suture material on small artery anastomoses. Surg Gynecol Obstet 107:79
Piza-Katzer H (1974) Mikrochirurgische Technik bei Gefäßen mit einem Durchmesser unter 1,2 mm (homologe Aortentransplantation). VASA 3:293
Poole JCF, Sanders AG, Florey HW (1958) The regeneration of aortic endothelium. J Path Bact 75:133
Poole JCF, Sanders AG, Florey HW (1959) Further observations on the regeneration of aortic endothelium in the rabbit. J Path Bact 77:637
Poole MD, Bowen JE (1977) Two unusual bleedings during anticoagulation following digital replantation. Br J Plast Surg 30:267
Popov DG, Trichkova PI (1977) A new technique for end-to-side-anastomoses in microvascular surgery. Plast Reconstr Surg 59:444

Reuter H (1970) Hemmung der Plättchenaggregation durch Acetylsalicylsäure. Dtsch Med Wochenschr 95:14
Rigg BM (1975a) Transfer of a free groin flap to the heel by microvascular surgery. Plast Reconstr Surg 55:36
Rigg BM (1975b) A micro-irrigator. Plast Reconstr Surg 56:349

Salmon PA, Assimacopoulos CA (1964) A pneumatic needle holder suitable for microsurgical procedures. Surgery 5:446
Salyer KE, Kyger ER (1973) Studies in rats of survival of composite homotransplants of skin and subcutaneous tissue with microvascular anastomoses. Plast Reconstr Surg 51:672
Samuels PB (1955) Method of blood vessel anastomosis by means of metal clips. AMA Arch Surg 70:29
Scharrer J (1969) Thromboseprophylaxe mit Aspirin. Der Einfluß von Acetylsalicylsäure auf die Thrombozytenaggregation in vitro und in vivo. Klin Wochenschr 47:1318
Schmidt-Tintemann U, Biemer E, Duspiva W (1976) Replantation abgetrennter Finger, Daumen und Hände durch Mikrochirurgie. Dtsch Ärztebl 73:1367

Schricker KTh, Raithel D, Juchelka L (1977) Einfluß von Aspisol auf die Plättchenfunktion bei gefäß-chirurgischen Eingriffen. Münch Med Wochenschr 119:961
Scoville WB (1966) Miniature torsion bar spring clip. J Neurosurg 25:97
Seidenberg B, Hurwitt ES, Carton C (1958) The technique of anastomosing small arteries. Surg Gynecol Obstet 106:743
Servant JM, Ikuta Y, Harada Y (1976) A scanning electron microscope study of microvascular anastomoses. Plast Reconstr Surg 57:329
Sigel B, Acevedo FJ (1963) Electro-coaptive union of blood vessels. A preliminary experimental study. J Surg Res 3:90
Smith JW (1966) Microsurgery review of the literature and discussion of microtechniques. Plast Reconstr Surg 37:207
Smith RL, Blick EF, Coalson J, Stein PD (1972) Thrombus production by turbulence. J Appl Physiol 32:261
Sterling JA (1964) The use of a simplified stapling apparatus for automatic suturing of small blood vessels. Angiology 15:246
Strauch B, Murray DE (1967) Transfer of composite graft with immediate suture anastomosis of its vascular pedicle measuring less than 1 mm in external diameter using microsurgical techniques. Plast Reconstr Surg 40:325
Swenson O, Gross RE (1947) Absorbable fibrin tube for vein anastomosis. Surgery 22:137
Szabo Z (1977) Microvascular surgical technique today In: Phillips JM (ed) Microsurgery in gynecology. Workshop for laparoscopy and microsurgical repair of the fallopian tube. University of California, Irvine

Takaro T (1964) The american and the russian vascular staplers. Arch Surg 89:536
Terzis J, Faibisoff B, Williams HB (1974) Use of polyethylene bag background in microsurgical repair of peripheral nerves. Plast Reconstr Surg 54:102
Thurston JB, Buncke HJ, Chater NL, Weinstein PR (1976) A scanning electron microscopy study of microarterial damage and repair. Plast Reconstr Surg 57:197
Todd AS (1958) Fibrinolysis autographs. Nature 181:495
Todd AS (1959) The histological localisation of fibrinolysine activator. J Path Bact 78:281
Todd AS (1961) The tissue activator of plasminogen and thrombosis. In: Walker W (ed) Thrombosis and anticoagulant therapy. Livingstone, Edinburgh
Todd AS (1964) Localisation of fibrinolytic activity in tissues. Br Med Bull 20:210

Urschel HC, Roth EJ (1961) Small arterial anastomoses: I. Nonsuture. Ann Surg 153:599

Vinazzer H, Pütter J, Loew D (1975) Influence of intravenously administered acetylsalicylic acid on platelet functions. Haemostasis 4:12

Warren BA (1964) Fibrinolytic activity of vascular endothelium. Br Med Bull 20:213

Williams CL, Takaro T (1963) Russian stapler in small artery anastomoses and grafts. Angiology 14:470

Zweifach BM (1959) Lansing A (ed) In the arterial wall. Williams and Wilkins, Baltimore, p 15

Part 2

Clinical Microvascular Surgery

A. Replantation with Microvascular Anastomosis (microreplantation)

The first cases of replantation were performed using the techniques and knowledge of vascular surgery. Using such techniques Hopfner (1903) successfully replanted canine legs and Lapchinski (1960) reported good results following replantation of canine extremities.[1] In 1966, Buncke and Schulz reported their results in experimental replantation of amputated rabbit ears. The previous year, the same authors had attempted replantation of middle-hand and digit amputations in rhesus monkeys, in which vessels of 0.7–1.2 mm in diameter were anastomosed. In a series of 10 cases, only one digit was successfully replanted.

The first successful replantation in a human is attributed to Komatzu and Tamai, who, in 1965, replanted a fully amputated thumb by microvascular anastomosis, although this case was not made public until 1968.

Reports on successful replantation of subtotal digit amputations came from Kleinert and Kasdan (1963, 1965), Kleinert et al. (1965), Kutz et al. (1965), Kutz et al. (1969), Cobbett (1969b) and Lendvay (1968).

Case reports on replantation following total amputation came from Chen, CW (1966), Lendvay and Owen (1970), Snyder et al. (1972), O'Brien et al. (1973c) and Biemer and Duspiva (1976b). A larger series of 31 cases was presented by O'Brien et al. in 1973(a). The "American Replantation Mission to China 1973" reported the replantation of 100 total and 100 subtotal digit amputations performed at "No. VI People's Hospital", Shanghai. Lendvay (1973) described a series of 63 cases of replantation following digit and middle-hand amputations. In the German-speaking world the first reported series was given by Owen (1975), at the "93rd Congress of the German Association of Surgery": he presented his experiences over a 10-year period, in which 213 replantations, following total and subtotal amputations, were performed. More recent reports have come from Schmidt-Tintemann, Biemer and Duspiva (1976c), Berger et al. (1976), Mandel et al. (1976), O'Brien (1977), Biemer (1977a) and Biemer et al. (1977).

By the end of 1976, the "Chi-Shui-Tan" Hospital in Peking could review 44 cases of replantation of totally amputated digits. At this time at the "No. VI People's Hospital", Shanghai, where the first totally amputated finger had been replanted in 1965, there were statistics on over 300 replantations in the hand region (1977). In 1977, Biemer et al. presented the, until then, largest series in Europe of 184 replantations in 132 cases.

1 These techniques, however, proved unsuccessful when dealing with vessels of less than 2 mm in diameter and it was only through the development of microvascular surgery that it became possible to replant peripheral parts requiring small vessel anastomosis (micro replantation)

I. Definitions and Nomenclature[2]

Replantation surgery is concerned with relatively new operational techniques, for which there were, until recently, no clear definitions in existence. Biemer (1977c) drew attention to the difficulties arising from this lack of precise definition and proposed a series of guidelines and criteria.

1. Replantation

The term "replantation" means the operative restoration of all structures important to the function of the amputated part, including the re-establishment of the circulation, following an amputation injury.

The length of time from the moment of amputation to vascular anastomosis is frequently termed the "ischaemic time". In amputation cases, however, there is a complete loss of blood supply to the amputated part, with total lack of oxygenation, and it is therefore more exact to talk of the "anoxaemic time". It is important to realize that the "anoxaemic time" extends from the moment of amputation until the restoration of arterial blood supply, not simply until the beginning of the operation!

2 The following definitions conform to the guidelines worked out by the Replantation Committee of the "International Society for Reconstructive Microsurgery" and adopted at their 5th Symposium in May 1979 in Guaruja, Brazil. In Vienna in December 1978, the "1st Symposium of the German-speaking Working-party on Microsurgery of Peripheral Nerves and Vessels" had already worked out definitions, which served as a working basis for the Replantation Committee

2. Amputation

"Amputation" is an injury in which all anatomical structures are totally or partially divided, and where the amputated peripheral part shows no sign of a circulation. It is therefore to be expected in such cases that, without vascular repair, the amputated part will not survive.

The terms "total" and "subtotal" amputation have been used to date in a haphazard fashion. Terminology has been further confused by the use of expressions like "as good as fully amputated" or "practically totally severed". The division into total and subtotal amputation is especially important, when assessing functionally successful late results of replantation surgery. In cases where there are intact tendons and nerves, for example, one would expect a more favourable result with regard both to movement and to sensitivity.

3. Total Amputation

The term "total amputation" is restricted to cases in which there is separation of all structures. If even the smallest fibre-connections or skin-bridges persist, then the injury must be classified as a "subtotal" amputation, unless the surgeon completely separates the parts prior to the commencement of the operation.

4. Subtotal Amputation

"Subtotal amputation" is an injury in which the most important anatomical structures, particularly blood-vessels, are separated and there is no longer any evidence of circulation in the distal part. If important anatomical structures remain intact, and there is a clear indication of residual blood flow, then such a case must be defined as a "serious combined injury with vascular impairment" (cf.: Revascularisation). In "subtotal amputation", the soft tissue connection may not be more than $^1/_4$ of the circumference of the part (see Figs. 66 and 67a, b).

In order to make a further clarification of "subtotal amputation" according to the re-

Fig. 66. Sub-total amputation of an index finger. Only the flexor tendons are retained; type III

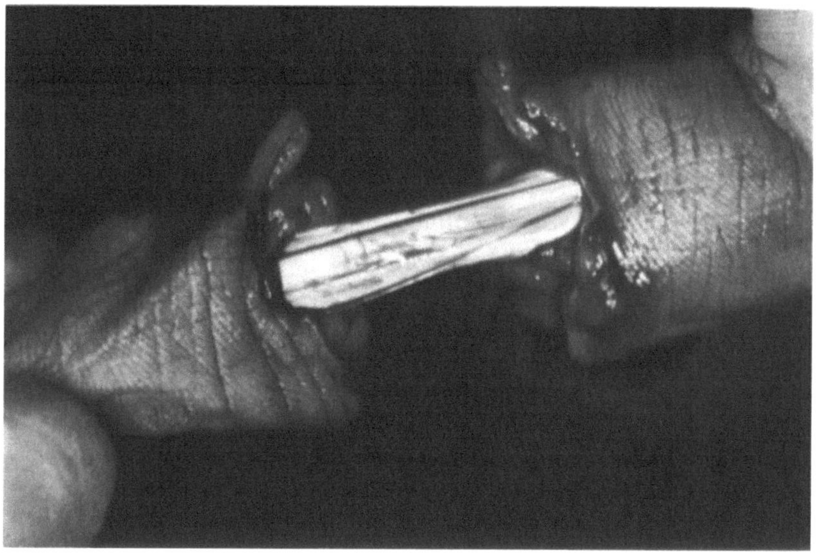

maining intact structures, Biemer (1977c) proposed the following classification:

Table 3. Classification of Subtotal Amputations

	Retained structures
Type I	Bone
Type II	Extensor tendon
Type III	Flexor tendon
Type IV	Main nerve connection
Type V	Skin bridge

Thus, a subtotal finger amputation, in which the digital nerves are intact, is classified as Type IV.

5. Revascularisation

This term is used to describe the restoration of the main vascular connections, in cases in which some or many of the important structures remain intact, and in which there is evidence of a circulation. The vascular anastomosis therefore serves only to improve the circulation of the peripheral part. This is the major difference between "revascularisation" and "subtotal amputation": in the latter case, without vascular anastomosis, necrosis would occur. An example of revascularisation is the injury of the volar surface of the wrist joint with division of the ulnar and radial arteries, not involving the bone, but with a broad dorsal skin-bridge persisting and providing vascular connection. The blood flow to the distal part is certainly grossly diminished but not entirely disrupted.

The distinction between total and subtotal amputation is more sharply defined in some centres, where the term amputation is restricted to total severance from the body, and the operative repair designated as replantation. All other cases, in which there are any structural connections with the body, are grouped under the heading of revascularisation (Lister 1977). In these centres, a case in which the smallest skin-bridge remains intact, is classified not as subtotal amputation but as revascularisation, even although the operative repair of all structures must be carried out just as in a total amputation. Since evaluation of the functional result of such a case is comparable with replantation, it is more meaningful to describe it as a subtotal amputation. Furthermore, although division into only 2 categories (replantation and revascularisation) avoids borderline difficulties between replantation of subtotal amputations and revascularisation, it masks the differences between so-called revascularisation and serious combined injury with vascular impairment.
Lastly, there is no comparison between two

so-called revascularisation cases, which present on the one hand with a small intact skin-bridge and on the other hand with intact tendons or nerves.[3]

6. Replantation: Macro- and Micro-replantation

Two groups of replantations are now recognised according to the level of amputation:

Table 4. Replantation

	Macro-replantations	Micro-replantations
Upper extremity	Proximal to the wrist joint	Distal to the wrist joint
Lower extremity	Proximal to the ankle joint	Distal to the ankle joint

In addition to the amputation level, the two groups differ in the relative importance of the three major points in replantation surgery:

1. Feasibility of replantation.
2. Indication for replantation.
3. Technique of replantation.

Macroreplantation:
1. Feasibility of replantation.
   a) General condition of patient.
   b) Anoxaemic period.
   c) Condition of the amputated part.
2. Indication for replantation.
3. Technique.

Microreplantation:
1. Technique (microvascular surgery).
2. Feasibility of replantation.
   a) Condition of the amputated part.
   b) Anoxaemic period.
   c) General condition of the patient.

3. Indication for replantation.

Experience has shown that the more central the level of amputation, and therefore the bigger the amputated part, the more important is the anoxaemic period, especially with regard to muscle-damage: therefore, there remains a shorter period of time at the disposal of the surgeon prior to replantation, despite cooling or perfusion. Furthermore, the life of the injured patient can be endangered by macroreplantation, through toxic renal damage leading to anuria, or by infections such as gas gangrene (Chen CW 1976). Thus the indications for macroreplantation require special consideration.

In practice, such life-threatening complications never occur in microreplantation surgery. The operative techniques in macroreplantation are of lesser importance than the indications, and they can be performed by adhering to the basic principles and well-known rules of accident surgery, vascular surgery and peripheral nerve surgery. In contrast, microreplantation requires the techniques of microvascular surgery with all its attendant problems. In this text, only the second group – microreplantation – will be discussed.

3 In accordance with the guidelines laid down by the Replantation Committee of the "International Society for Reconstructive Microsurgery" at their 5th Symposium in Guaruja, Brazil, in May 1979

II. Classification of Amputations in the Hand

The majority of admissions with peripheral amputations are hand injuries, with only a few exceptions (cf. Chap. XII).

Amputations in the hand are classified in the following manner: (an exact description of the zone-divisions and related technical problems is to be found in Chap. VI, 1) (see Fig. 74).

Hand amputations (Zone V):
The amputation line lies between the wrist joint and the arterial palmar arch. To re-establish circulation, it is sufficient to anastomose 1 artery and 2 veins, and the vessels normally have a diameter of more than 3 mm.

Middle-hand amputation (Zone IV):
The amputation line in this area passes through the common digital arteries and, consistent with the anatomy, one arterial anastomosis will arterialise two digits.

Digit amputation (Zones I, II, III):
The amputation line here passes through the palmar digital arteries.

In accordance with the above division of the hand, replantations are counted in the following way:
Hand and middle-hand amputations count individually as one case, whereas the fingers are counted singly, even when they are connected to one another by skin-bridges.

III. Indications for Replantation

After the initial shock following an amputation injury, it is a natural reaction on the part of the patient to seek replantation at any price. Generally the patient has the misconception that through replantation the amputated part will be restored fully, e.g. in hand amputation, that the appearance and function will return to normal. It must be specifically explained to the patient that this goal is seldom achieved. In addition, it is essential to discuss with the patient the probable functional result: the necessary treatment plan, including the lengthy operation, time in hospital, post-operative management and incapacity to work etc.

There is universal agreement that there is a clear indication for replantation in thumb and multiple amputations. Furthermore, there is no question that, in middle-hand and hand amputations, a replantation should always be attempted. Also, there is always an indication for replantation in all children, because of the more favourable results (see Fig. 93).

The decision becomes more difficult when considering a single digit or part of a digit, and here it appears from various discussions that there is less agreement. In the hand, amputations which are relatively unimportant for overall function in most occupations, and thus have a low rating on the insurance and compensation scales, may or may not be considered for replantation.

Because of these difficulties, several authors have attempted to give clear indications for replantation, e.g. O'Brien and Miller (1973) took age, profession and the wishes of the patient as indications for replantation of the ulnar 3 fingers. Owen (1976) spoke out against single digit replantation: similar references as to the indications for replantation were reported from China (American Replantation Mission to China 1973).

In many places strong opinions are expressed

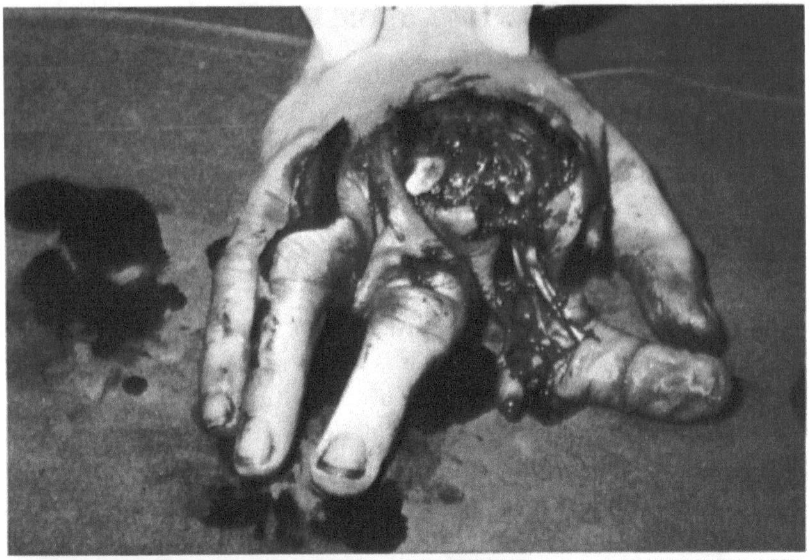

a

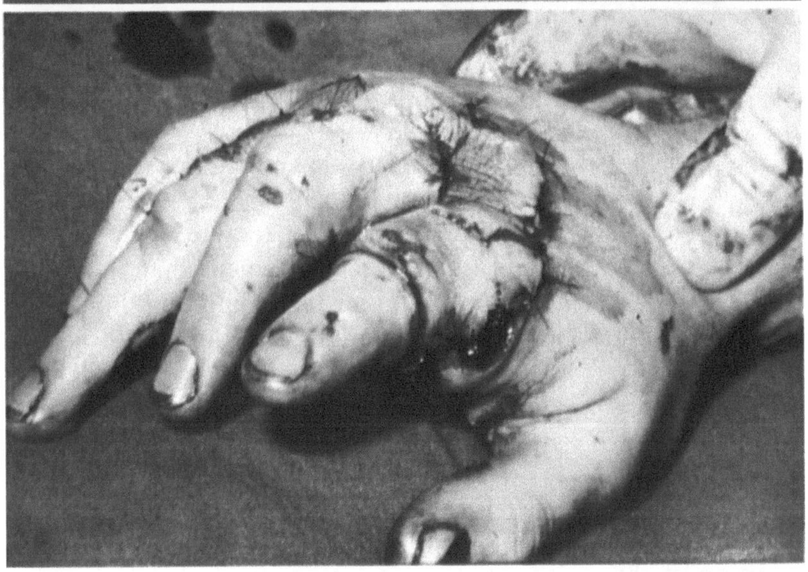

b

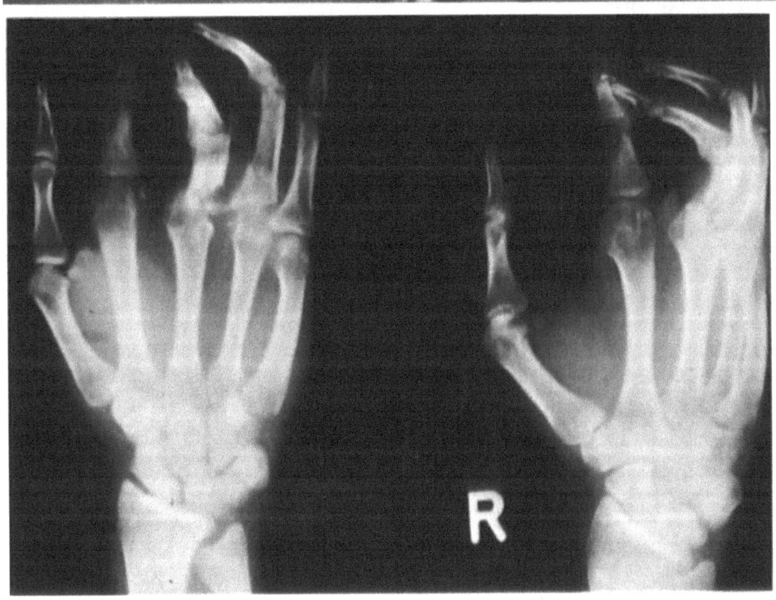

c

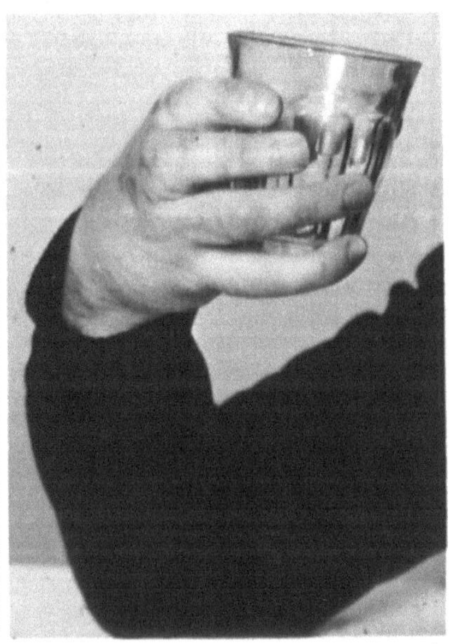

d

Fig. 67 a–d. 23 year-old railwayman with a sub-total amputation of the index and middle fingers caused by a locomotive injury. Replantation of the index finger was only possible following resection of the entire proximal phalanx. The shortened index finger is excluded from the majority of gripping actions and in such cases, therefore, the indication for replantation should be limited. In such a case, replantation should only be performed when there are special considerations or a justifiable request on the part of the patient

Table 5. Indication plan for replantation on the hand

Amputation → Replantation

Condition of the amputated part | Condition of the patient

Absolute indication	Relative indication	No indication
Thumb	Thumb: distal to the IP joint	–
Index finger: missing D-III	Index finger: retained D-III Index finger: distal to the DIP-joint	Index finger: destroyed MP-joint
	Artificial joint ←	
Middle finger: missing D-II	Middle finger: destroyed PIP-joint	Middle finger: destroyed MP-joint
Remaining fingers: multiple amputations	Remaining fingers: retained D-II & D-III	Remaining long fingers: distal to the DIP or destroyed MP-joint
All amputations in children		
Mid-hand, Hand	← Aesthetics Profession occupation Hobby	← Aesthetics Profession/ occupation Hobby

Request from the patient after comprehensive discussion

against the replantation of the distal phalanx: Likewise, the imposition of an age-barrier of around 60 years is considered (Millesi 1976). When one considers the good functional results obtained in patients over 60 years of age, the authors can see in age no contra-indication to replantation (see Fig. 80). Also the mechanism of injury in amputation does not provide an absolute criterion for replantation. This is especially true of severe injuries such as heavy crushing injuries or avulsion injuries, where the first impression on examination can be entirely different from the detailed picture seen at operation. Furthermore, the final functional result is largely dependent upon the subjective attitudes of the patient, and his efforts in the post-operative period. Therefore, the indication for replantation must always be assessed individually, according to an exact knowledge of the facts of each case and after discussion with the injured patient.

It is important to explain the full consequences of replantation for the patient, e.g. long operating time, anaesthetic risk, protracted hospitalisation, subsequent operations, lengthy absence from work, etc. Such explanations should be more comprehensive, the more "unimportant" the amputated part is for the function of the hand.

In summary, the following criteria should be taken into account, when considering the indications for replantation:

1. Objective Points.

A. Importance of the amputated part for general hand function.

B. Probable functional result.

C. Feasibility of replantation:
   a) Condition of the amputated part and technical feasibility of the replantation.
   b) Anoxaemic period.
   c) Condition of the patient.

D. Risk of the replantation for the patient: (anaesthesia, medication, previous medical history, incapacity to work, etc.).

2. *Subjective Points.*
   A. Special importance of the amputated part for the individual patient: (profession, occupation, hobbies and activities).
   B. Desire for replantation.
   C. Aesthetics.
   D. Psychological motivation.
   E. Personal motivation.

3. *Organisational Considerations.*

4. *Economic Considerations.*

Indication-plan for replantation of the hand (see p. 61, Table 5)

The above plan is based on functional results after replantation and should serve as a guide for the doctor who first treats and advises the patient. It should not be used to exclude certain amputation injuries from replantation when giving advice over the telephone. The explanatory discussion with the patient is always essential and should only be undertaken by the experienced replantation surgeon.

IV. Guide-lines for the Primary Treatment of Amputation Injuries

The consideration for replantation is greatly influenced by the first-line treatment. This initial treatment is primarily concerned with maintaining the vital functions of the injured person, according to the rules of general accident surgery, e.g. control of respiration, maintenance of circulation, treatment of shock, etc. Since amputations in the hand area are most commonly isolated injuries, the general condition of the patient is normally good – in contrast to macroreplantation – and the above points seldom enter into consideration.

It is important that the amputated part is found and brought with the patient, a point which is not so obvious, as it at first appears. Manipulation of the stumps, such as cleaning, disinfection, clamping or ligation, should be avoided. A pressure-bandage is *always* sufficient to stop bleeding. The injured patient, with the amputated part, should be transported as fast as possible to the appropriate replantation centre. The amputated part should be cooled at ca. 4° Celcius, especially if the period of transportation is lengthy. This is most readily achieved by using two plastic bags placed one inside the other. The inner bag contains the amputated part packed in compresses and the outer bag contains ice-cubes – so-called "dry-cooling" (Biemer 1977e).

This reduction in temperature effectively lengthens the survival time, and thus the feasibility of replantation, of a digit up to almost 24 hours (O'Brien and Miller 1973). The authors themselves have successfully replanted a digit cooled in this manner after 16 hours.

V. Replantation Technique

The general rules of suture technique in microvascular surgery (see Chap. "Suture technique in microvascular surgery") are valid in the clinical situation, but should be supplemented by the following points:

1. Maximum care and uncompromising accuracy during all steps of the operation.
2. Maximum exposure.
3. Anastomosis of undamaged vessels (as far as it is possible to judge under maximum magnification).
4. Avoidance of any tension at the site of anastomosis.
5. Anastomosis of vessels of equal diameter whenever possible.
6. Avoidance of blood-stasis, following free blood-flow through anastomosis.
7. Exact pre-operative planning.
8. Strict adherance to the operation plan.
9. Good arm-rests and comfortable seat.
10. Continual post-operative monitoring.

On admission of the patient with an amputation injury, the general feasibility of replantation is first assessed. This embraces the following points:

Condition of the Patient (previous medical history, associated injuries, level of amputation).

Anoxaemic time

Condition of the amputated part (type of storage).

Life-threatening associated injuries always take precedence over a replantation.

Following a clear indication for replantation, a careful pre-operative examination is essential. In addition to chest X-ray and E.K.G., which may be required, X-rays of both the proximal amputated stump and the distal amputated part are necessary. In addition, blood samples are taken for serum electrolytes, grouping, cross-match and coagulation studies. Haemoglobin and haematocrit-estimation go without saying, and naturally tetanus prophylaxis is carried out.

In contrast to other replantation surgeons (O'Brien et al. 1973c; Tamai 1974; Bowen et al. 1975; No. VI People's Hospital Shanghai 1976), the authors do not routinely use a tourniquet. They are of the opinion that pulsating vessel-stumps are more easily identified and that only thus can the free blood-flow be assessed properly. The same is true regarding venous function: after arterial anastomosis in replantation, the venous reflux allows an easier and more meaningful identification of the vein stumps. Those veins with the strongest reflux are then chosen for anastomosis.

Furthermore, the release of a tourniquet, following successful vascular anastomosis, allows breakdown-products to flow into the already anoxaemic-damaged amputated part, whereas free venous outflow allows these products to be washed out of the replanted part.

The cleaning and disinfection of the amputated part must be performed with meticulous care, so that no cleaning fluid reaches the vessel-stumps, since all disinfectant products lead to epithelial changes and "intimal" damage.

Despite the abundant visible dirt in injured hands and amputated parts, nearly all preoperative bacteriological specimens are found to be sterile. In view of this, disinfection does not appear to play a significant role. It is important, however, that all foreign bodies, such as sawdust, grass, etc., should be removed under loupe magnification.

On both the amputated part and on the stump, all structures which are to be repaired, with the exception of the veins, are identified and marked: the arteries with clips, the nerves and tendons with sutures of different thickness. This identification and marking is best performed under loupe magnification ($\times 4$) since this offers a better operating field than the microscope (see Fig. 68).

The neurovascular bundles are to be found lateral and palmar to the flexor tendon: the arterial stumps are recognised by the blood clot at their severed ends and this clot can readily be expressed by light pressure. The identification and preparation are performed using microsurgical instruments, in order to avoid fur-

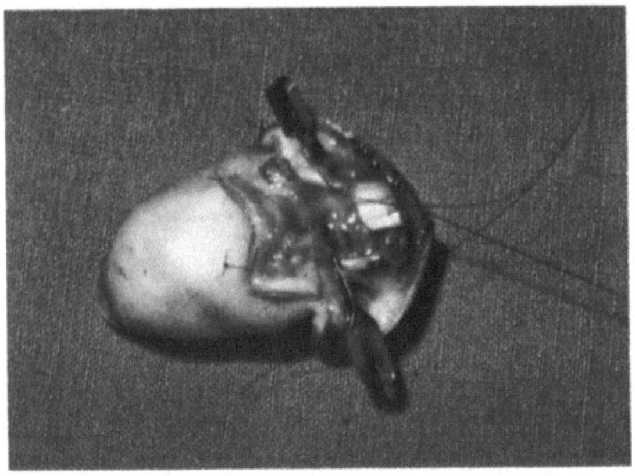

Fig. 68. The amputated part fully prepared, with the vessel stumps and nerves marked and the incision edges sutured back

ther injury to the tissues and especially to the vessels.
A 1 cm long skin incision is made over the neurovascular bundles and the skin edges on both sides are sutured back, so that identification (and later, the anastomosis) is made easier. These incisions also serve to interrupt the circular scars, especially in clean-cut guillotine amputations, which are prone to develop contracture.
In practice, both volar arterial stumps are always prepared, even when, for technical reasons, only one anastomosis is performed. A replantation should never commence before all structures are clearly identified and marked.
After osteosynthesis, for example, it is almost impossible to find an unmarked nerve, which has retracted.

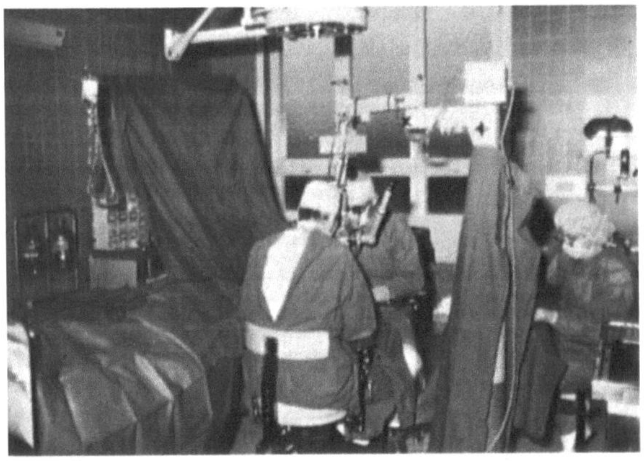

Fig. 69. Replantation in the hand

The overriding principle of replantation surgery is that all steps must be performed in a most precise manner, according to an appropriate and strictly adhered to operation plan.
For this reason, the complete operation should be performed by one surgeon without relief.
All structures must be clearly marked prior to wound debridement, otherwise important structures could easily be shortened unintentionally.

1. Wound Debridement

Sufficient and careful wound debridement is vital in replantation surgery. All devitalised structures must be excised and this is especially true in crushing and avulsion injuries. Necrosis in the area of anastomosis leads without fail to thrombosis, or alternatively to infection with subsequent vessel occlusion. A free skin graft as a covering is always to be preferred to skin necrosis.
An important rule is that one may only replant "healthy" on "healthy" tissue.
Extensive tendon damage leads to deformity, and a secondary or primary tendon procedure or the insertion of a silicone rod is to be preferred in such situations. The excision of damaged tissue and the shortening of the vessels are performed under the stronger magnification of the microscope, and this is discussed in the section on vessel anastomosis.

2. Bone Shortening

The aim of bone shortening is twofold:
1. To provide favourable conditions for the safe and effective osteosynthesis, by the removal of bone splinters and straightening of alignment.
2. To allow anastomosis of vessels and nerves without tension.
The proportion of shortening is a matter of individual judgment. In the thumb, however, every effort should be made to preserve the length and the joints, as far as possible.

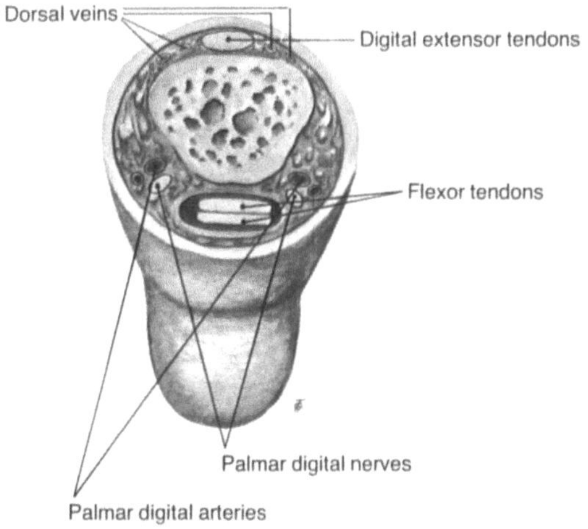

Fig. 70. Cross section of a finger showing all structures requiring connection

Vessel defects per se are no indication for further bone shortening, since the deficiencies can be overcome by the use of vein grafts (see Chap. "Microvascular grafts").

Perfusion or *preoperative angiography* have little to offer, since they fail to give additional information or improve conditions at the start of operation, and can in fact cause additional vessel damage.

The actual replantation is performed in the following order (see Fig. 76):

1. Osteosynthesis.
2. Repair of the flexor digitorum profundus or alternatively flexor pollicis longus in the thumb, and if necessary flexor digitorum superficialis.
3. Repair of the tendon sheath, if possible.
4. Anastomosis of both volar digital arteries.
5. Anastomosis of both volar digital nerves.
6. Repair of extensor tendons.
7. Anastomosis of veins.
8. Loose skin closure.

3. Osteosynthesis

There are four main requirements for osteosynthesis:

1. It should be able to be performed quickly and simply.
2. It should provide good stability.
3. It should leave the adjacent joints freely mobile.
4. The materials used should be capable of easy removal.

The four most commonly used techniques at this time differ in the fulfilment of these requirements (see Fig. 71).

a) Central Kirschner Wire

Advantages: This is the simplest and fastest technique and can be carried out in every situation. It is especially simple to use in fractures near joints and comminuted fractures. In addition, the material can easily be removed. It allows rotation of the replanted part and this often simplifies vessel anastomosis.

Disadvantages: This technique fails to provide good stability, especially with regard to rotation. Furthermore, the adjacent joints are normally fixed by the central Kirschner wire.

b) Two Short Crossed Kirschner Wires

Advantages: This technique allows greater stability and prevents rotation. It is also relatively easy to perform and simple to remove, while leaving the adjacent joints freely mobile.

Disadvantages: There is greater danger of damaging the neurovascular bundles or tendons. One cannot slide the fragments together, since the crossed wires tend to block approximation. This method is only suitable for amputa-

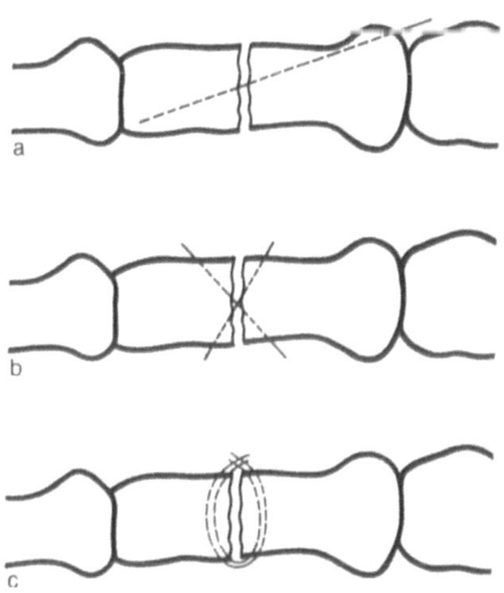

Fig. 71 a–c. Osteo-synthesis techniques most commonly in use in replantation surgery of the hand. **a** axial, intramedullary K-wire **b** crossed K-wires. **c** trans-osseus wire sutures tions at some distance from a joint. Furthermore, crossed Kirschner wires cannot be used in comminuted fractures.

c) Trans-Osseous Wire Sutures

Advantages: This technique provides a stable osteosynthesis and also allows for a possibility of compression at the fracture site while leaving the neighbouring joints free. The two wire sutures must be passed on both dorsal and volar sides and can be combined with a temporary Kirschner wire.
Disadvantages: This technique is more difficult and more time-consuming to perform and requires wide exposure of both bone ends. The technique is unsuitable for fractures occurring very near joints and comminuted fractures. The material used can only be removed with difficulty, if at all, and there is a danger of metalosis.

d) Central Intra-Medullary Screw

Tamai (1977) proposed the use of a single intra-medullary screw (a screw without a head) in total amputation injuries.
Advantages: This technique provides absolute stability while leaving the neighbouring joints free and also allows for the possibility of compression at the fracture site. In addition, it is a relatively simple technique to perform.
Disadvantages: The technique is only suitable in total amputations and is not suitable for fractures close to joints or compressed or comminuted fractures. The screw cannot be removed and therefore the metal body has to remain in the finger with the possible danger of metalosis.
Osteosynthesis using plates and screws of the small fragment AO instruments is used only occasionally in replantation surgery in the mid hand. A screw can be used to provide a stable osteosynthesis in smooth oblique amputation injuries, particularly the thumb. From the variety of techniques the most suitable method of osteosynthesis for each replantation should be chosen. In the authors' experience of amputations, the majority of cases involving fracture or comminuted fractures were treated using the central Kirschner wire osteosynthesis. In addition, about 45% of amputations show involvement of a joint, or alternatively the amputation line itself passes directly through a joint. The lack of rotational stability of the osteosynthesis technique is shown following suturing of the extensor and flexor tendons.

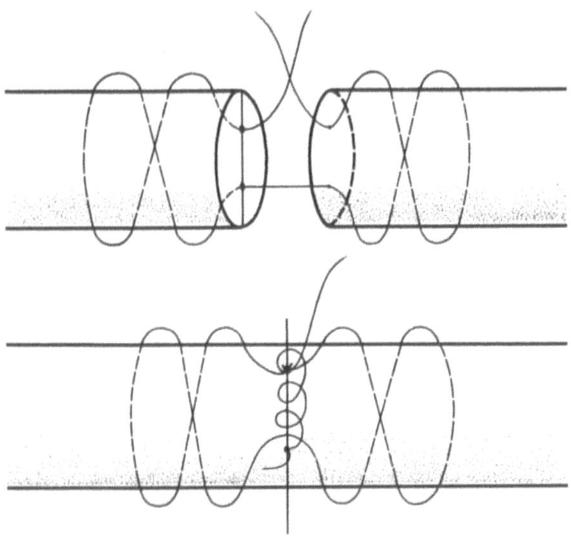

a

Fig. 72. a Modified Bunnel suture, with fine adaptation according to Kleinert. **b** Modified Kessler suture

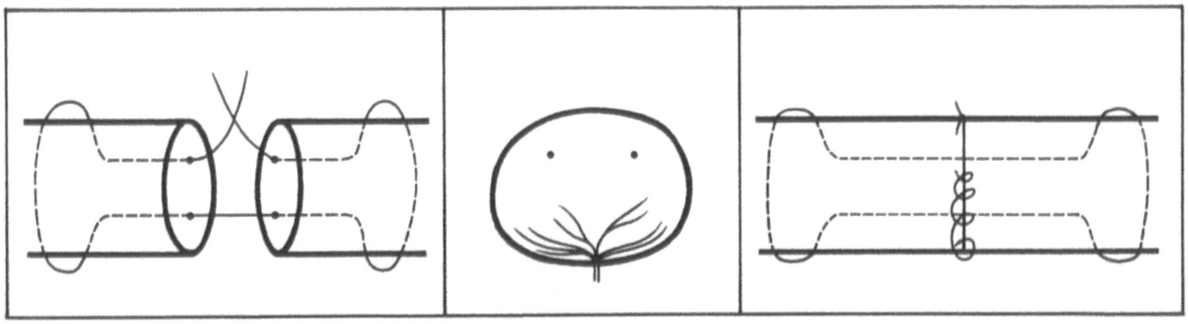

b

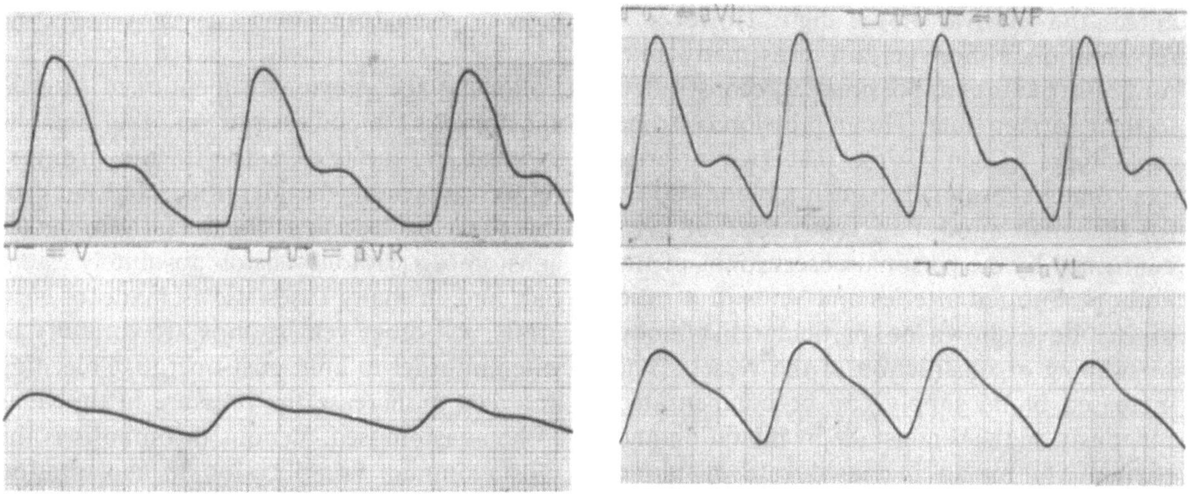

Fig. 73. Pulse curves in fingers. Top row – contralateral, healthy finger; bottom left – replanted digit with repair of single digital artery; bottom right – replanted digit with repair of both digital arteries

This instability however can be turned to great advantage where vascular anastomosis is difficult to perform. Often by appropriate rotation of the replant, the anastomosis can be greatly simplified. In damaged limbs a primary arthrodesis is performed in the functional position and here the techniques using a pulley or a screw have proved beneficial.

4. Suturing of the Flexor Tendon and Tendon Sheath

The superficial flexor tendons are resected when the damage is extensive e.g. heavy crushing. In guillotine-type amputations, the techniques for re-positioning and suturing are the same as for the deep flexor tendons. The flexor tendons are carefully trimmed to the undamaged tissue and sutured using the Bunnel suture (shoe string suture) or Kessler-suture with 4-0 or 5-0 monofilament nylon (see Fig. 72). An additional continuous oversew using 6-0 monofilament nylon is performed to obtain fine adaptation at the suture site. The two ends of the tendons are fixed using two number 18 needles so that the suturing can be performed free of tension. In addition, the tendon sheath should always be repaired, where possible, using 6-0 monofilament nylon.

5. Arterial Anastomosis

Prior to suturing the arteries, it is essential that the patency of the arterial stumps is checked. A perfect anastomosis becomes meaningless if the proximal vessel lumen is occluded by a thrombus. Shortening of the vessel ends is particularly important and should be performed until no changes in the vessel walls are observed under microscopic magnification. A large proportion of *early thrombosis,* occurring intra-operatively or shortly after reconstitution of blood flow, originates from residual vessel wall damage (Acland 1973; Biemer and Duspiva 1976b). Furthermore, the anastomosis must always be performed without tension and, if necessary, extensive microvein grafts should be inserted. The suturing of the anastomosis is performed in the manner previously described. It is important, as in all microsurgical treatment, that there is good exposure: this is achieved using the previously mentioned small lengthwise incisions over the neurovascular bundles. Following blood-flow through a patent arterial anastomosis, a strong venous reflux should set in within a few minutes. Only following a prolonged anoxaemic time of over 10 hours is there delay, and profuse bleeding from the veins occasionally takes 10 to 20 min. Where possible both volar arteries are sutured, although a single patent anastomosis also guarantees the survival of the digit. However a replantation is more certain, if as many anatomical structures as possible are reconstituted to their former state. The impression of some replanteurs (Chen 1976), that two arterial anastomoses result in too great a blood supply for the small number of veins, has not been confirmed by the personal observations of the authors. Sutured arteries and veins in a ratio of 2:1 have shown no particular likelihood to swelling or obstruction of the vessels. The increased blood supply can be compensated obviously on the venous side by dilatation and particularly by an increased rate of blood flow. For this reason, following full arterialisation the venous reflux is concentrated into only one or two vessels, and by tying off all other venous stumps an almost arterial spurting reflux is achieved. This increased venous pressure and greater rate of blood flow act as a good prophylaxis against frequently occurring venous thrombosis.

6. Nerve Suturing

The nerve is repaired using an epi-perineurial or perineurial suture of 10-0 monofilament nylon. Usually two to three interrupted sutures are sufficient for a digital nerve.

The nerve must be repaired without tension, suturing only undamaged tissue. To facilitate nerve repair, two number 18 needles are inserted into the epineurium (analogous to the technique used in tendon rapair) thus transfixing the nerve stumps.

7. Management of the Extensor Tendon Apparatus

Extensor tendons are repaired using 4-0 nonabsorbable monofilament nylon inserted as horizontal mattress sutures. Final adaptation can be achieved using 6-0 monofilament nonabsorbable nylon. Wherever possible the entire extensor tendon apparatus should be repaired.

8. Vein Anastomosis

Following the previously mentioned arterial anastomosis, bloodlessness of the area is avoided and the two veins with the strongest reflux can readily be identified. The lack of soft tissue protection of the dorsal vein makes anastomosis without tension absolutely essential, and in many cases use is made of vein grafts. All other vein stumps are carefully ligated in order to limit post-operative bleeding and also to increase the pressure in the veins to be anastomosed. Venous thrombosis is the most common complication in replantation surgery. It is therefore essential that the venous anastomosis is performed with the greatest care and exactitude. The arterial anastomosis is performed prior to suturing the veins for the following reasons:

1. It shortens the anoxaemic time.
2. It permits all metabolic products to be flushed out.
3. It permits a more precise control of the patency of the venous stumps.
4. It allows for the selection of veins with the greatest reflux.

In contrast to this, O'Brien and Miller (1973) and Chinese replanteurs (Chen 1976) give preference to primary vein suture, even they agree that it is often very difficult and time consuming to localise vein stumps on the amputated part prior to replantation (China 1976). The blood lost through open veins is, in a 1–3 finger replant, insignificant. In a 4–5 digit replantation of a hand or mid-hand amputation, blood loss may reach a sufficient proportion to make blood replacement necessary. In mid-hand and hand amputations, therefore, it is often more advantageous to repair one or two veins prior to opening up the arteries. In these cases, the veins are found without difficulty.

9. Skin Closure

Skin closure must be as loose as possible to avoid pressure on the vessel anastomoses. On the other hand, the vessels require a safe covering and it is sometimes necessary to perform local transverse skin flaps or free skin grafting to obtain cover. It has been shown that it is often less risky to leave an anastomosis uncovered than to force closure by stretching the skin. 4–6 interrupted sutures are sufficient to close a circumferential wound of a digit. As a basic principle, replantation aims at completing repair in one stage. This means that in addition to vessel anastomosis, functional structures are simultaneously repaired. This is certainly technically simpler than secondary operations such as those proposed by Snyder (1972) and Mandl (1976) for subsequent tendon or nerve reconstruction.

The successful replantation of total amputations of the thumb without venous anastomosis have been described by Snyder et al. (1972) and Chen (1976). Similarly, Tamai (1974) described a case in a 20-month old infant, but in the experience of the authors such cases are isolated examples. In the authors' series, two amputations in three and four year old children were replanted but no venous anastomosis was possible. Only one of these cases survived in part, despite a full course of heparinisation and repeated scarification. The large scale anticoagulation of the blood as well as the severity of the blood loss, which has to be replaced, must be weighed against the expected results. The authors allow bleeding out from the extremities for up to eight days and thereafter obviously sufficient spontaneous venous connections have formed. In contrast to this treatment plan, is their personal observation that venous thrombosis occurring on the 10th post-operative day has led to complete necrosis of a replant.

10. Dressings

The dressing must be absorbent and loosely applied and should contain no circumferential turns which might lead to constriction. Splintage, which requires an elastic bandage fixation, is therefore excluded following replantation. The replanted part must remain free so that it can be observed at all times for determination of vascularity on the basis of colour, temperature and capillary filling. The extremity is supported in a slightly raised position. Particularly in a finger replantation, a free venous back-flow can be obtained by maintaining the hand in a supinated position.

11. Medicinal Treatment

The main aim of medicinal treatment in microvascular surgery is to inhibit thrombus formation. Initially all replanteurs undertook full heparinisation with 20,000–30,000 units/ 24 hours (O'Brien 1973; Lendvay 1973; Tamai 1974) and these authors still carry out this procedure today. This anticoagulation of the blood, however, leads to grave blood loss and careful management requires precise and relatively costly supervision. A reduction in the dose of heparin, and subsequently a full abandonment of heparinisation, produced equally high success rates (Biemer 1977a). Similarly, Acland (1972), in animal experiments, failed to demonstrate a significantly lower thrombosis rate using heparinisation. The following medicinal treatment is now currently employed by the authors:

Pre-operatively

1. Shock treatment.
2. 20 mg Dipyridamol I.V. [4]

Per-operatively

1. Four hourly 20 mg Dipyridamol[4].
2. 500 ml low molecular Dextran [5].
3. 3,000–4,000 units heparin I.V. (about 50 units per kg body weight in adults) prior to release of the clamps following arterial anastomosis (this burst of heparin is used only in crushing injuries, post-thrombectomy cases, difficult anastomoses etc.).

Post-operatively

1. 2 × 75 mg Dipyridamol orally daily for 14 days.
2. 1 G. Acetyl salicylic acid [6] orally daily for 14 days.
3. 500 ml low molecular Dextran [5] I.V. for 6 days.

Dipyridamol and Acetyl salicylic acid can now be given orally as a mixed preparation. [7]

---

4 Persantin, Thomae
5 Rheomacrodex, Knoll
6 Colfarit, Bayer
7 Asasantin, Thomae

All replantations are treated with prophylactic antibiotics using a combination preparation of Oxacillin and Ampicillin[8]. The shock treatment is particularly important in multiple amputations and where there are severe associated injuries. Hypovolaemia, with the natural response of centralisation, offers very unfavourable conditions for the successful replantation of an extremity.

8 Totocillin, Bayer

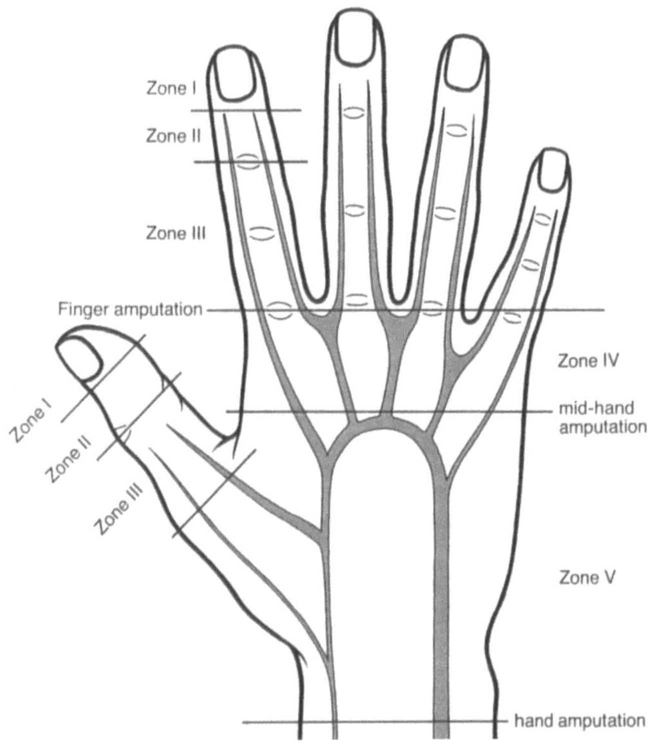

Fig. 74. Division of the hand into zones according to the level of amputation

VI. Considerations of Differing Levels and Mechanisms of Amputation[9]

1. Levels of Amputation in the Hand

Zone I: Zone I extends from the finger tip to the root of the nail. Loss of this part does little to impair the basic function of the hand and this is expressed in the attitude of Insurance Companies. Nevertheless, after such an injury, the finger is robbed of its refined sensibility and from an aesthetic point of view there is loss of the nail-bearing segment. Certain occupations, e.g. music-making, are no longer possible. Proximal to the nail bed the veins are formed from the capillary area of the finger pulp so that dorsally no veins suitable for anastomosis are found. Occasionally a volar vein is available. In contrast, the arteries at this level are still well formed and in most cases can be anastomosed. The nerves have already branched out towards their functional end organs. Because of all these factors, replantation is mostly not possible and in fresh clean cut amputations the possibility of using the amputate as a composite graft should be borne in mind. In 16 cases of clean cut amputations in Zone I, 12 amputates were applied as composite grafts and showed successful healing (Werber and Biemer 1978; see Fig. 75).

Zone II: Zone II extends from the base of the nail to the distal interphalangeal joint. The arteries at this level are well formed but the veins in contrast are often very small in calibre and thin-walled. Attention should be turned to the availability of volar veins: arthrodesis

9 The classification of the levels of amputation and the mechanisms of amputation conform to the guidelines of the Replantation Committee of the International Society for Reconstructive Microsurgery drawn up at the 5th Symposium in May 1979 in Guaruja, Brazil

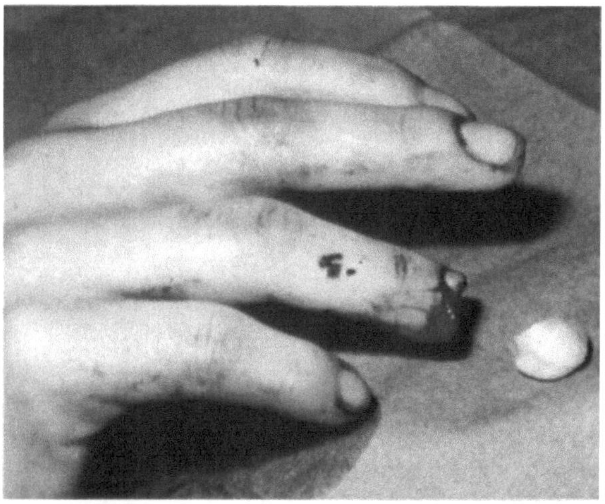

75a

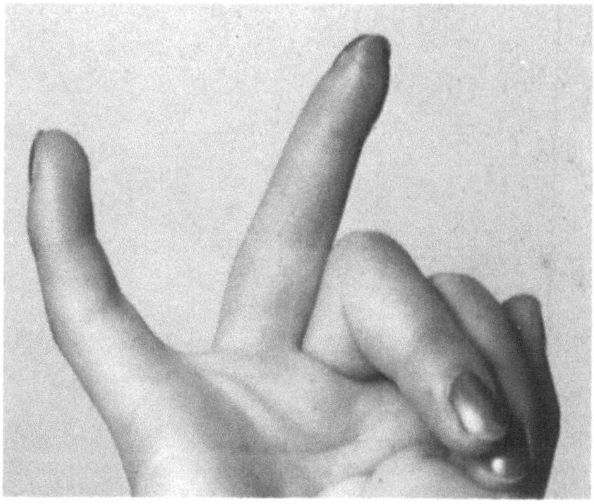

75b

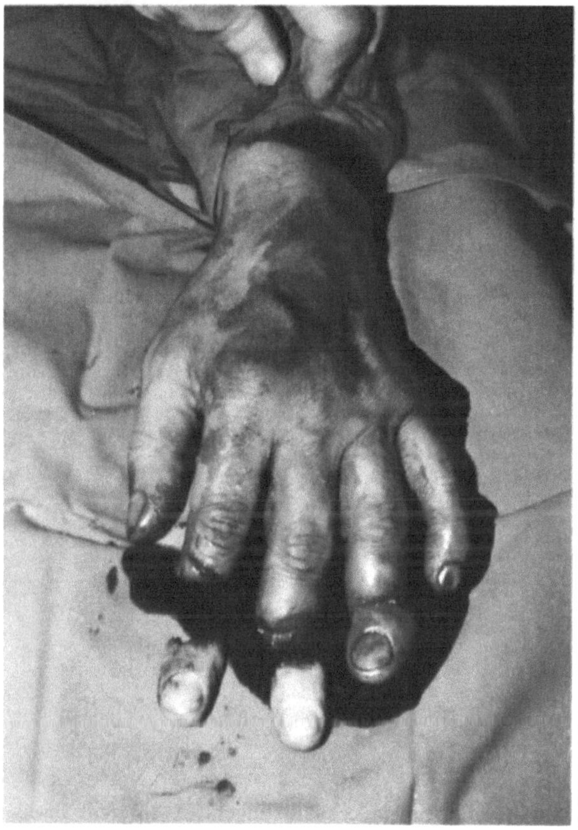

76a

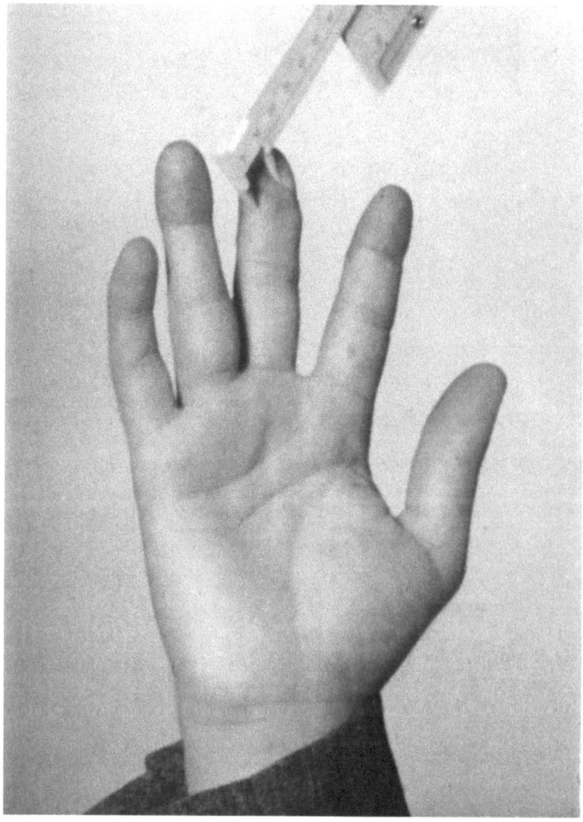

76b

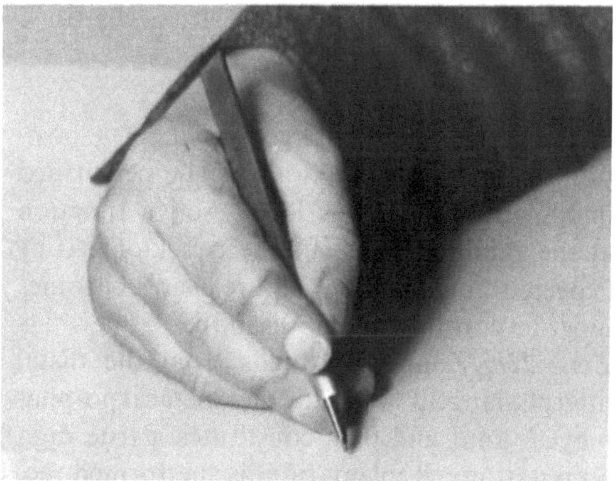

76c

Fig. 75 a, b. Replantation of a finger tip as a composite graft without vascular connection

Fig. 76 a–c. 34 year old man with total amputation of the distal joints of the index and middle fingers in zone II following a circular saw injury. Five months post-operatively there is already a 2 point discrimination of 10 mm a 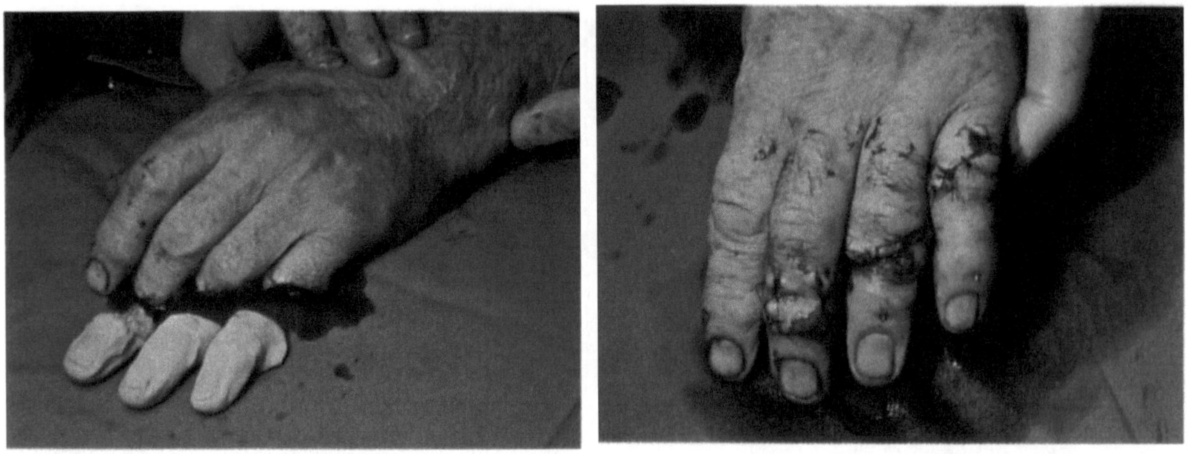 b

c 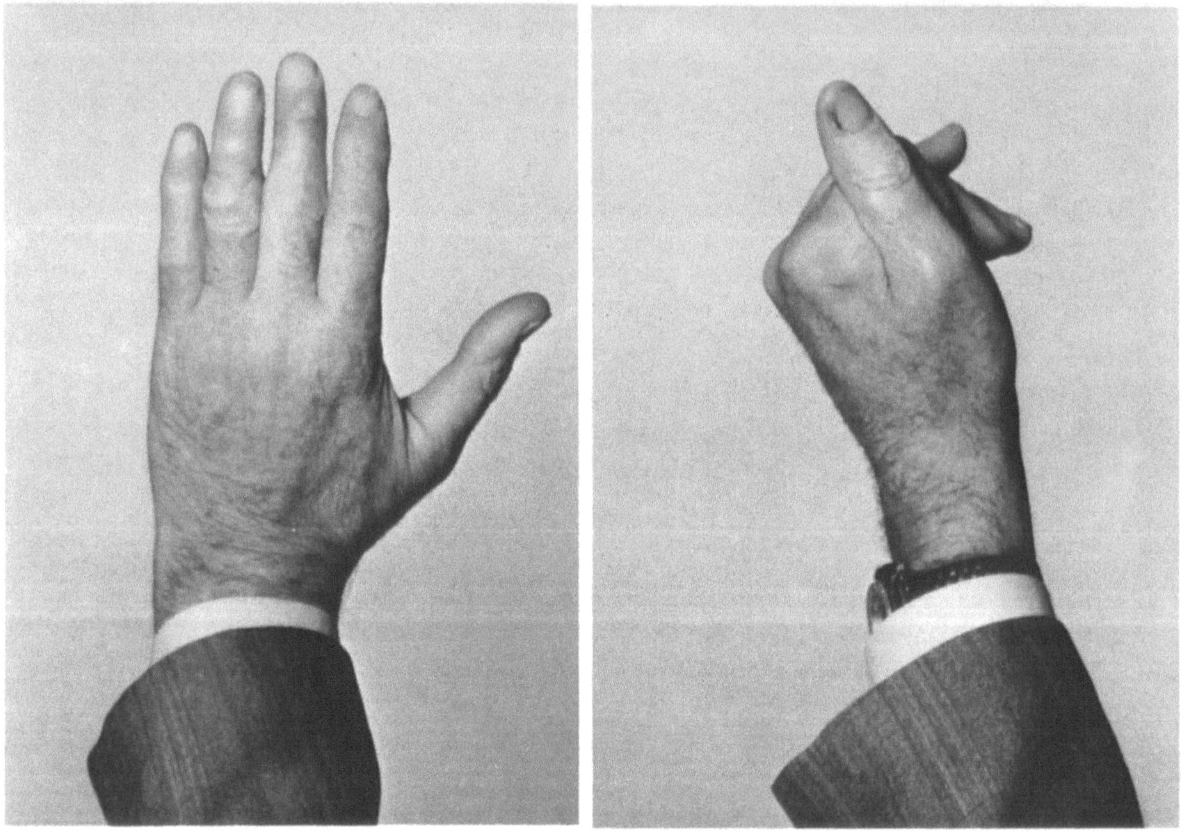 d

Fig. 77 a–d. 58 year old man with a total amputation of the middle, ring and small fingers at different levels in zone III, following a wire snare injury. A primary arthrodesis was performed in the proximal joint of the little finger

of the distal interphalangeal joint, in a position of function, should always be performed in replantation at this level. Active function at the retained joint surface is seldom to be expected and tendon suture here becomes most important for stabilisation.

Zone III: Zone III extends from the distal interphalangeal joint to the metacarpo-phalangeal joint and thus constitutes a true digit amputation. Replantation is performed according to the criteria and techniques mentioned in the previous chapters. Destruction of the metacarpo-phalangeal joint greatly reduces the functional result of the replantation. The indication for replantation in such cases, particularly single finger amputations, becomes narrower although attention can be focussed on replacing the joint with a prosthesis (see Chapter "Primary Replacement of Destroyed Joints"). In the thumb, the ulnar artery

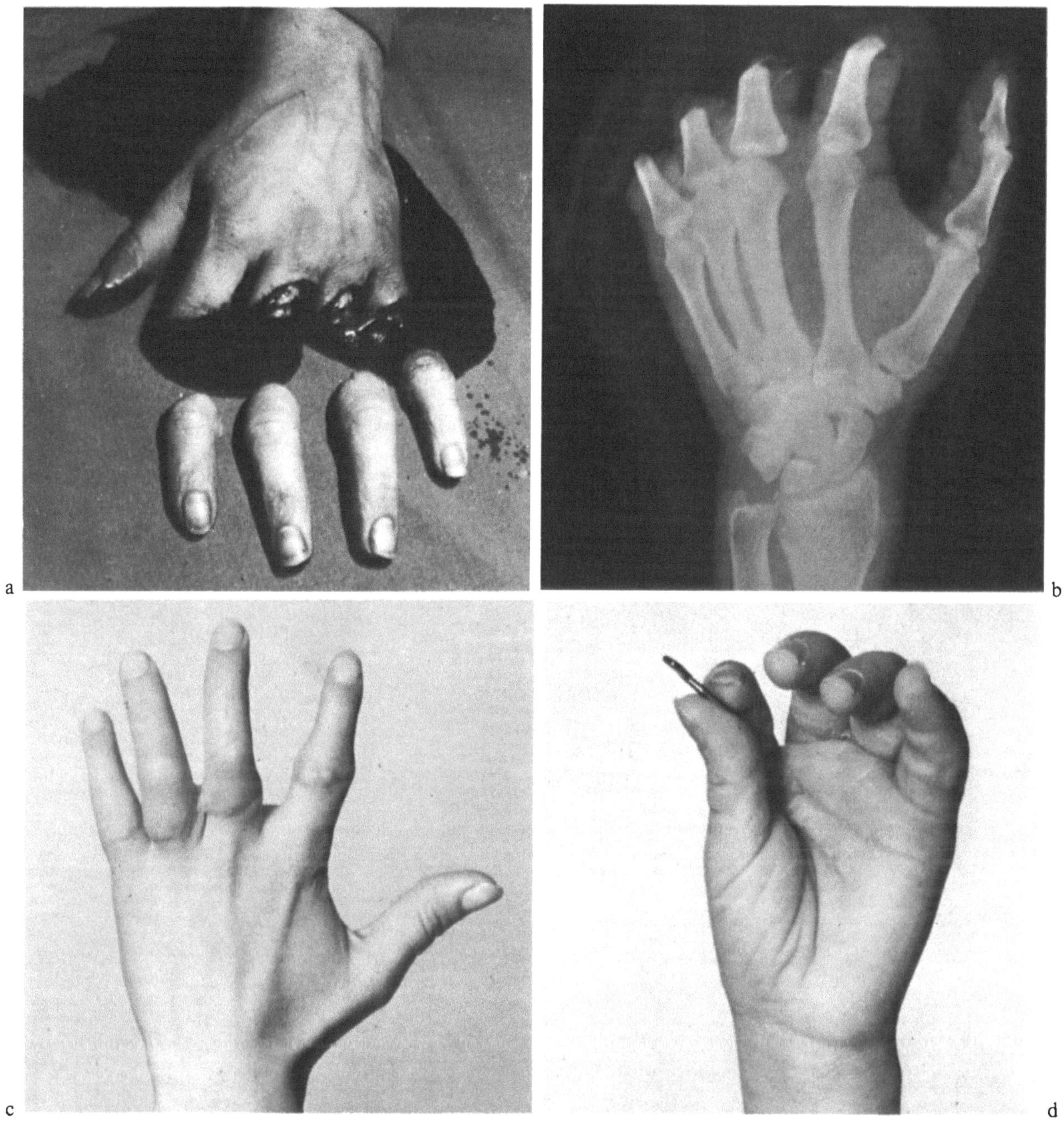

Fig. 78 a–d. 26 year old woman with a guillotine amputation of all four long fingers following an injury in a paper-cutting machine. Functional result two months post-operatively

is almost always the dominant vessel best suited for an anastomosis. Equivalent findings are observed in the index finger where the radial vessel is frequently very delicate and may even be completely absent.

Zone IV: Zone IV extends from the metacarpophalangeal joint to just proximal to the arterial palmar arch. Amputations in this zone are often termed mid-hand amputations where the communal digital arteries are severed. Thus, with a single arterial anastomosis, two digits can be arterialised. The dorsal veins on the back of the hand are resilient and because of their numerous netlike connections, two venous anastomoses will suffice for the four long fingers. The small muscles of the hand, which are either destroyed or not capable of revascularisation, must be sacrificed.

Zone V: Zone V encompasses the area between the palmar arch distally and the wrist

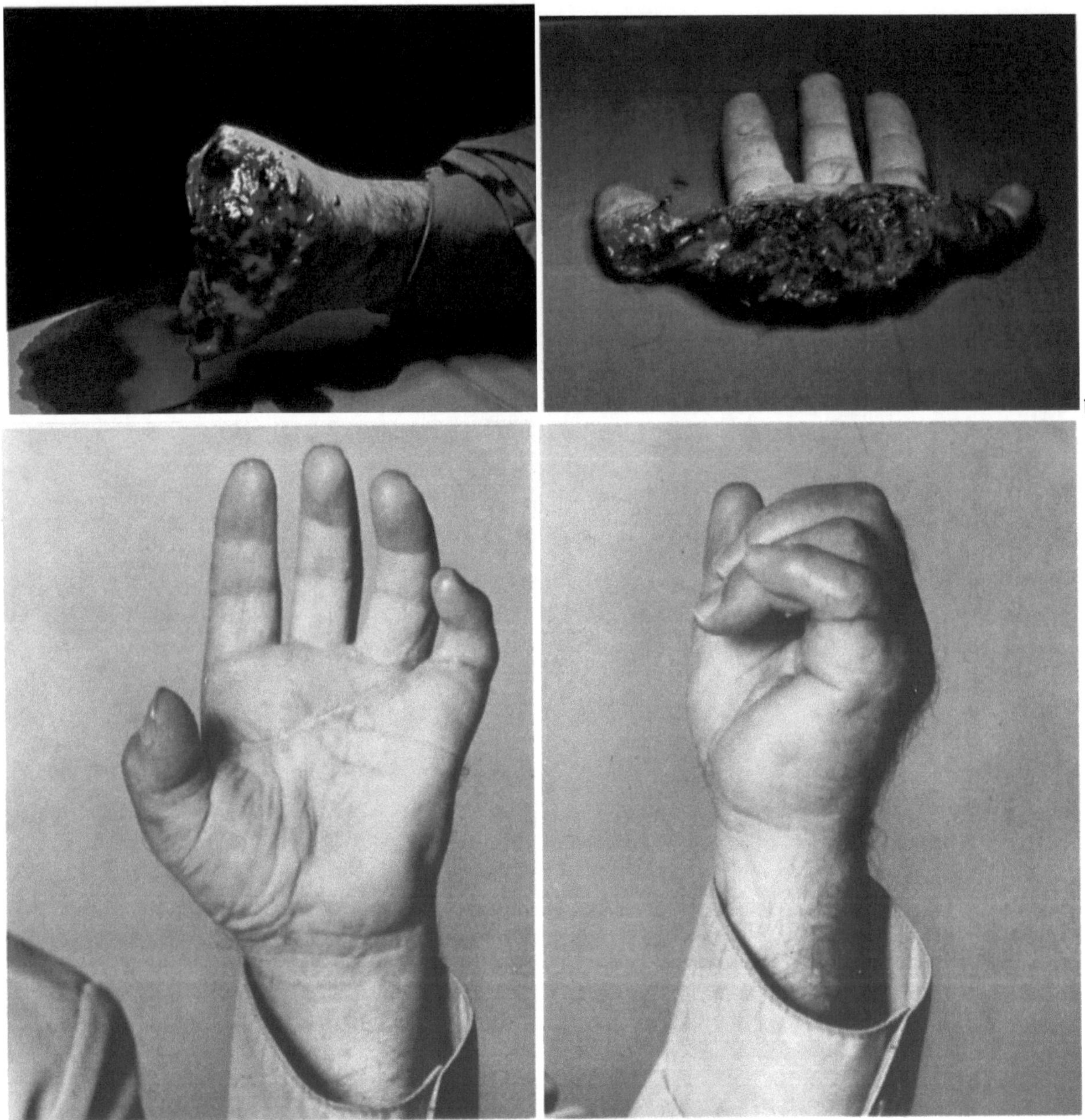

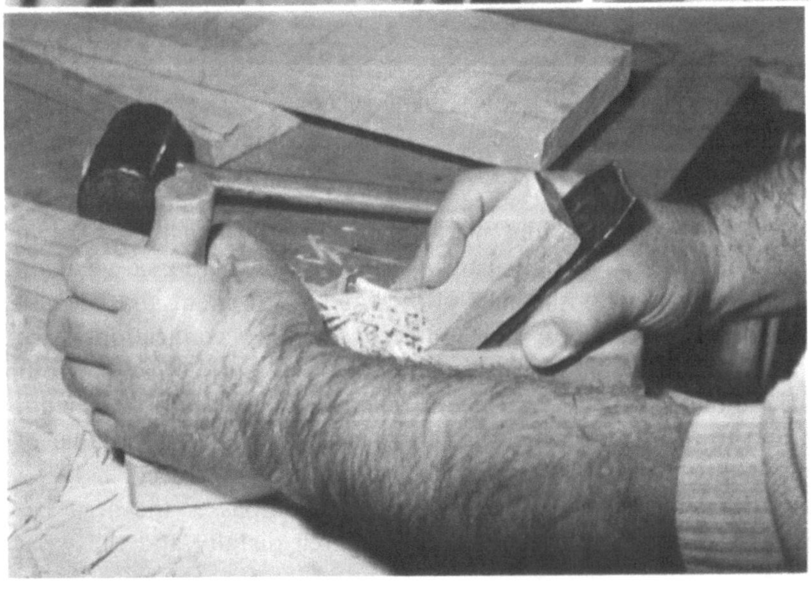

Fig. 79 a–e. 59 year old man who sustained a circular saw injury resulting in total amputation through the mid-hand (zone IV). **c–e** Post-operative result at six months

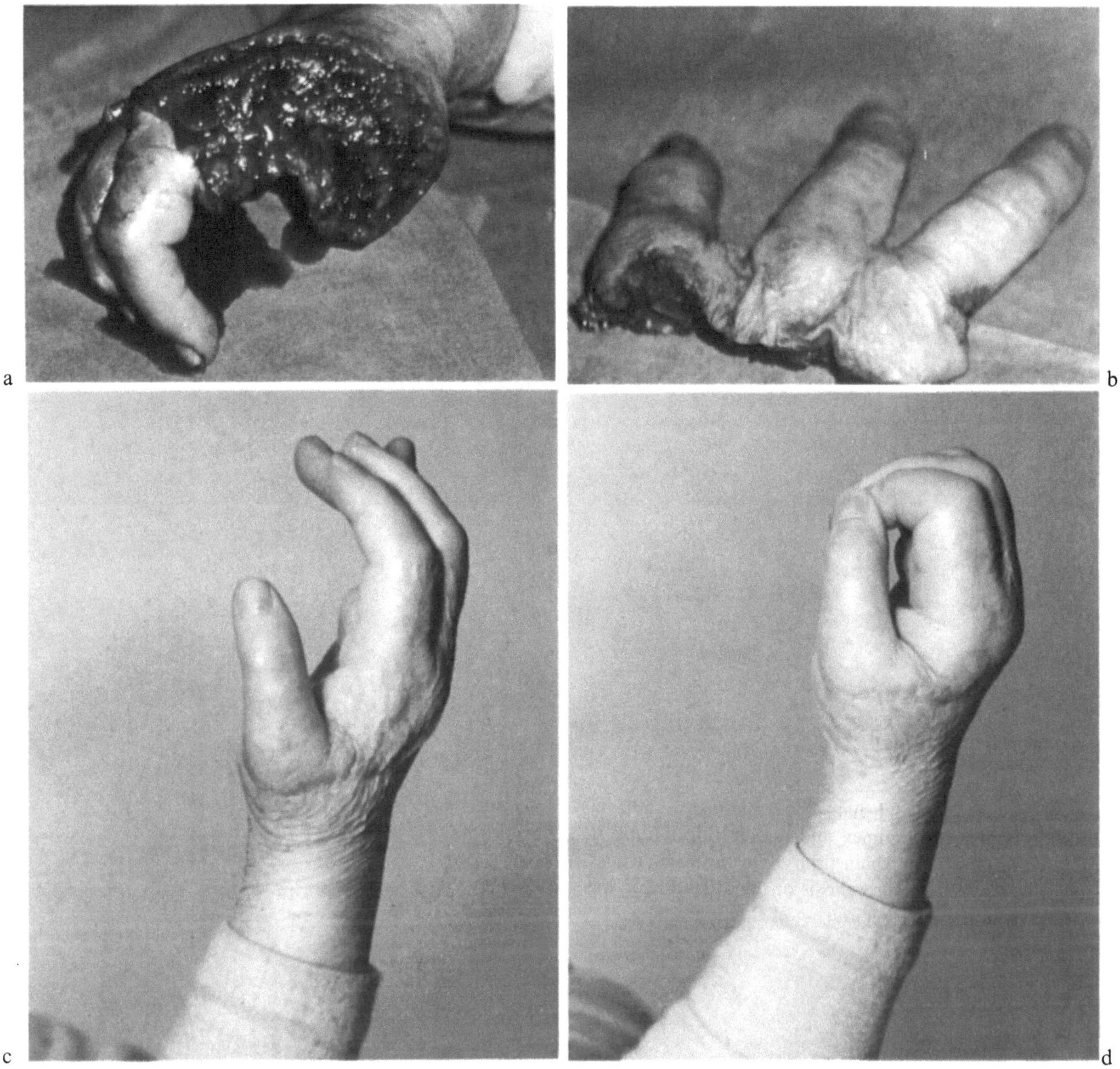

Fig. 80 a–d. Circular saw injury in a 72 year old woman resulting in 'en bloc' amputation of the thumb, index and middle fingers. The functional result at 9 months post-operatively is shown

joint proximally. Re-establishment of the palmar arch suffices for arterialisation. The more important ulnar artery is anastomosed to the superficial palmar arch. A complication in this region is division of the mixed motor and sensory median and ulnar nerves. In amputations in this region the carpal tunnel should always be split to avoid obstruction and pressure damage.

2. Guillotine Amputations

Smooth cut amputations offer the best conditions for replantation. The extent of the tissue trauma is negligible, requiring minimal debridement and shortening of the vessel stumps (see Figs. 76–78). Under guillotine amputations, the authors include circular saw amputations, since generally only a few millimetres of tissue damage is found.

3. Crushing Injuries

In crushing injuries precise management of the vessel stumps is necessary so that an appropriately wide debridement extending to absolutely healthy tissue is carried out. The wide-

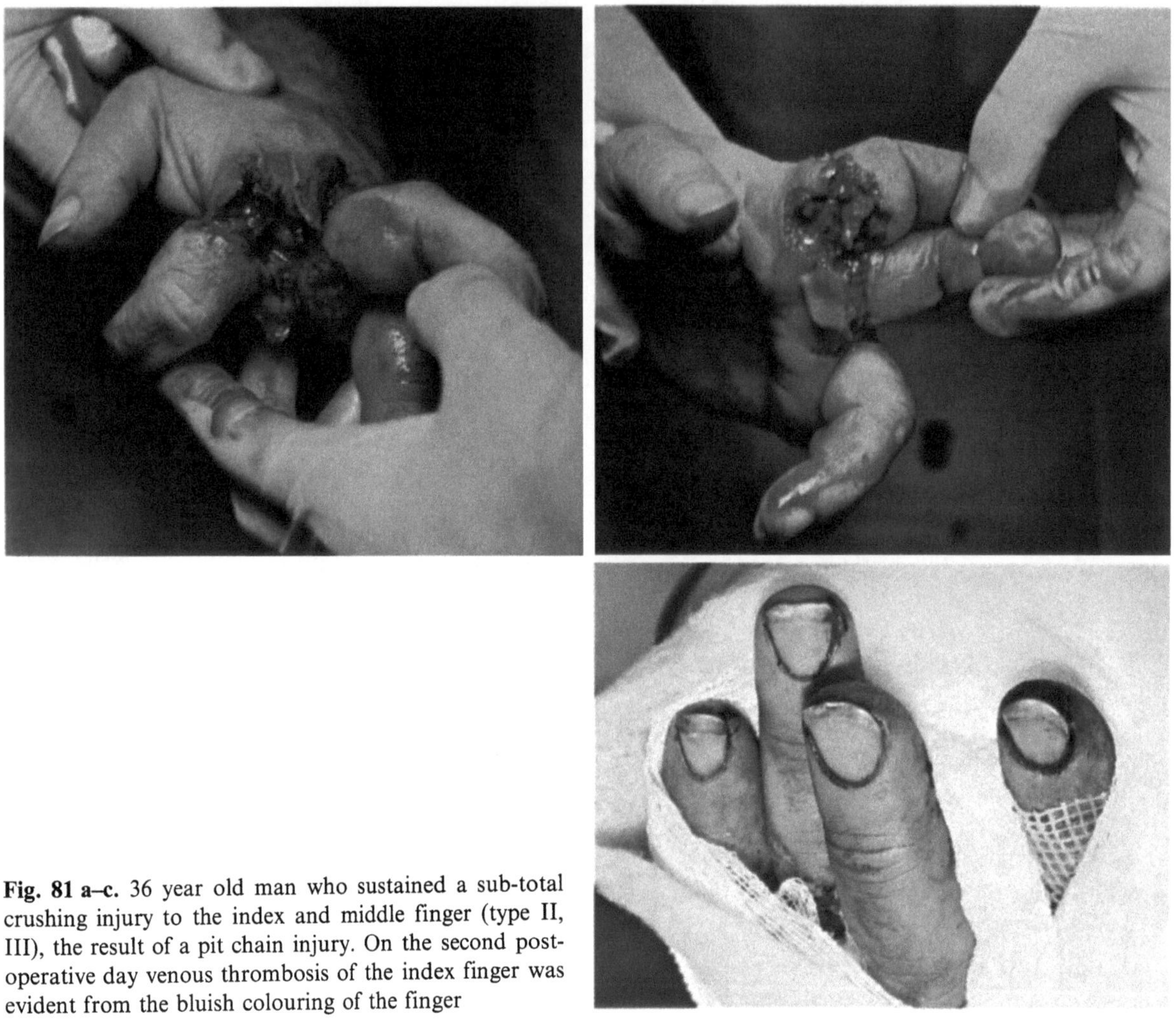

a b c

Fig. 81 a–c. 36 year old man who sustained a sub-total crushing injury to the index and middle finger (type II, III), the result of a pit chain injury. On the second post-operative day venous thrombosis of the index finger was evident from the bluish colouring of the finger

spread use of vein grafts inhibits an over-enthusiastic tendency to shorten the extremity. Blunt instruments most often cause this type of injury and frequently lead only to subtotal amputations. The retained structures are often so severely damaged, however, that it is more sensible to convert a subtotal crushing injury into a total guillotine amputation and then, only after appropriate shortening, carry out the replantation (see Fig. 81).

4. Severe Crushing and Combination Injuries with Damage to the Amputated Part

A very precise inspection of the tissue is required in such cases, but a full resection of all damaged tissue is mostly not possible because of the extent of the damage. Subsequently, complications are frequent, such as thrombosis resulting from damaged intima or secondary necrosis. It is amazing that vein grafts which have been uncovered in extensive areas of necrosis are functional and can survive. Careful perfusion with heparinised Ringer solution can occasionally give information about the patency and continuity of vessels in the amputated part. Since, in the majority of cases, the actual extent of tissue damage cannot be determined at first, it is difficult to assess the functional result that can be achieved, and such severely traumatised amputations remain a problem with regard to the indication for replantation (see Fig. 82).

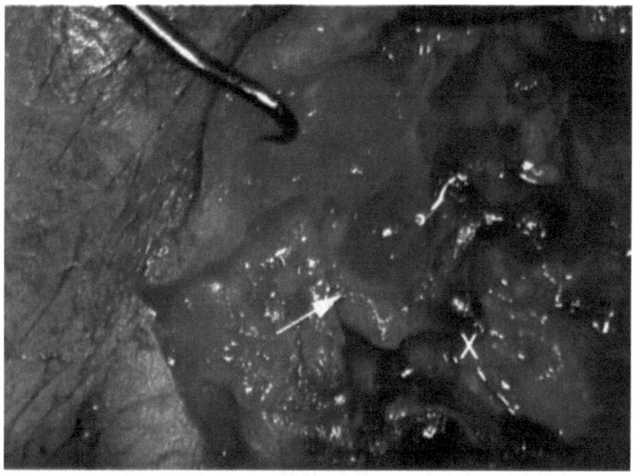

d

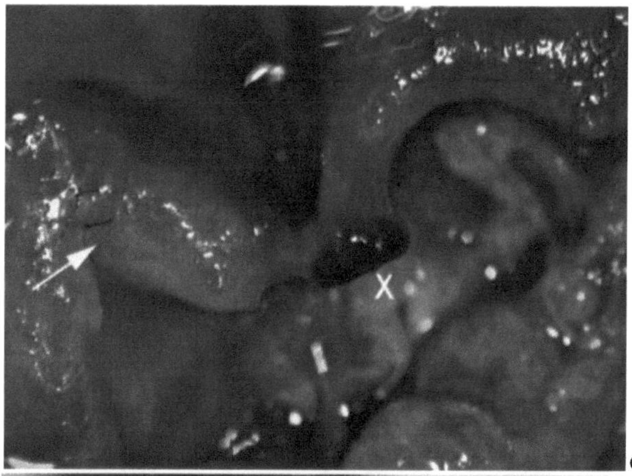

e

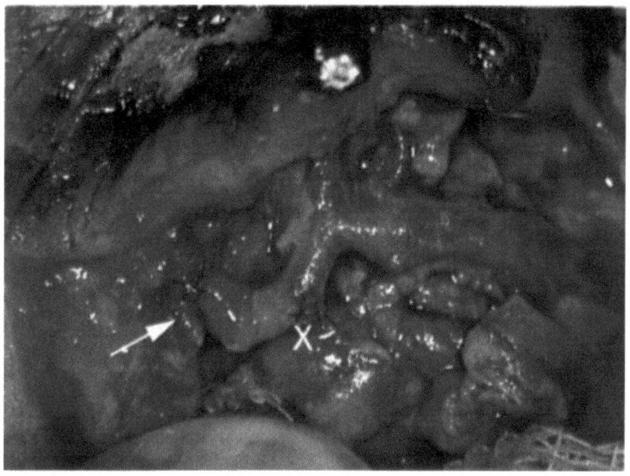

f

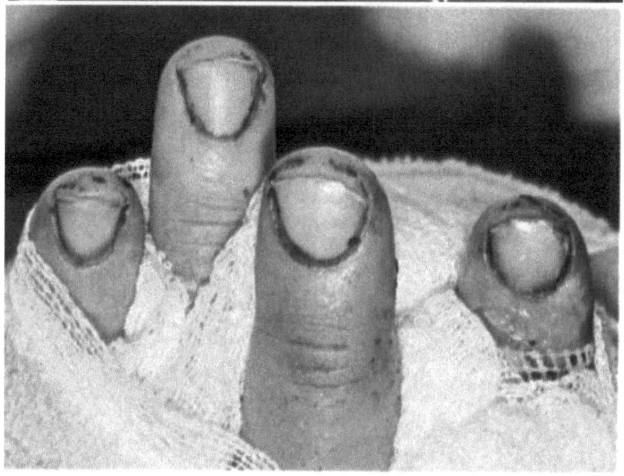

g

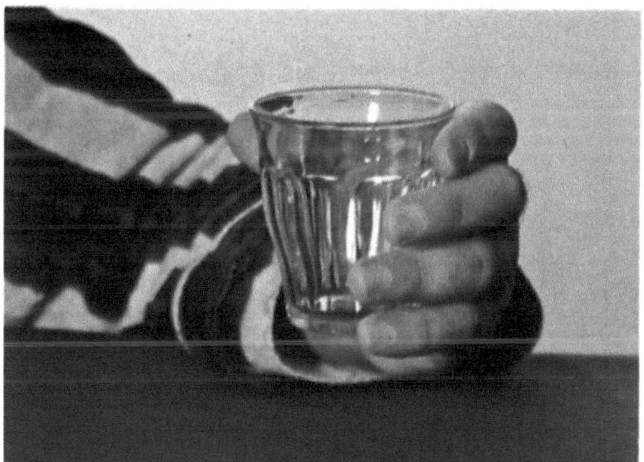

h

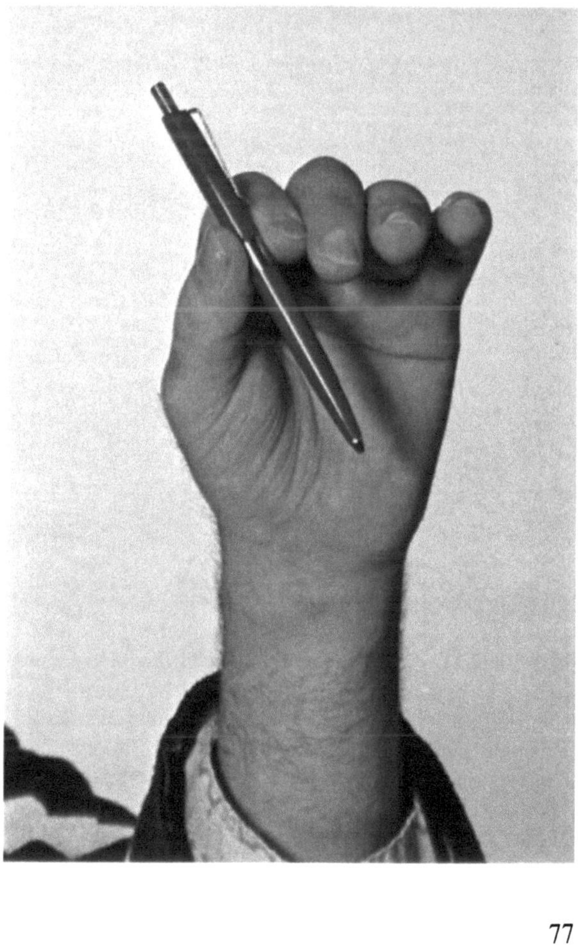

i

Fig. 81 d–i. At re-operation, a thrombosis was found in the area of the crushing injury and not at the anastomosis (arrow demonstrates patency of the anastomosis site). A thrombectomy was performed via a side-branch, which is marked with an 'X' **h, i.** Result three months later

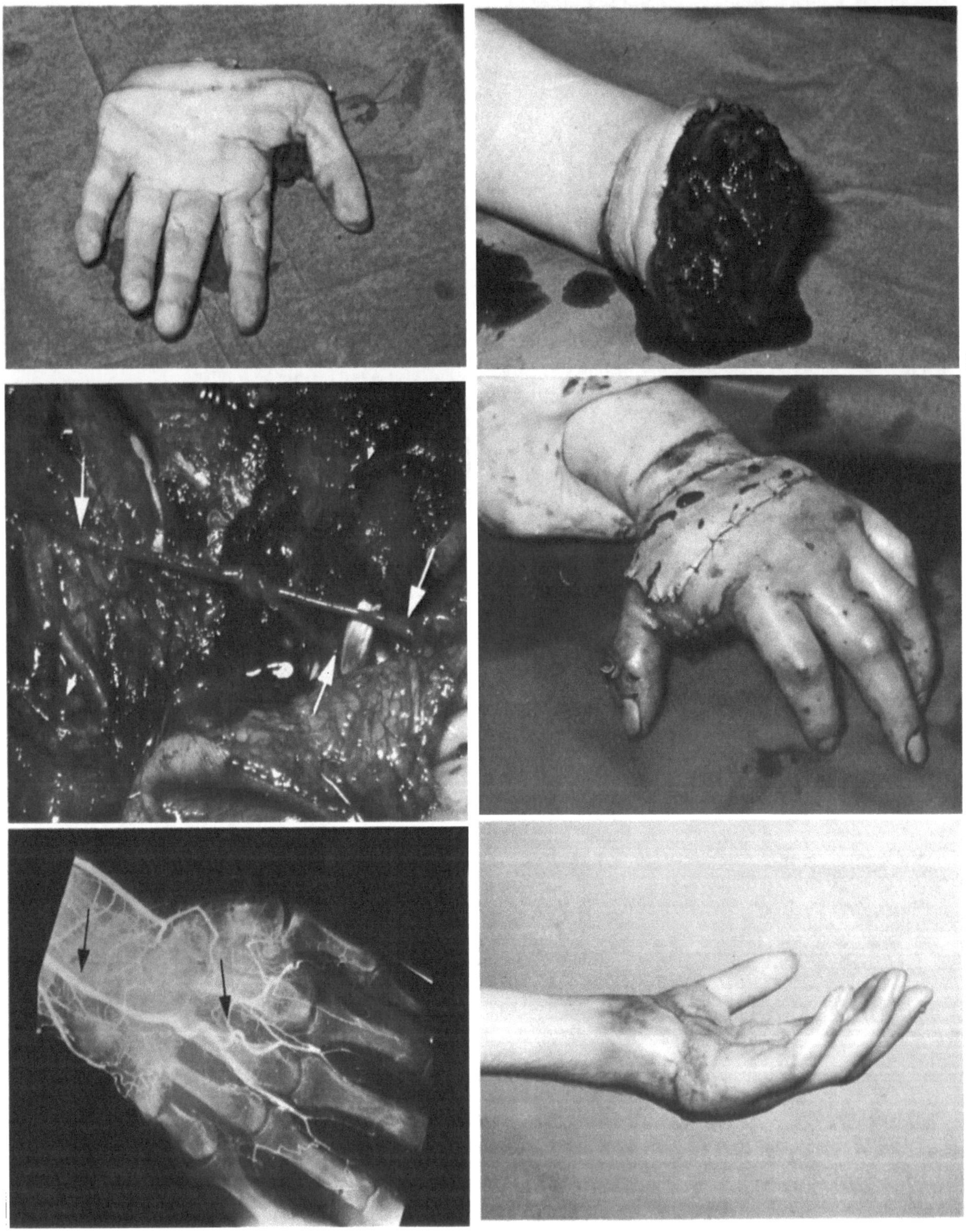

a b c d e f

Fig. 82. a, b Total crushing amputation in the hand (zone V), in a 28 year old woman; the result of an injury from a punching machine. Broad zones of crushing are easily recognised and there is additional evidence of crushing of the amputated part and forearm. **c** The arterial supply was connected using a 7 cm long 'Y' shaped vein graft between the ulnar artery (left) and the superficial and deep palmar arteries (right). The arrows show the sites of the anastomoses. **d** The appearance at the end of the replantation. The areas of crushing were extensively resected and the skin replaced using split skin grafts. **e** At six months post-operatively, the vein graft remained patent (arrows at the anastomoses sites). **f** The result at five months following replantation, with some return of sensation already evident

5. Avulsion Injuries

The group of avulsion amputation injuries in the majority of cases offers the most unfavourable conditions for replantation. The problem lies with the differing levels of separation of the different structures. In the authors' experience, the flexor tendons are most commonly ripped out from the forearm musculature, whereas the extensor tendons are divided at the level of the bone fracture. The neurovascular bundles are avulsed at a variable distance, with the nerves frequently divided further proximally than the vessels. The dorsal veins, on the other hand, are severed in line with the edge of the skin and the separation of the skin can be quite variable. Avulsion injuries of the thumb are most common (Biemer et al. 1977). In the majority of cases the reconnection of the arterial supply is possible by using vein grafts. Avulsion of the artery frequently results in circumferential detachment of the intima and this must be carefully sought.
Where this occurs, obviously the whole segment of the vessel must be sacrificed and replaced. Reconstruction of the flexor tendon, when it is pulled out from the forearm musculature, is not possible and replacement in the thumb can be obtained by transferring the superficial flexor tendon of a long finger. However, the thumb will give an astonishingly good result without a flexor tendon, i.e. without active bending of the metacarpophalangeal joint or the interphalangeal joint. This is because the thumb alone, by its carpometacarpal saddle joint and movements due to the thenar musculature, can retain sufficient mobility. The nerve reconstruction in avulsion amputations must be individually solved. Frequently, grafts are also required and occasionally a 'Y'-connection, using only one central stump, is expedient (Figs. 83, 84).

6. Degloving Injuries

Degloving injuries are recognisable by the retention of the skeleton tendon apparatus. It is the soft tissue coat alone which is stripped off or amputated. Fingers caught in a roller and pulled into a machine suffer degloving of the soft tissue coat of the fingers, as the injured person moves in a counterdirection.
Another typical mechanism is the catching of a ring, resulting in stripping of the skin coat from the ring finger. As these mechanisms of injuries demonstrate, additional severe trauma of the amputated part must always be expected, either the result of crushing by rollers or through telescoping together by ring avulsion.
The peripheral bone can occasionally be divided at a variable length from division of the skin.
Aesthetically, as well as functionally, such degloving injuries are very difficult to manage, but the successful replantation of the skin coat can yield very good results (see Figs. 85 and 86).

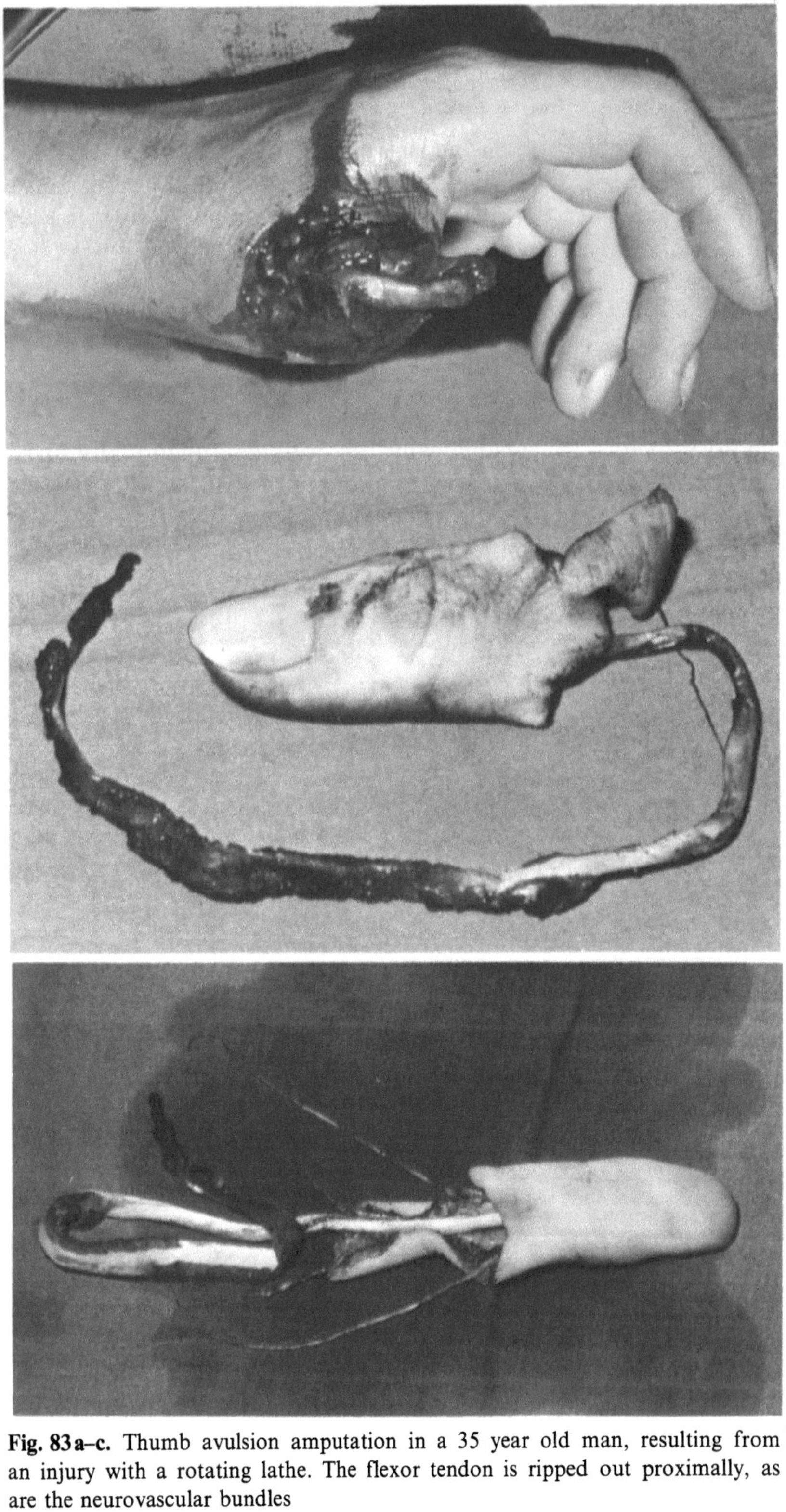

a

b

c

Fig. 83a–c. Thumb avulsion amputation in a 35 year old man, resulting from an injury with a rotating lathe. The flexor tendon is ripped out proximally, as are the neurovascular bundles

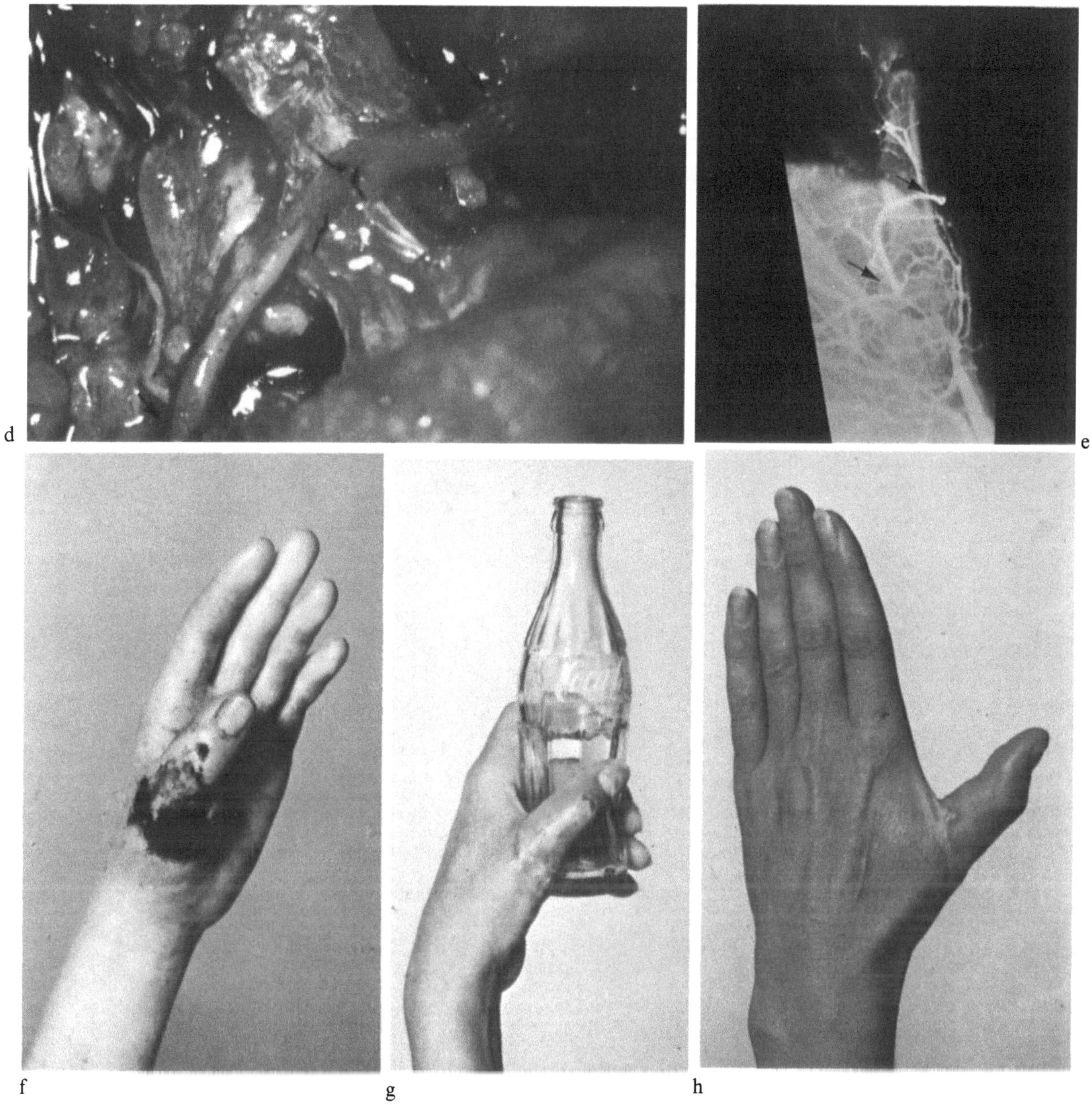

Fig. 83 d–h. The arterial supply was connected using a vein graft running diagonally over the flexor tendon. The area at the base of the thumb, which was short-circuited by the vein graft, subsequently showed superficial skin necrosis which, however, healed spontaneously (*arrows* demonstrate the site of anastomoses). **g–h** Post-operative result eight months following replantation a 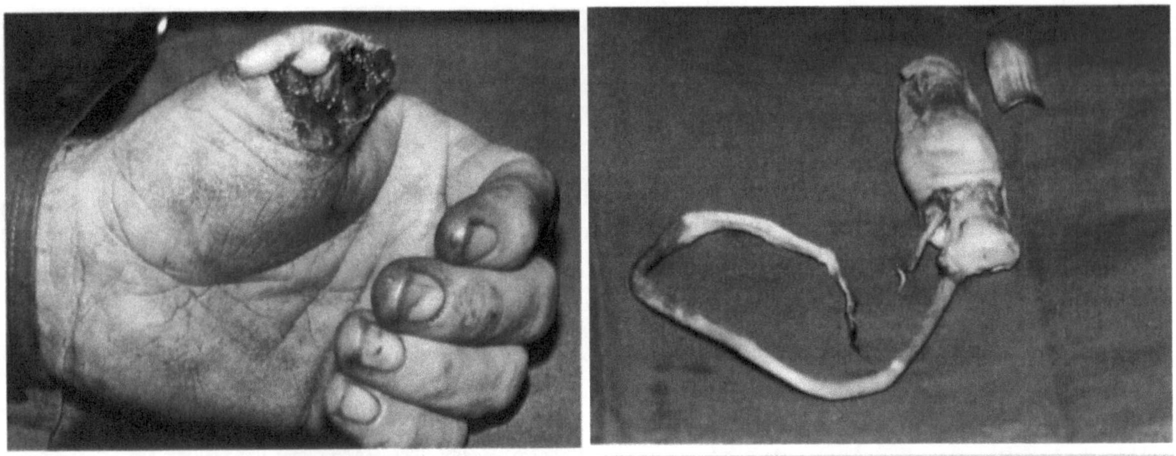 b

c 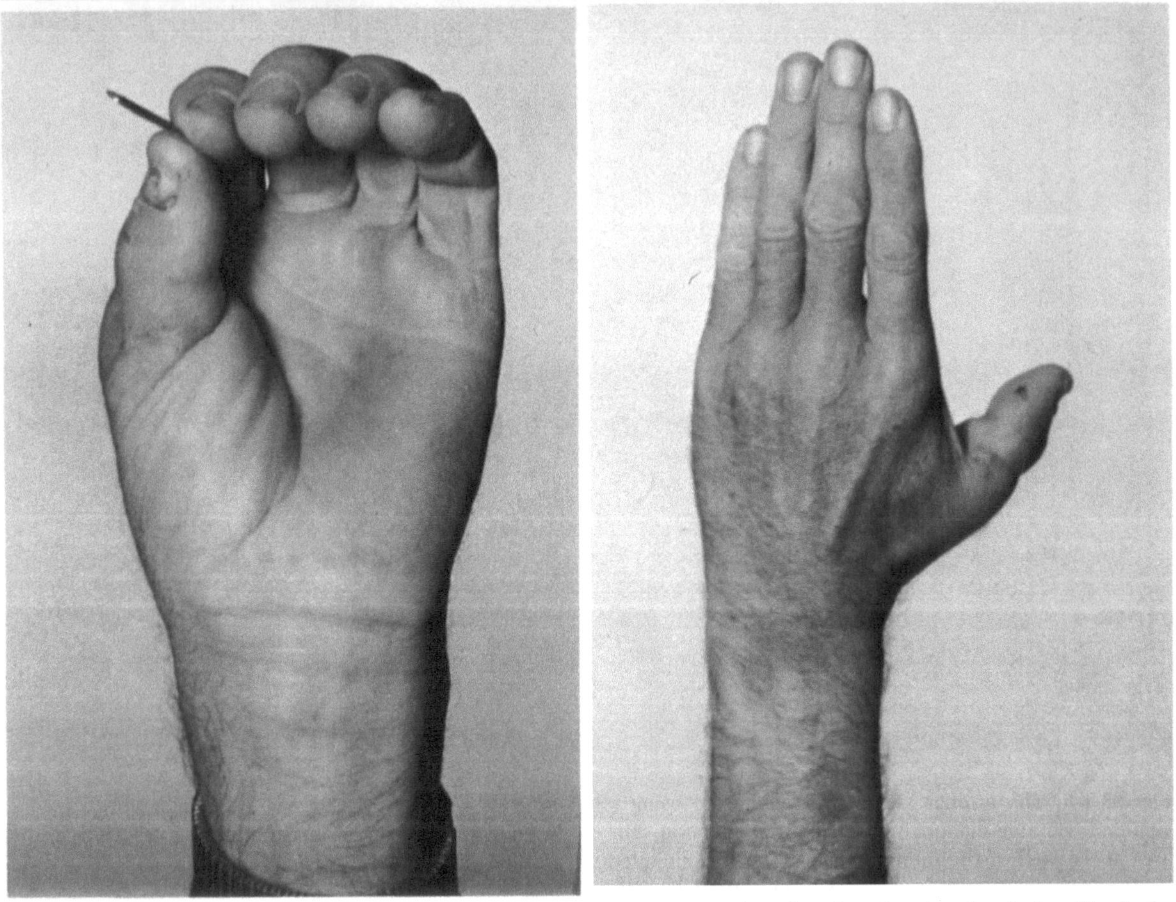 d

Fig. 84 a–d. A tap axle injury in a farmer resulting in an avulsion amputation with additional damage of the amputated part. Post-operative result is shown at 6 months and there is a functional arthrodesis of both the interphalangeal and metacarpophalangeal joints of the thumb

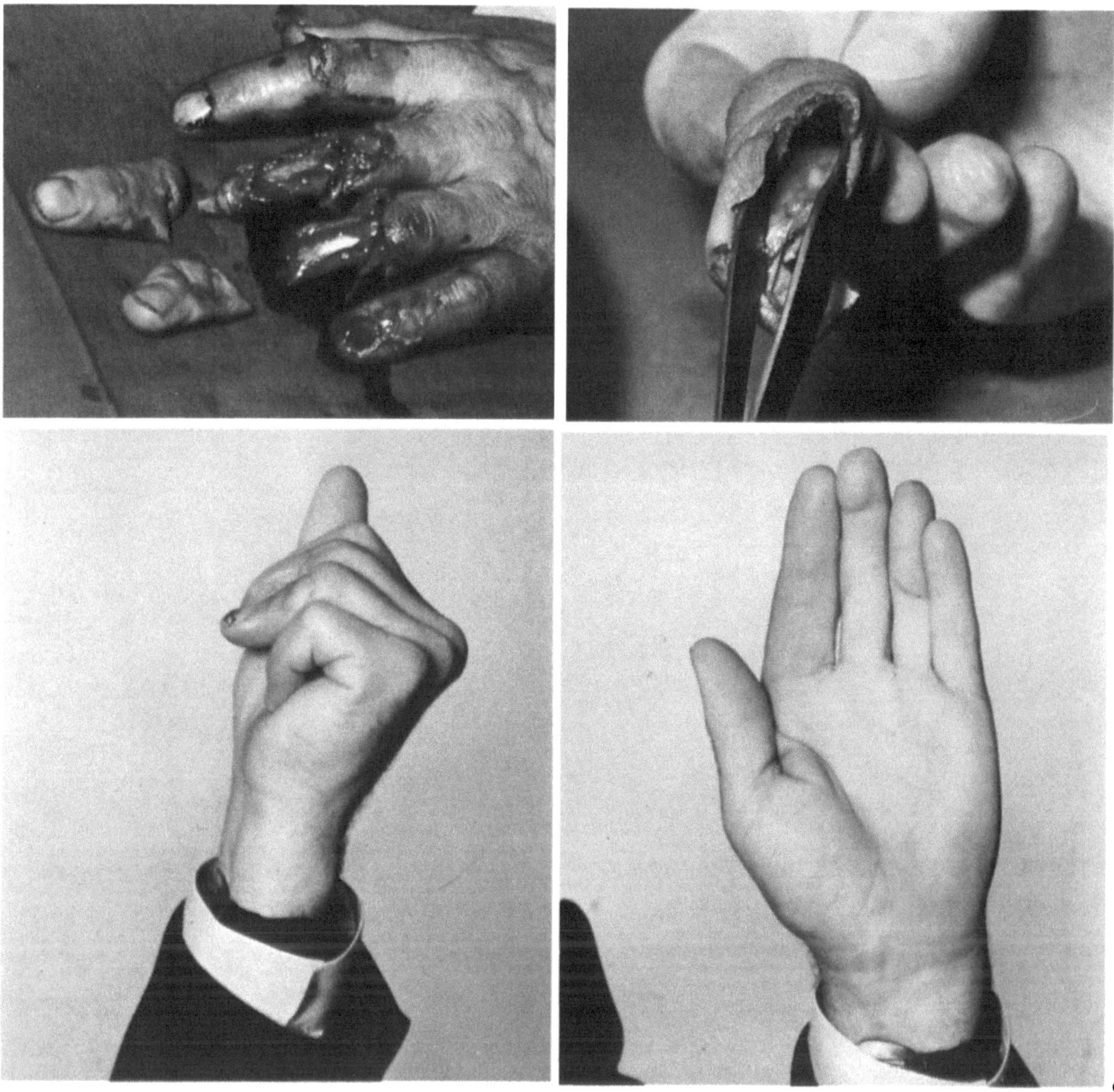

a b c d

Fig. 85 a–d. Roller injury resulting in a degloving amputation of the middle and ring fingers. The soft tissue covering is completely empty and there is additional crushing. Post-operative appearance at seven months following replantation

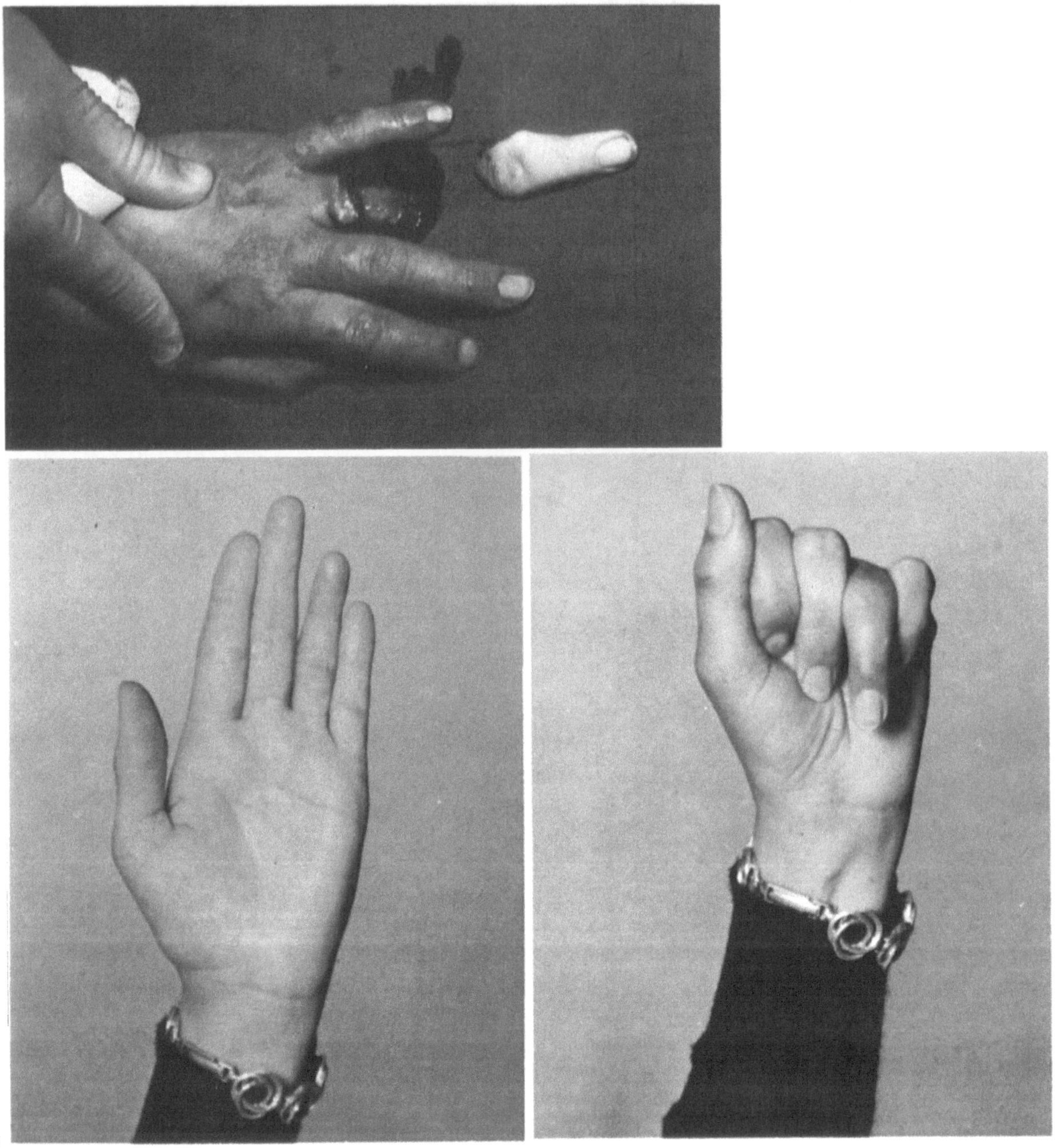

a b c

Fig. 86a–c. 44 year old woman who sustained a wedding ring injury resulting in degloving of the ring finger. A good aesthetic and functional result was achieved

VII. Primary Replacement of Destroyed Phalangeal Joints

Duspiva et al. (1979) reported that in about 45% of cases the level of amputation led to injuries or destruction of the joints of the finger. An arthrodesis of the distal interphalangeal joint is relatively unimportant from a functional point of view.

In contrast, the loss of a proximal interphalangeal joint leads to considerable impairment, which varies according to the occupation of the injured party. Since, in any replanted finger, a partial restriction of movement in the proximal and distal interphalangeal joints is to be expected, an arthrodesis of the metacarpophalangeal joint frequently results in total incapacity of the digit. Thus, replanted index fingers with destroyed metacarpophalangeal joints or interphalangeal joints are subsequently mostly left out of gripping and grasping, and the pinch grip is then performed between the thumb and the middle finger (see Chap. 'Indications').

Primary implantation of a joint prosthesis can help improve such functional loss. The authors use the Niebauer-Cutter prosthesis[10] (see Fig. 87) or the more sensitive St. George joint prosthesis.[11]

Particular indications for the implantation of an artificial joint exist where the metacarpophalangeal joint is destroyed in the index and middle finger, and possibly in the ring finger. Replacement of the proximal interphalangeal joints should only be performed when there are special indications.

Primary joint replacement is only possible in clean-cut injuries and where there is sufficient soft tissue covering for the prosthesis. Any adverse effects on the microanastomosis in such cases has not been established (s. Fig. 88).

---

10 Cutter

11 Link, Hamburg

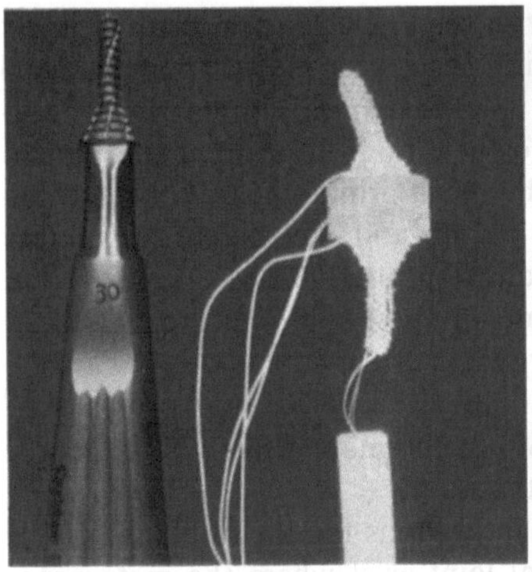

87

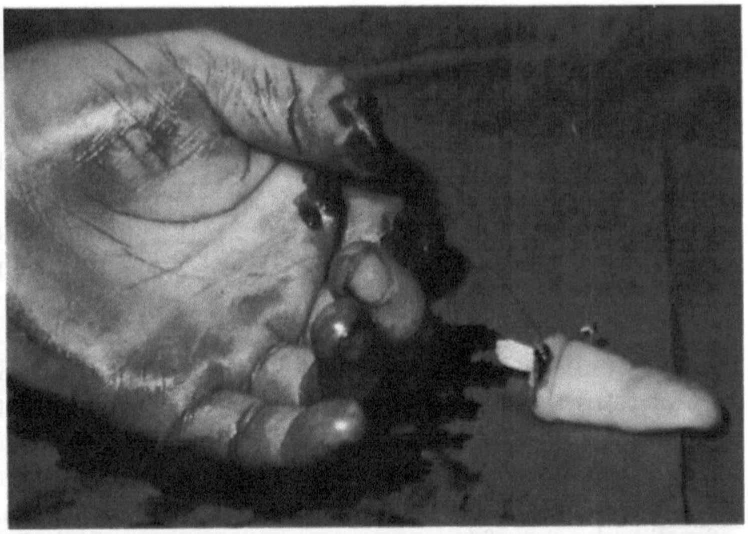

88a

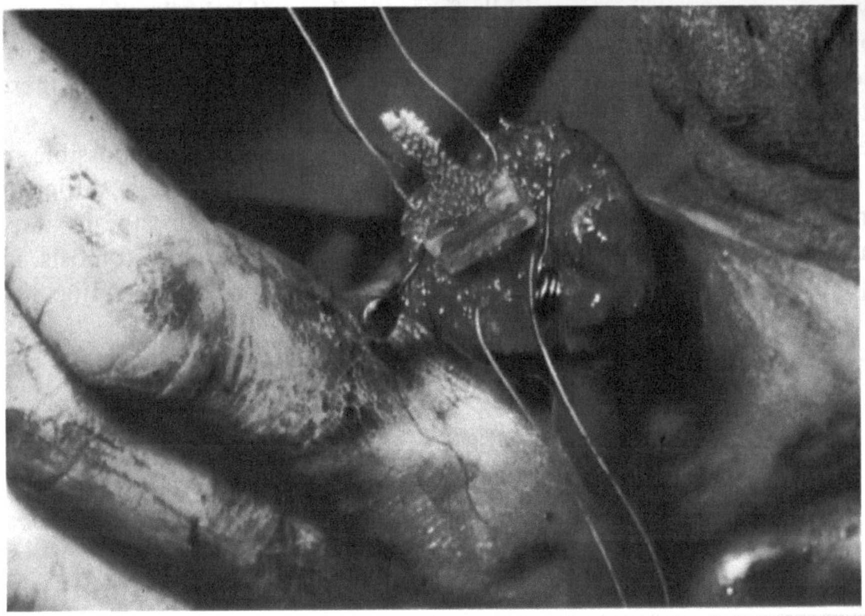

88b

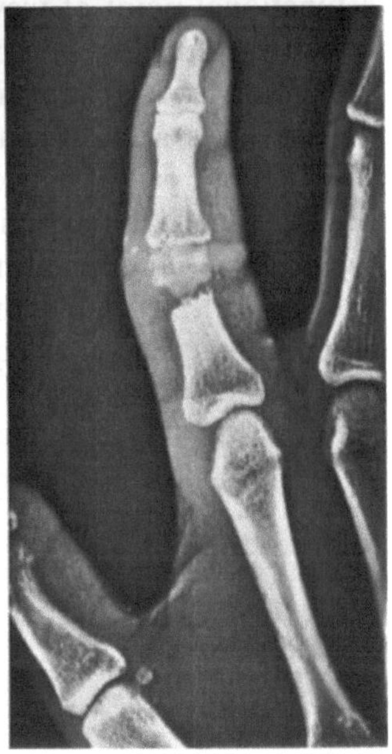

c

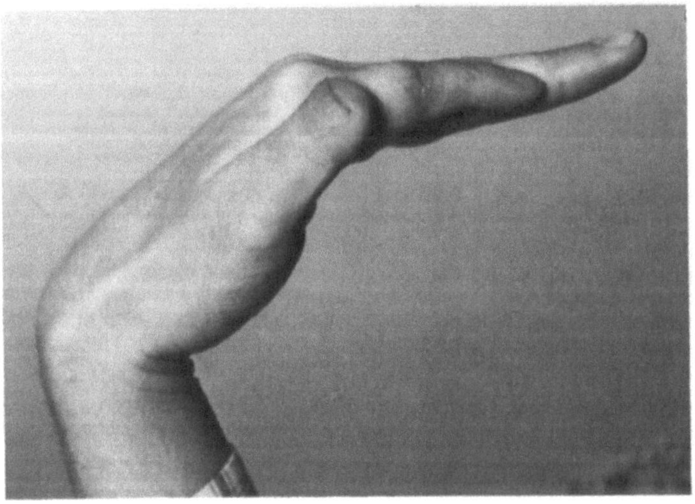

d

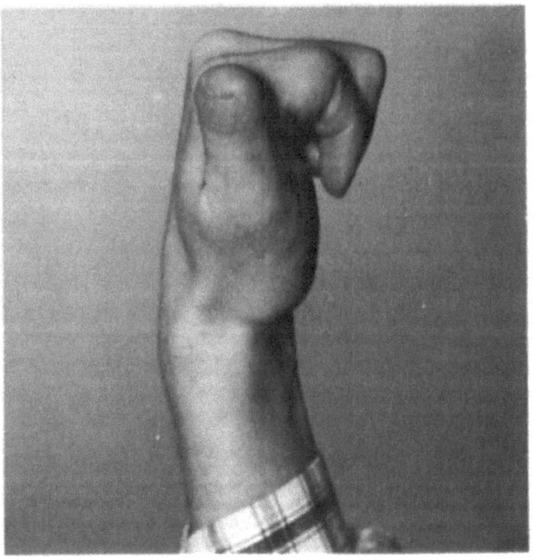

e

Fig. 87. Niebauer finger joint prosthesis (Cutter), with suitable punch for insertion

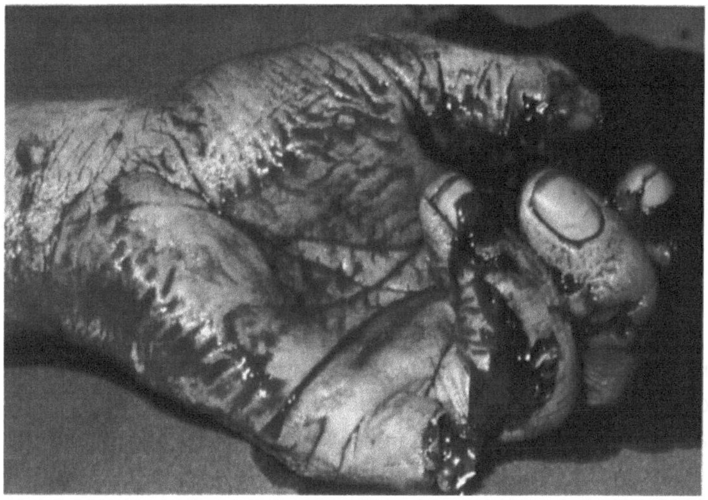

89a

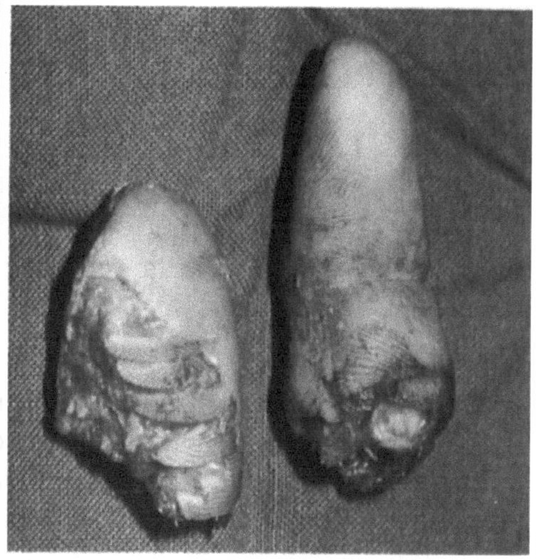

b

◀ **Fig. 88a–e.** Circular saw injury in a 19 year old man, resulting in total amputation of the index finger with destruction of the proximal interphalangeal joint. The destroyed joint was replaced at the time of replantation using a Niebauer-Cutter prosthesis. Following tenolysis, full function in this joint was achieved. **c–e.** X-ray of the index finger showing the joint prosthesis and functional result 8 months following replantation

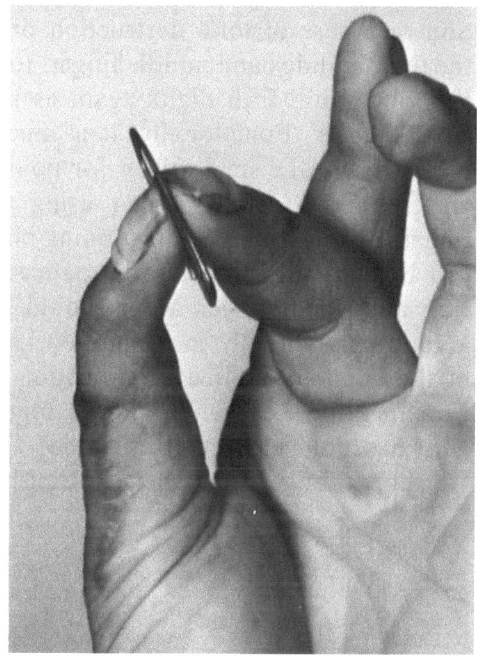

c

Fig. 89 a–c. Total amputation of the thumb in zone II with marked destruction of the amputated part and total amputation of the little finger in zone III. Since replantation of the thumb was not possible, the amputated part of the small finger was transplanted primarily onto the thumb stump

Fig. 90 a, b. Total amputation of the middle, ring and little fingers, as well as total amputation of the thumb in zone III. There was an additional sub-total amputation of the index finger. Because of the severity of the destruction of the amputated parts, it was only possible to use the ring finger replanted as a thumb, thus achieving a good gripping function

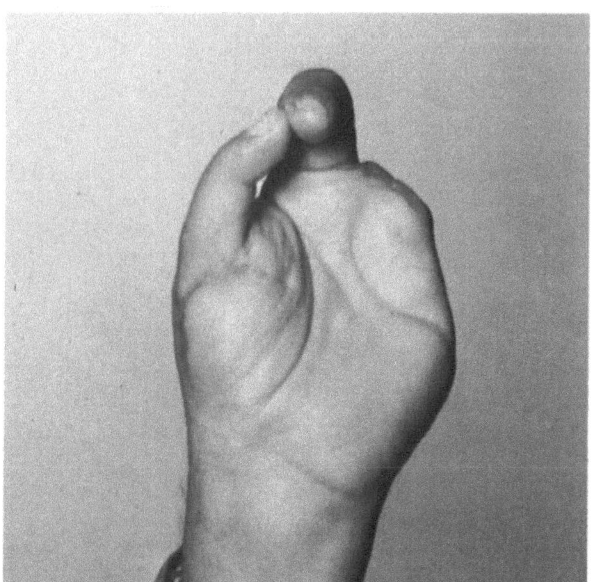

90a

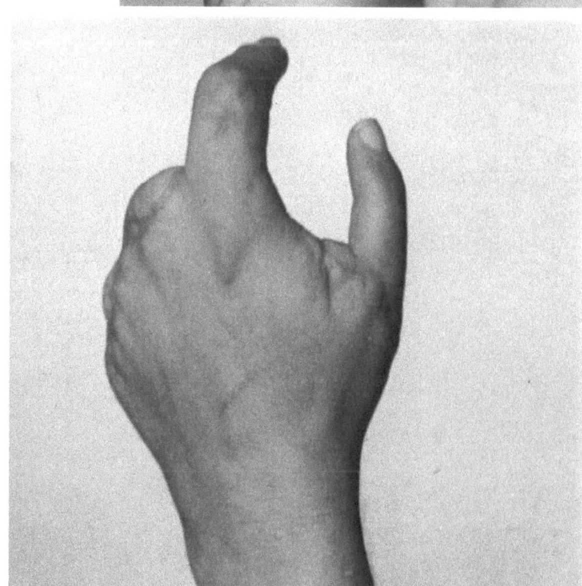

90b

VIII. Primary Finger Transplantation

In multiple amputations and cases where there is total destruction of individual fingers, the aim is to build a hand with an optimal gripping function out of the available, replantable digits. It is of no value in a five finger amputation or a case of total destruction or loss of the thumb, index and middle finger, to replant the fourth and fifth digits again as ring and small fingers. Functionally, it is much more useful to use the small finger for pollicisation and rebuild a middle finger using the ring finger. By this means, a functioning pinch grip can be achieved, whereas the patient with a ring and small finger alone would have to accept an essentially more limited usefulness of the hand. A unified classification for this primary 'finger exchange' in replantation surgery has not yet been formulated. The term 'finger exchange', equivalent to transposition, or pollicisation, was until now used to describe a function-improving operation, in which one digit was transferred on its neurovascular bundles.

Since, however, following a total amputation, a free tissue transplantation is performed, the difference here is analogous to that between skin flaps and skin transplantation, see B II 'Definitions and nomenclature'; where all criteria for the description 'transplantation' are given. Another possibility would be to use the term 'heterotopic finger replantation'.

The basic principles for primary finger transplantation are:

1. Reconstruction of a thumb with, where possible, a normal length. Amputated long fingers with destroyed metacarpophalangeal joints are especially suited for this purpose. Alternatively, amputated parts of digits can be used to lengthen the thumb stump.
2. Reconstruction of the middle finger. It is functionally more important to build a competent middle finger rather than an index finger, since the possibility of grip between thumb and middle finger is greater.
3. Following reconstitution of competent 'pincers', the remaining amputated parts can be used to complete the hand, as appropriate (see Figs. 89 and 90).

IX. Post-operative Management

Replantation cases are generally regarded as requiring intensive supervision post-operatively. On the one hand, this is because of the continuous monitoring of patency and the early recognition of thrombosis, and on the other hand because of the medical treatment involved. This is particularly true when heparinisation is performed.

For the first three days, the patency of the vessels in replants must be checked every half hour to one hour. Here the parameters are – colour (rosy, pale, bluish), temperature (normal or lower than the comparable finger on the opposite side), turgor (blocked up, filled to bursting, empty) and capillary filling by nail or skin pressure (strengthened, normal, absent). Deviation of any one of these criteria from the norm, when noticed by the nursing staff monitoring the case, should be notified immediately to the replantation surgeon on duty.

In the clinical situation, routine and constant monitoring using the Doppler apparatus, photoelectric pulse meters or percutaneous PO_2 measurements, is still not proven.

1. Arterial Thrombosis

When there is an arterial thrombosis, the digit is pale and empty and the skin temperature falls to at least 5 °C lower than the healthy opposite side. Furthermore, there is no capillary filling following pressure exerted on the nail or skin. Failure to bleed following piercing of the skin is the surest criterion and Doppler investigation or percutaneous PO_2 measurements can provide further proof.

2. Venous Thrombosis

The replanted part is bluish, bursting and shows an increased capillary filling. Piercing of the skin produces mostly a spurt of blood which, subsequently through continuous bleeding of the digit, leads to a brightening of the bluish colouring (see Fig. 91). The skin temperature is similarly lowered to about 5 °C lower than the opposite side and the amputated parts quickly develop blistering (see Fig. 92a). When there are signs of a circulatory disturbance as described above, the splintage and dressings must be carefully examined to eliminate any obstruction or compression of the vessels. Thereafter the skin sutures should be inspected and removed as necessary. Should these measures fail to lead to an improvement or normalisation with 2 hours, then a thrombosis must be presumed and there then exists a clear indication for reoperation.

Such secondary operations can most commonly be performed under local anaesthesia, since the incisions and approach are predetermined, and the handling of the vessels is not painful. Following thrombectomy, a vein graft is nearly always required (see Chap. 'Microthrombectomy and vein grafts'), since the former anastomosis must be excised (see Fig. 91).

The replanted part must be maintained in a slightly elevated position and the maintenance of the hand in a supine position allows ready observation and an unrestricted venous outflow from the fingers. In contrast to hand surgery in general, where dressings are changed as seldom as possible, replantation surgery requires dressings to be changed as frequently as possible. Blood encrusted dressing material must be carefully removed after soaking with hydrogen peroxide H_2O_2, since dried-out dressings act as armour-plated splints.

The post-operative medicinal treatment has already been outlined (see Chap. 'Medicinal treatment'). It is important to monitor circulation intensively, since a fall in blood pressure or centralisation can easily lead to a thrombosis. Personal observation has shown a reduction of smoking is not necessary. It is of great importance to discuss the details of the operation, as well as the possible complications, with the patient. Only then, can the otherwise healthy patient understand and follow the surgeon's directions.

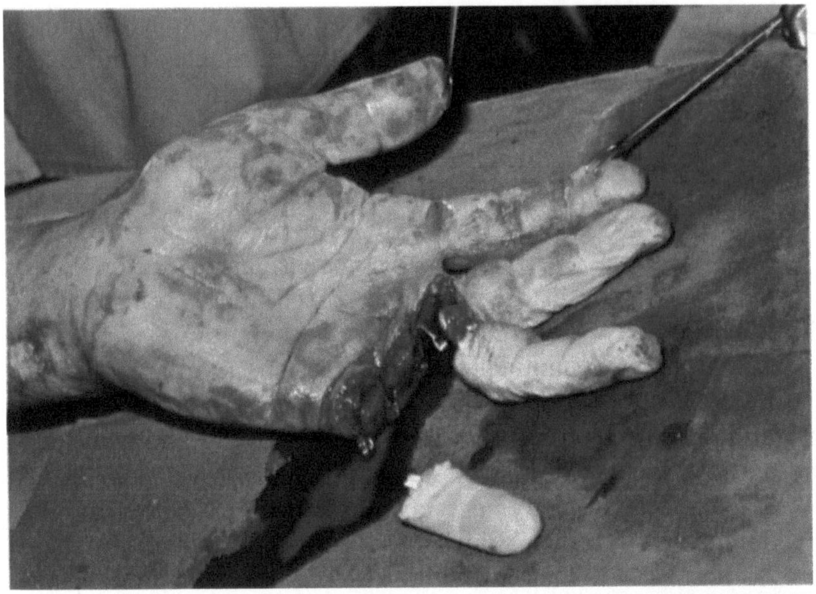

a

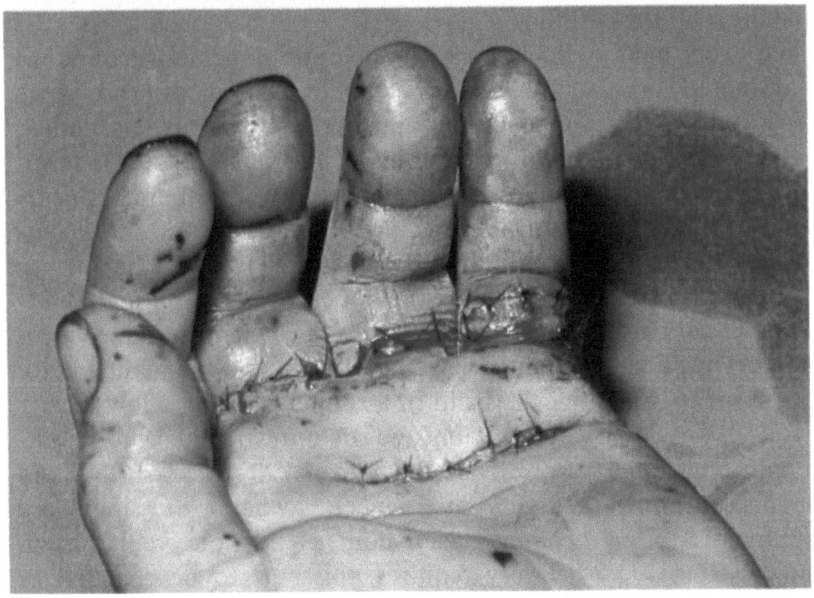

b

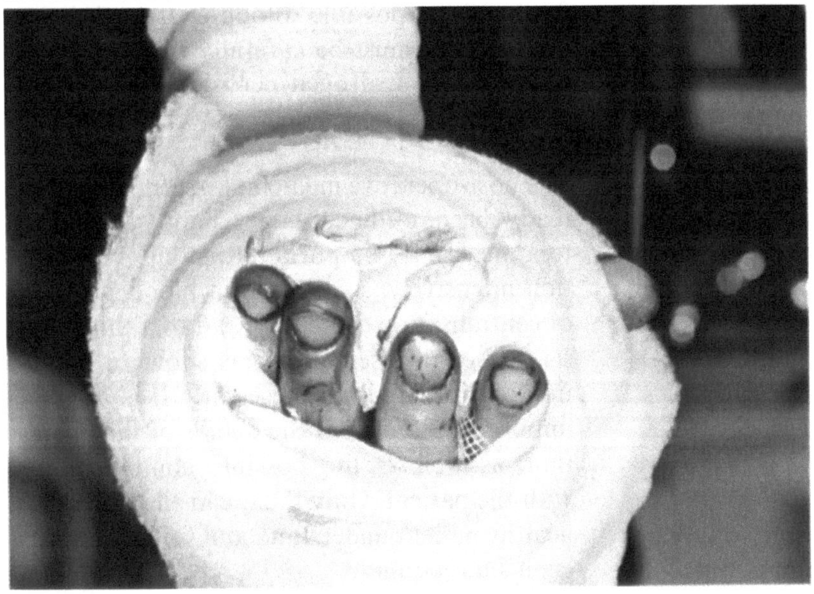

c

Fig. 91. a Sub-total amputation of the middle and ring fingers and total amputation of the small finger. **b–d** Initial replantation was free from complications but after 24 h, there was evidence of a venous thrombosis in the ring finger. Fig. d shows the typical thrombus appearing proximal to the site of anastomosis. **e, f** Following thrombectomy and direct suturing of the veins, the colour of all fingers returned to normal. Following removal of the thrombus, there is evidence of a strong stream of blood and high pressure in the venous system (see Fig. e)

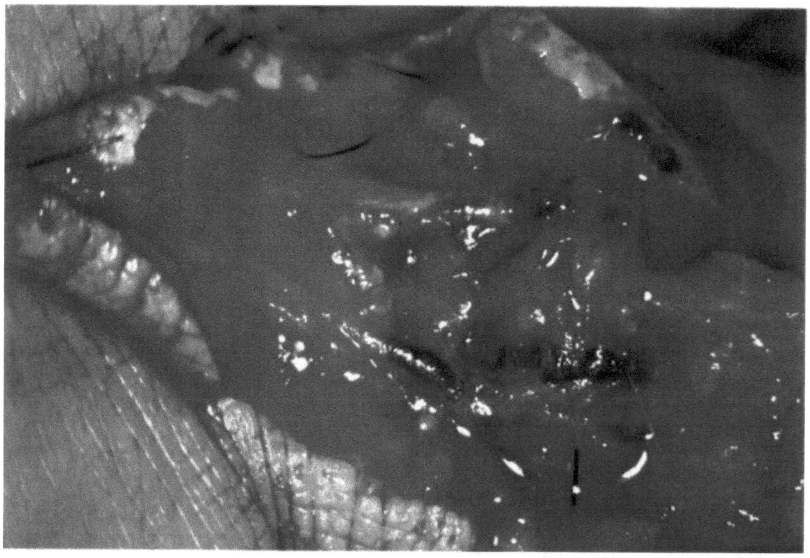
d

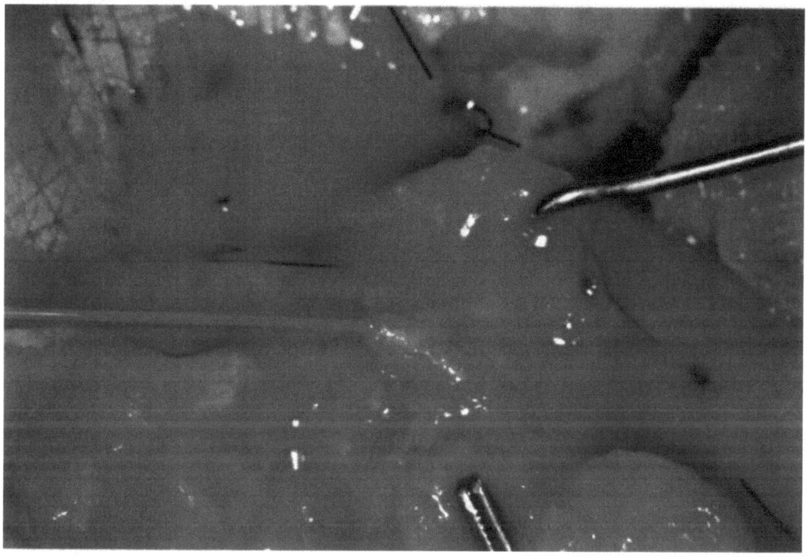
e

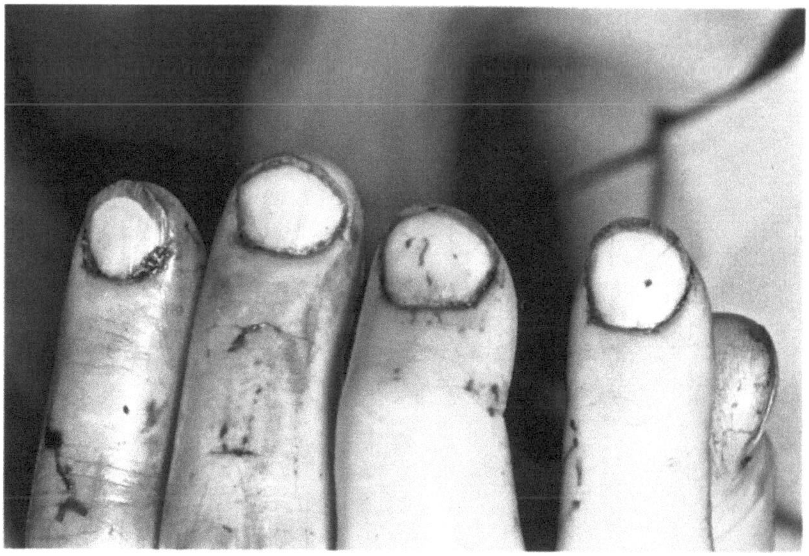
f

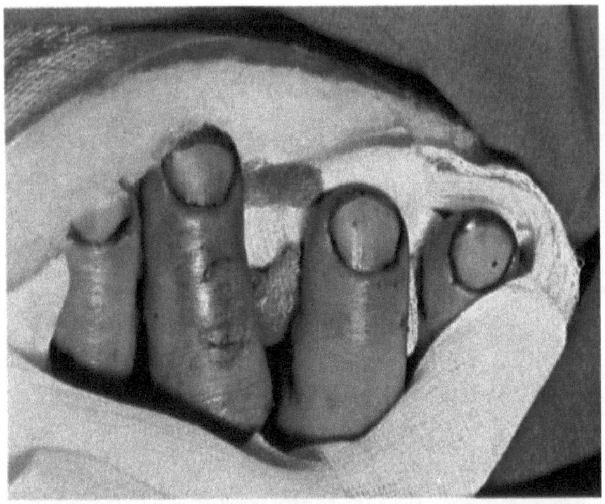

g

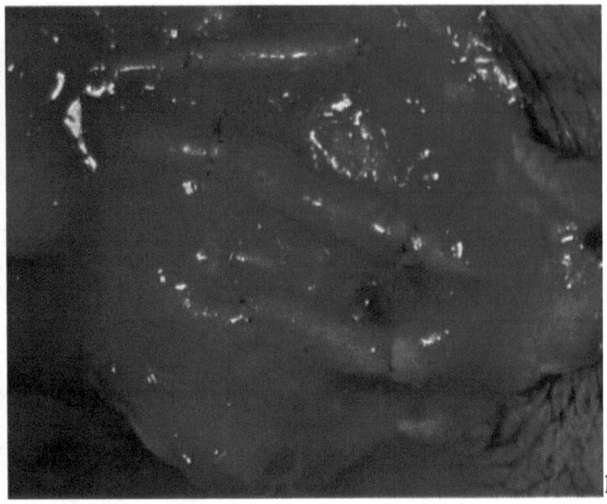

h

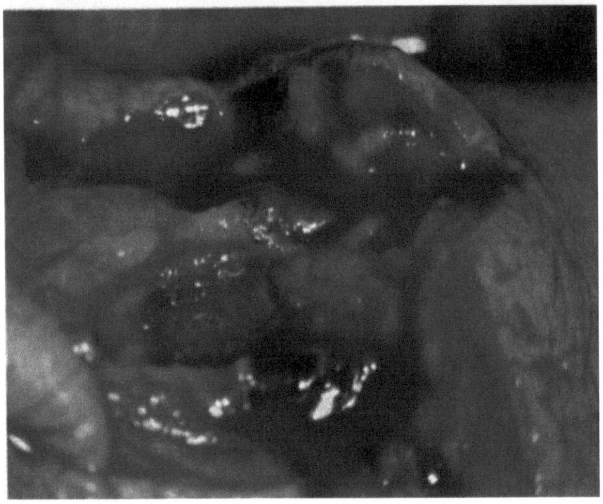

i

Fig. 91 g–k. 24 hours later, there was renewed venous thrombosis in the ring finger and re-exploration again showed the typical appearance of thrombosis at the site of anastomosis. There was a suspicion of too much tension at the site of the anastomosis, resulting in thrombosis and therefore three separate 5 mm long micro-vein grafts were inserted. **j, k** Following the two thrombectomies, the ring finger healed well and the appearance at two months following replantation is shown

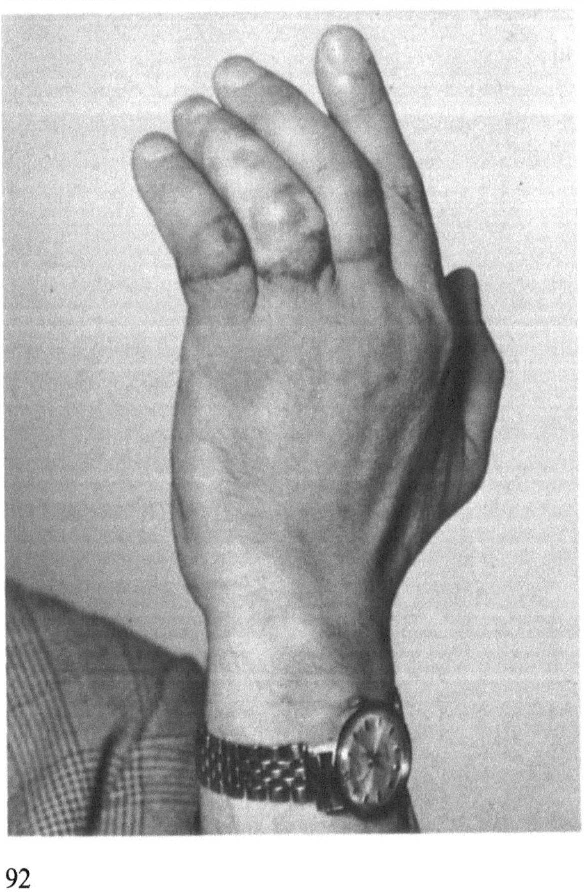

j

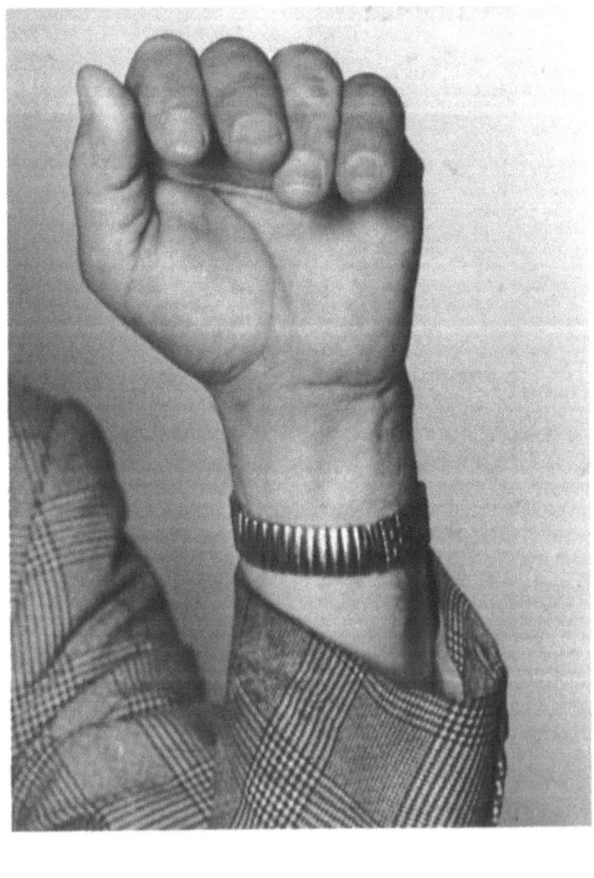

k

Fig. 92 a, b. Replanted index finger following total amputation, resulting from a lawnmower injury. A venous thrombosis has existed for two days and severe changes in the finger can be seen. Despite this, thrombectomy and perfusion is successful, as shown by the recognisable pink colour of the digit. The new anastomosis is covered with a split thickness graft

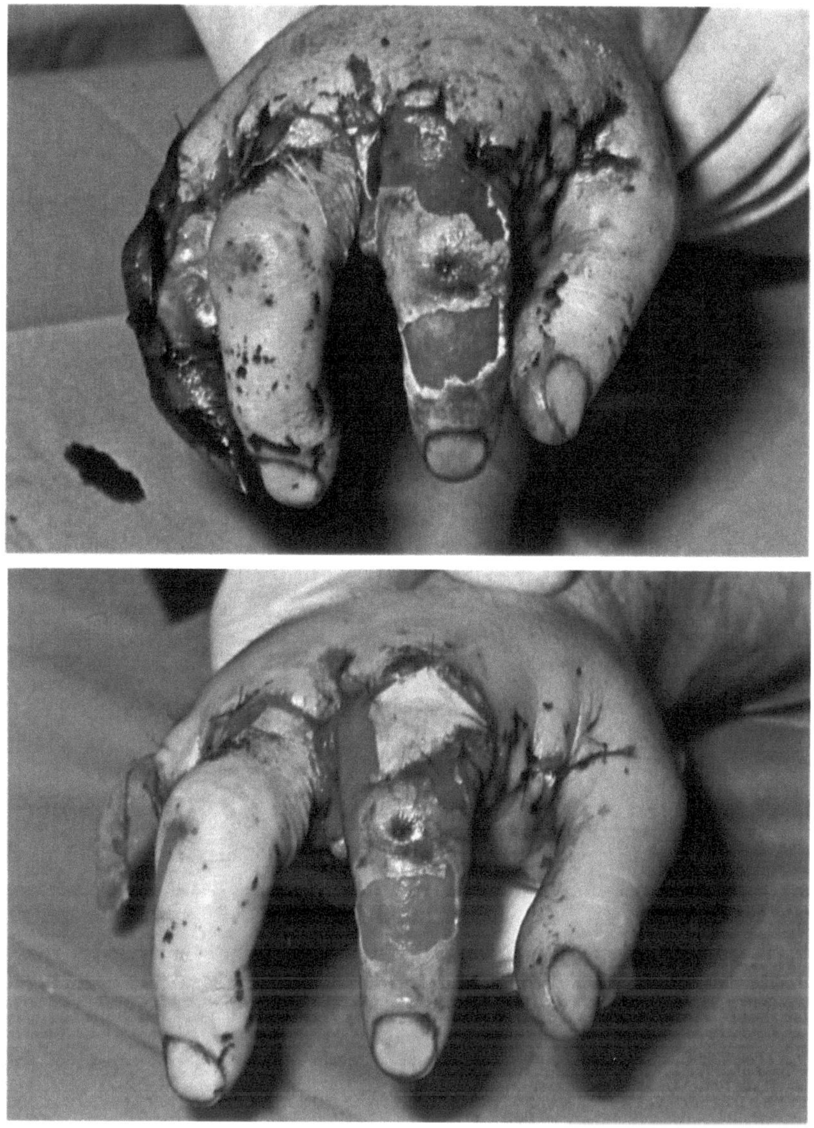

a

b

X. Physical Management

As in all severe hand injuries, the physiotherapist and occupational therapist play an exceedingly important rôle in post-operative management. Physiotherapy commences on the 2nd to 3rd post-operative day with careful passive exercise and treatment of all non-fixed joints. A close collaboration with the appropriate departments is essential to understand and discuss each individual case. Active exercise of all free joints commences from the 3rd week. After radiological union of the fractures is noted and the oesteosynthesis material is removed, the whole hand, particularly all replanted parts, are actively and passively exercised twice daily. The occupational therapy leads to the collective use and coordination of the replantation and retained limbs, so that functionally optimal action is achieved. A functionally good result of this post-operative treatment can only be achieved when the patient actively and consistently supports the treatment. Therefore, whenever possible, this early treatment should be performed in hospital under the control of the replantation surgeon. The shortage of beds, however, frequently results in patients being discharged from hospital as early as possible, and post-operative management is passed to the local hospital or general practitioner and their physiotherapists. In these circumstances, the personal attitude and initiative of the patient is shown most clearly. It is frequently difficult to overcome the patient's fear that the fingers could again 'break off'. For this reason, the exercises and the extent of movement should be fully explained to the patient prior to his discharge from hospital. It is important to dispense with every splinted dressing as early as possible, so that the restrictions of use of the extremity are not additionally emphasised. Accustomed alterations in grip should be avoided, e.g., the pinch-grip between thumb and middle finger, following an index finger replantation. The problems of post-operative management, which to a great extent depend on the character of the patient, exist in all forms of hand surgery, but come particularly clearly into play following replantation.

XI. Secondary Operations

Secondary operations on replanted extremities are often technically more difficult operations, since they must be performed most commonly in close proximity to the vascular anastomosis and in an area of scar tissue. Here, there is always a possibility of vessel or nerve injury because of the difficulty of surveying these structures, or because of atypical vessel connections. In order to reduce the number of secondary operations to a minimum, all structures should be reconstructed primarily, i.e. at the time of replantation. Secondary operations, however, are certainly not avoidable and the authors' personal experience is that they have proved necessary in 40% of replantations.

The most frequently performed secondary operation is tenolysis. Because of the long period of immobilisation of individual joints by osteosynthesis, extensive adhesions occur in the tendon suture area. In certain cases, even post-operative treatment cannot solve or stretch these adhesions. Suture dehiscence likewise leads to long areas of scarring, particularly the flexor tendons. This can only be repaired by means of two-stage flexor tendon surgery. Early mobilisation, which may lead to the avoidance of tendon adhesions or joint stiffening, can, on the other hand, cause pseud-arthrosis. In such cases, secondary operations are not avoidable, although occasionally, the unsteady movement of such unstable fractures, proves to be functionally favourable. This is particularly true when the neighbouring joint is destroyed.

All these secondary operations are performed according to the general techniques used in hand surgery. The only important difference is that an exact knowledge of the position of the vessel anastomosis is useful and it is therefore important that such secondary operations are carried out by the original replantation surgeon.

Table 6. Level of bone injury (amputation) in 194 cases

Mid carpus	total=37		
Thumb	total=34		
		MP joint	10
		Proximal phalanx	11
		IP joint	11
		Distal phalanx	2
Fingers	total=123		
		MP joint	30
		Proximal phalanx	38
		PIP joint	27
		Middle phalanx	15
		DIP joint	11
		Distal phalanx	2
Fractures involving joint			89
Fractures not involving joint			105

Table 7. Results and complications in 194 bony injuries (amputations)

Fractures – total=105		Fractures involving joint with partial division of the joint – total=89	
Good or satisfactory position, bone firmly united	68	Good or satisfactory position, bone firmly united with restoration of joint function	25
Bone firmly united with shortening of over 2 cm, angulation or rotation of over 10°	21	Arthrodesis (stable)	21
Pseud-arthrosis	16	Artificial joint	6
		Non-consolidated arthrodesis (not a true pseud-arthrosis according to the definition)	4
		Severe arthrosis of the affected joint	16
		Bone strongly united with angulation or rotation of more than 10° or shortening of over 2 cm	17

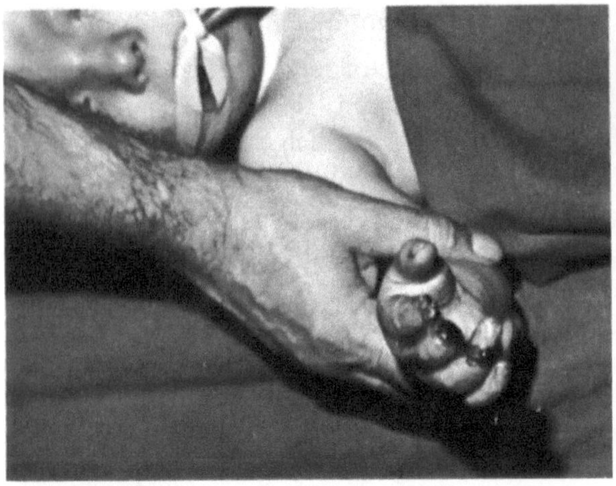
93a

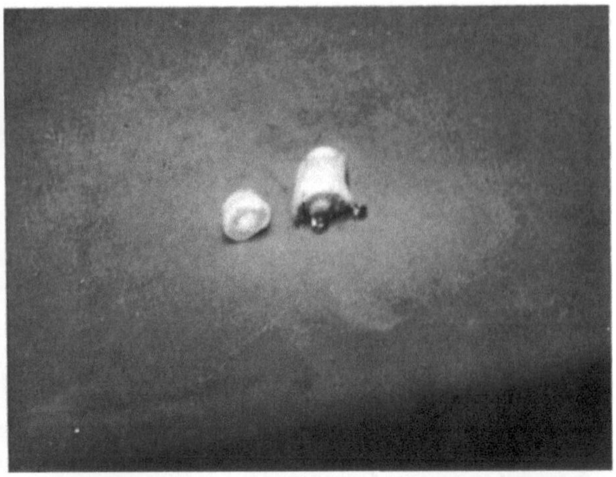
b

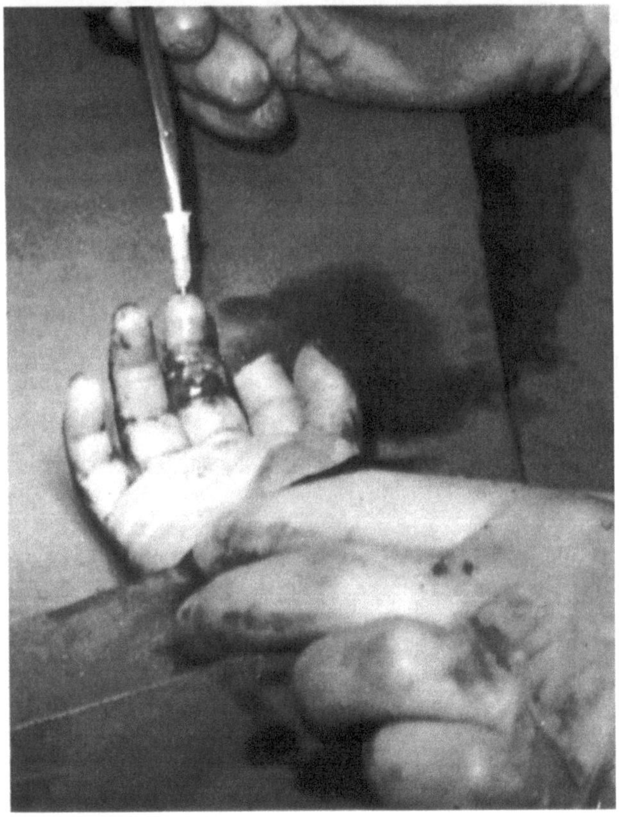
c

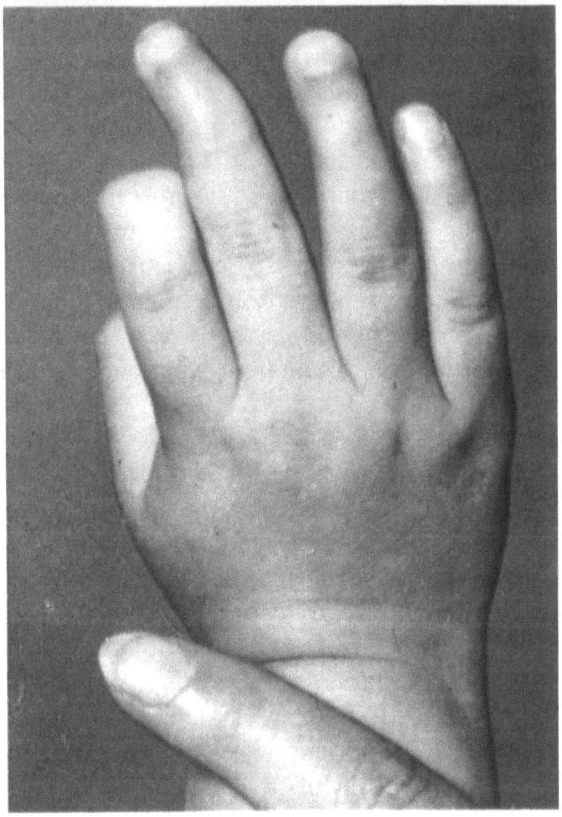
d

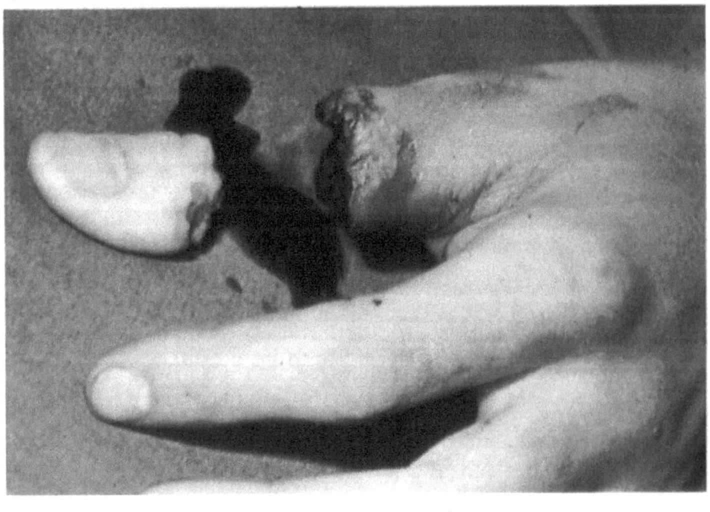
94a

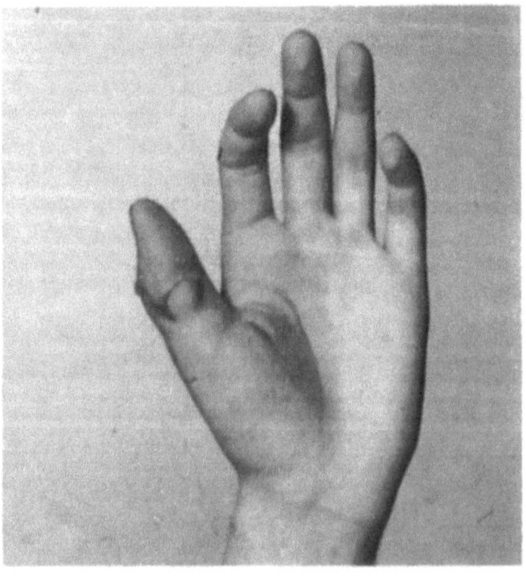
b

XII. Results

When considering the results of replantations, one must differentiate between the survival rate and the late functional results.

1. Survival Rate

The survival rate holds good whether the amputated part was partly or wholly healed. It is a measure only of the function of the vessel anastomosis. The results of replantation surgery in the literature have, until now, almost exclusively dealt with only the survival rate (see Tables 8 and 9). The age distribution ranged from 16 months to 76 years and the authors could not establish significant differences in the results due to age.

2. Late Functional Results

Assessment of the late functional results involves a variety of points of view which must be taken into account.

a) Objective Considerations

The function of the whole hand and of the individual joints of the replant, sensitivity, circulation and aesthetic appearance, can all be assessed objectively.

◀ **Fig. 93a–d.** 16 month old infant who sustained a hatchet injury resulting in total amputation of the index finger in zone I, and total amputation of the middle finger in zone II. The middle finger was successfully replanted, anastomosing an artery and a vein of 0.4 and 0.3 mm diameters respectively

◀ **Fig. 94 a, b.** Circular saw injury in a 22 year old patient, resulting in total amputation of the thumb in zone II

b) Subjective Considerations

Included in this are particular abilities which the replanted part confers on the patient (e.g. an early return to work or a return to previously pursued hobbies), personal discomfort (pain, cold sensitivity), functional disadvantages of the replantation which become more noticeable with the passage of time, and a wide variety of psychological aspects.

c) Socio-Economic Considerations

Treatment costs, sickness benefits and postoperative management costs etc. must all be considered. When appraising the replantation it is absolutely essential to take into account the initial condition. Where the joints are primarily destroyed or there is additional damage to the amputated part, the functional outcome must be presumed to be severely limited. Despite this, a replantation with this kind of background can give a functionally good result, if the basic grip functions can be reconstructed. In addition, aesthetic and psychological aspects should be incorporated into the assessment. The authors have performed an

Table 8. Results from different authors

	Time span (years)	Case numbers	Success rate
Lendvay (Sydney 1973)	4	63	45%
No. VI People's Hospital Shanghai 1973	10	200	56.3%
No. VI. People's Hospital Shanghai 1976[a]	1	31	93.5%
O'Brien, Melbourne 1977	5	103	69.9%
Mandel et al., Vienna 1976	2	31	74.2%
Owen, Sydney 1975	10	243	69%
Tamai, Nara, Japan 1974	10	135	88%
Berger et al., Vienna 1977	2	30	67%
Ikuta, Hiroshima, Japan 1977	5	110	79.1%
Own results	3	450	87.3%

[a] This number refers to one year (1973) following introduction of the operating microscope and stricter indications

Table 9. Results of replantations performed at the clinic "Rechts der Isar", of the TU Munich

Replantations of the upper extremity in 27 months total = 363

Replantations	363	Number of patients	245
Total amputations	204		
Subtotal amputations	159		
Success rate	87.9% = 319		

Type of amputation	Mechanism of amputation	Amputed part		Success rate	
Total amputations					
Total: 204	Guillotine: 147	Fingers	109	Fingers	91
Success rate: 172 = 84.3%		Thumbs	35	Thumbs	32
		Mid-hands	2	Mid-hands	2
		Hands	1	Hands	1
	Crushing: 30	Fingers	25	Fingers	19
		Thumbs	5	Thumbs	4
	Heavy crushing or severe injury to the amputated part: 10	Fingers	9	Fingers	5
		Hands	1	Hands	1
	Avulsion: 12	Fingers	4	Fingers	4
		Thumbs	7	Thumbs	7
		Arms	1	Arms	1
	Degloving: 5	Fingers	5	Fingers	5
Subtotal amputations					
Total: 159	Guillotine: 100	Fingers	72	Fingers	69
Success rate: 147 = 92.5%		Thumbs	22	Thumbs	22
		Mid-hands	3	MidHands	3
		Hands	3	Hands	3
	Crushing: 32	Fingers	26	Fingers	24
		Thumbs	5	Thumbs	4
		Hands	1	Hands	1
	Heavy crushing or severe injury to the amputated part: 23	Fingers	19	Fingers	14
		Thumbs	2	Thumbs	1
		Mid-hands	1	Mid-hands	1
		Hands	1	Hands	1
	Avulsion: 4	Fingers	4	Fingers	4

investigation of 103 replants performed on 53 patients using the following criteria for assessment:

1. *Pinch grip:* between thumb and replanted finger.
2. *Crude grip:* clasping an object with a diameter of 5 cm.
3. *Fist closure:* the distance between the end of the digit and the palm of the hand was measured; less than 3.5 cm = good; greater than 3.5 cm = poor.
4. *Joints:* whether the phalangeal joints show evidence of destruction or not.
5. *Condition of amputation:* guillotine, crushing, avulsion.
6. *Sensitivity:* temperature differentiation; 2-point discrimination; less than 20 mm = good; greater than 20 mm = poor.
7. Follow up varies from 3–9 months after replantation.
   The age of patients investigated varied from 4–67 years and the series comprised 44 men and 9 women with 48 total and 55 sub-total amputations.

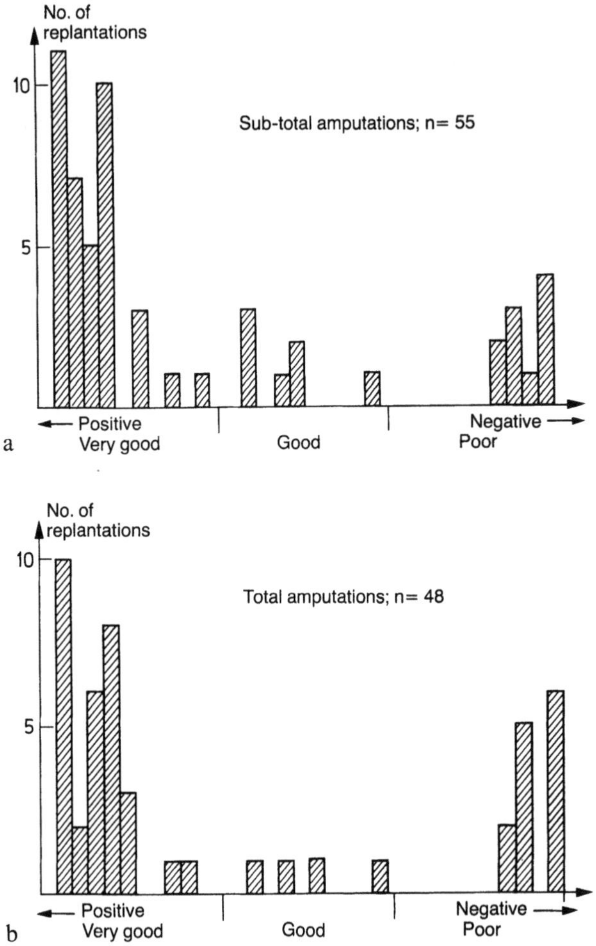

Fig. 95 a, b. Functional results following digital replantation (see text)

The overall results are demonstrated as a histogram (see Figs. 95a, b). In addition, patients with objectively poor functional results always regard the replantation as beneficial to themselves in follow up investigation and, in the same situation, they would, without exception, choose replantation. The recovery of sensitivity in the replant is very good. Amputation at the level of the metacarpophalangeal joint in zone 3 showed a return of some temperature differentiation and 2-point discrimination in almost all patients after 3–4 months. Amputations in zone 1 and zone 2 could achieve a 2-point discrimination of 10–15 mm in this time. Nail growth was, in all cases, fully inconspicuous except for the development of a groove in the nail-bed, the result of the anoxaemia. The growing nail, however, is normal. O'Brien believes that a faster nail growth is observed (1977).
Secondary amputation for functional reasons was necessary on only two occasions in 363 replantations performed in the hospital.

XIII. Microreplantation of Other Parts of the Body

(e.g., toes, ears, scalping injuries and penile amputations)

1. Toe Replantation

Toe replantations have not yet been described in the literature. This probably arises from the fact that, on the one hand this injury seldom occurs, and on the other there is frequently no indication for replanting a toe.
Large toe replantations, however, should be considered when technically possible. Functional and in particular aesthetic considerations serve as indications for surgery. The techniques and medication are identical to those used in finger replantations. It has been evident that, following completion of the arterial anastomosis, there is a delay in venous backflow, which is significantly longer than that seen in the upper limb. Because of the deeper situation of the plantar toe vessels, the arterial anastomosis can be performed more easily when the patient is in the prone position.
In an 'en bloc' amputation of the first and second toe, anastomosis of the dorsalis pedis artery is easier to perform, and arterialisation is sufficient. In an oblique 'en bloc' amputation of the large toe and the second and third toes, anastomosis of the dorsalis pedis artery can achieve complete arterialisation of the whole replant. In this case, however, for additional safety, the plantar arteries of the large and third toes were anastomosed (see Fig. 97).

2. Ear Replantations

Total amputation injuries of the ear occur very seldom. The authors have replanted a totally amputated ear with arterial and venous microanastomosis, but a venous thrombosis which developed on the third post-operative day, led to total necrosis of the ear. Technique and medication are the same as for finger replantation, bearing in mind the different anatomical factors.

3. Scalping Injuries

There is a specific indication for replantation of the scalp with vascular anastomosis, since the scalp skin, with its hair, cannot be replaced following tissue loss. Miller et al. (1976) first described the successful replantation of the scalp using vascular anastomosis. Anastomosis here was only possible using vein grafts but, because of the general heparinisation, there was considerable blood loss.
Biemer (1978), reported a case of replantation following total amputation of the scalp with additional crushing of the amputated tissue. Arterial anastomosis was performed on both sides using branches of the temporal artery. It proved comparatively difficult to find the veins which lie between the gallea and the epidermis in the subcutaneous fatty tissue. This case demonstrated that the blood supply passes across the midline of the scalp and that an arterial anastomosis performed on one side could supply the entire scalp. The patient was not heparinised, but otherwise the medication was similar to that used in finger replantation (see Fig. 99).

4. Amputation of the Penis

Penile amputations are extremely rare and world-wide, until now, there have been three reported cases of replantation following total amputation of the penis; the first in June 1976 in Japan by Tamai et al. (1977); the second in August of the same year at the Massachusetts General Hospital in Boston (Cohen 1977) and the third in April 1977 at the Helen Fuld Medical Center in Trenton, New Jersey (personal communication).
The vessels are relatively large and in the described cases could be anastomosed without difficulty. Anastomosis of the dorsal artery of the penis only is not enough to obtain full arterialisation of the glans penis. This was noted by Tamai et al. (1977) who advised that an additional deeper lying artery had to be anastomosed. To date there have been no reports as to the ability to attain an erection, following replantation of the penis.

5. Other Replantations Using Microvascular Surgical Techniques

In theory, any part of the body with a supplying artery and draining vein can be replanted following anastomosis. An example of this is the case of a 4 year old girl who sustained a combined amputation comprising the whole upper lip and the lower third of the nose as the result of a dog bite. The case was successfully treated following arterial anastomosis of the labial artery and three venous anastomoses: the diameter of the vessels was around 0.3–0.5 mm. There was superficial necrosis in the areas of the dog bite marks; otherwise complete healing was achieved (see Fig. 100 a–d).

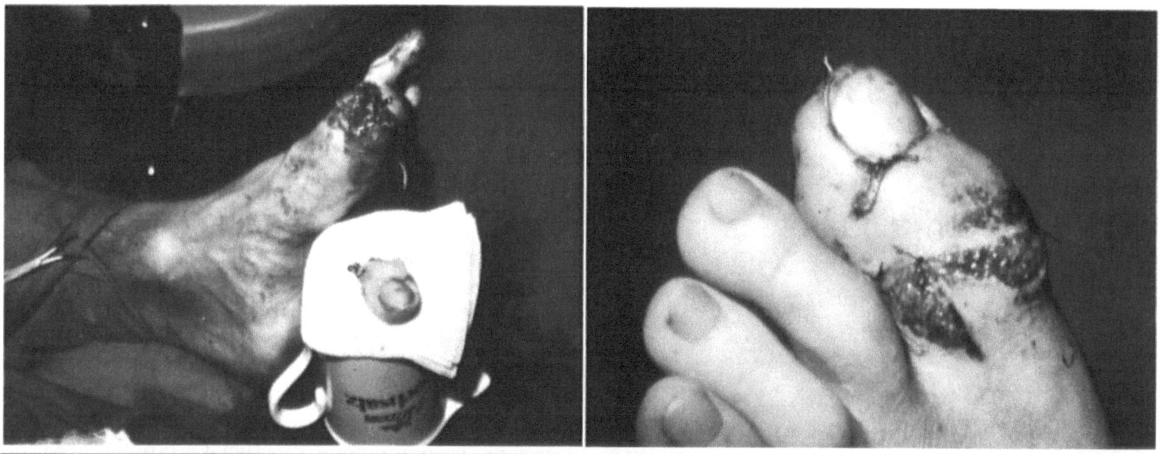

96a b

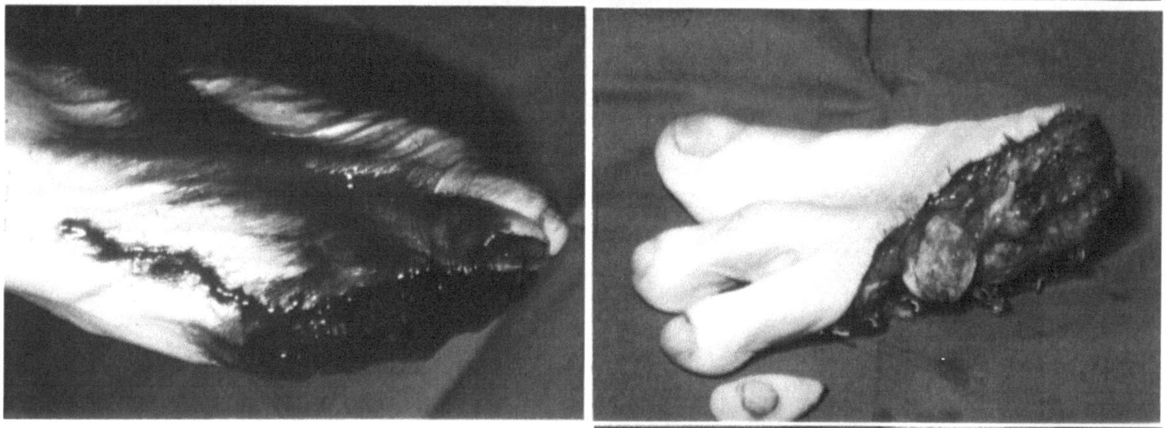

97a b

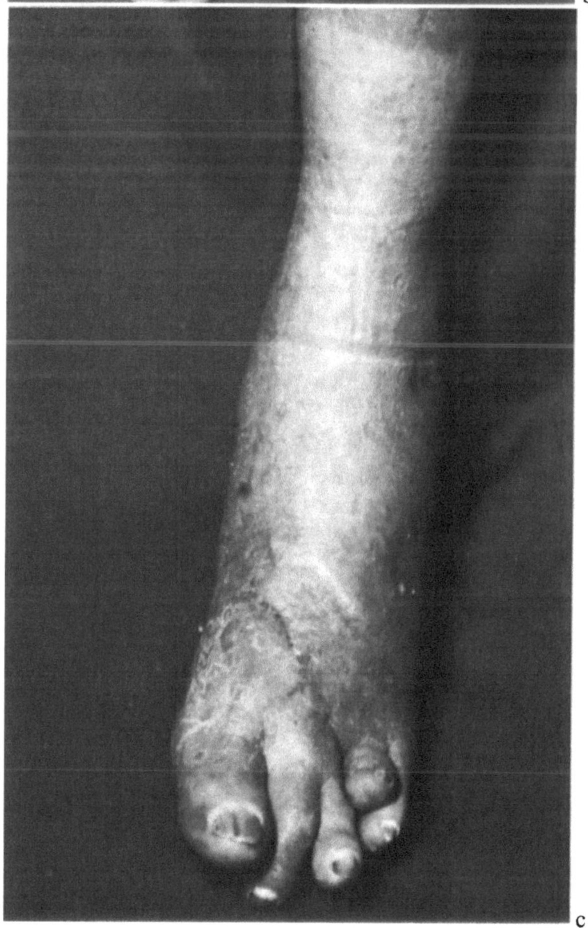

c

Fig. 96 a, b. Total amputation of the large toe resulting from a lawn-mower injury

Fig. 97 a–c. Mid-foot amputation in a 46 year old man resulting from an injury with a paper-cutting knife. **c** Six months following replantation. The patient can again walk normally

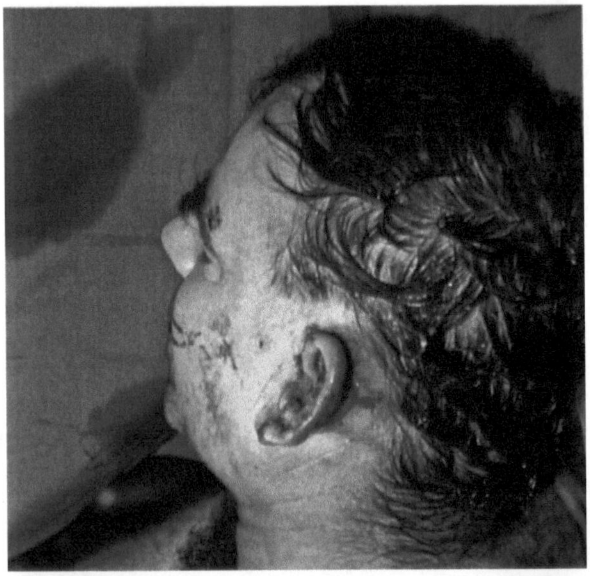

98

Fig. 98. Appearance two days post-operatively following initial successful replantation of a totally amputated ear. Subsequent venous thrombosis on the third day, which could not be cleared, led to later necrosis

Fig. 99 a–d. Accident involving a printing press resulting in a total scalping injury in an 18 year old woman. The amputated part shows additional evidence of crushing in the centre. **d** Both temporal arteries were anastomosed and three veins anastomosed in the temporal and frontal regions. There was some superficial necrosis in the centre of the replant in the area of crushing, but this healed spontaneously. Eight months following successful replantation, there is normal hair growth

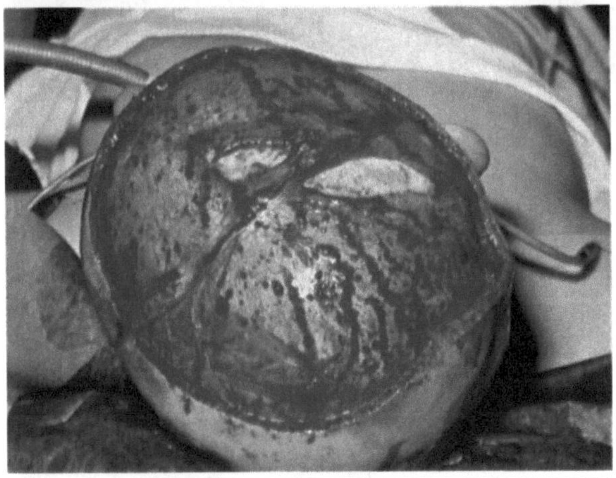

99a

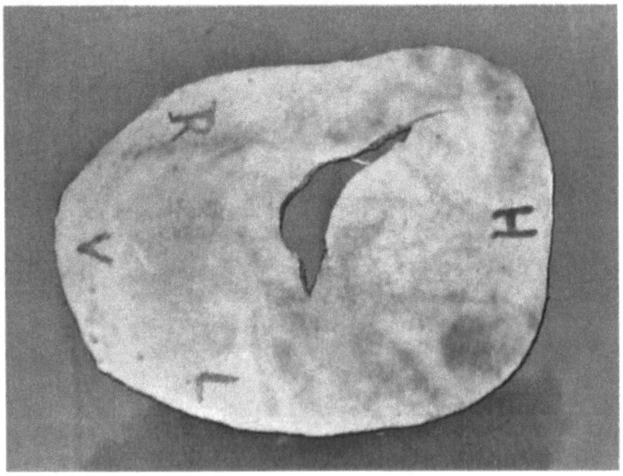

b

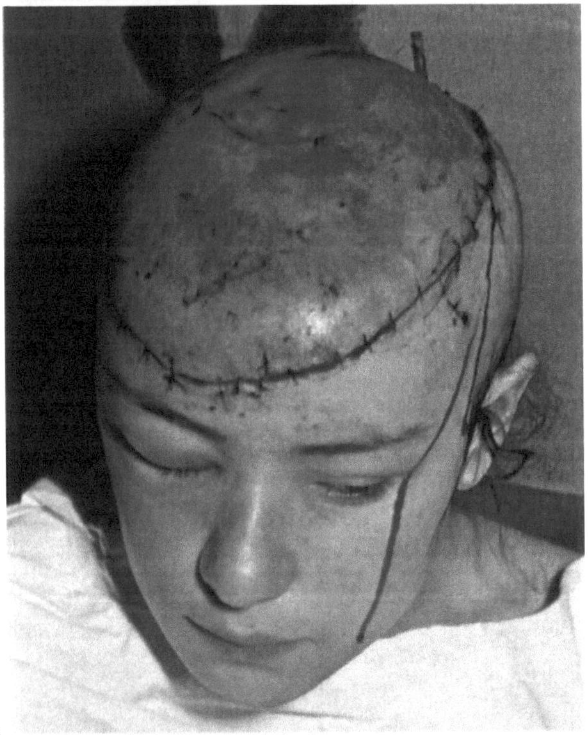

c

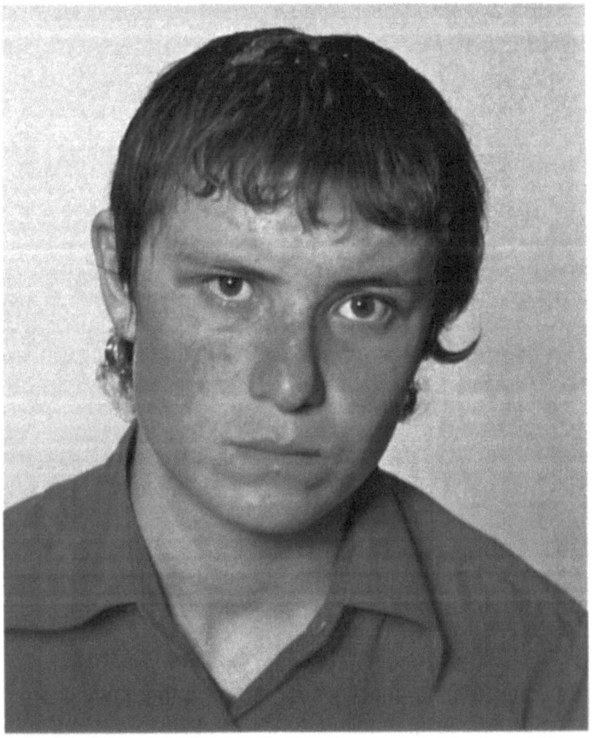

d

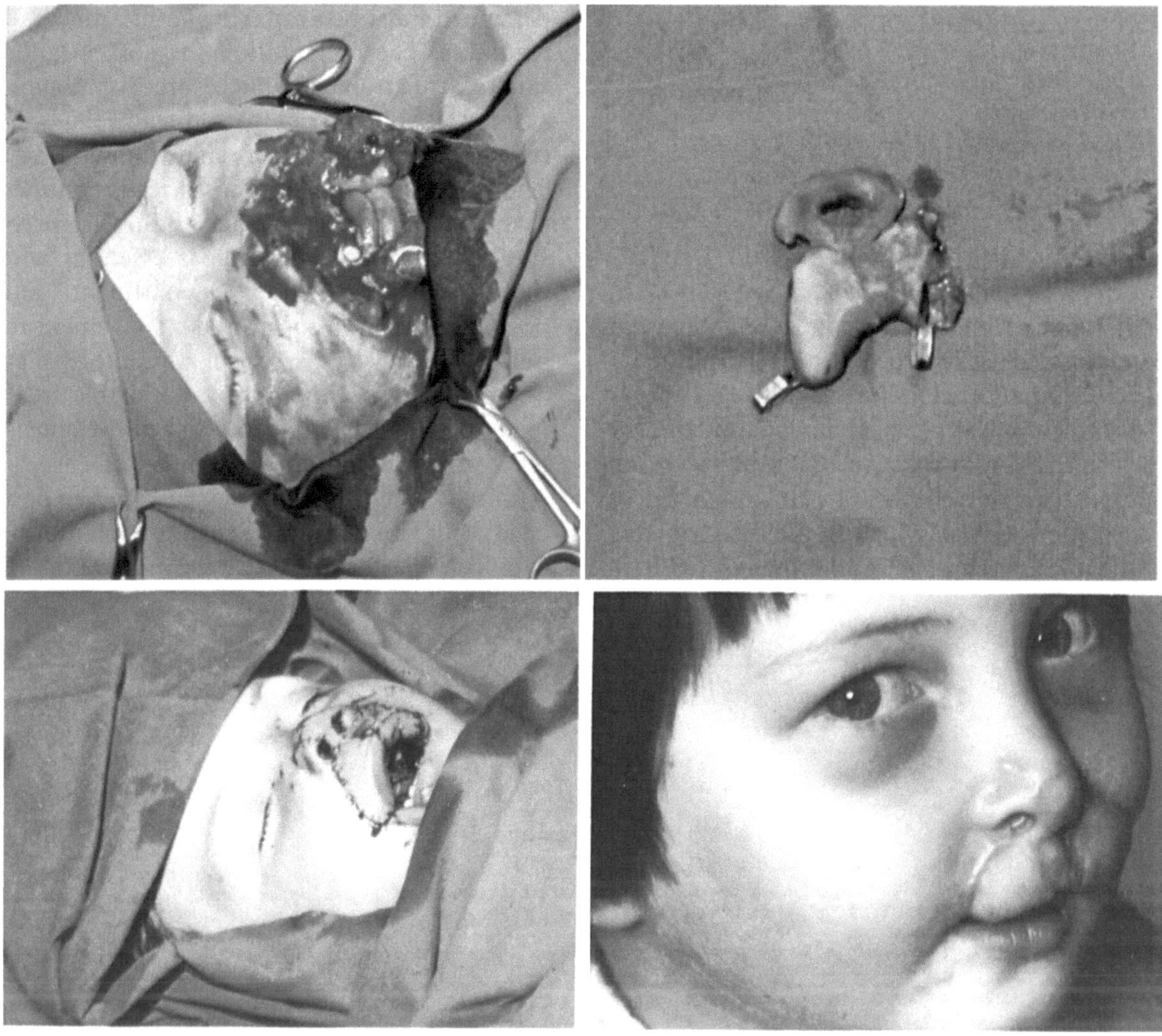

a b c d

Fig. 100 a–d. Four year old girl who sustained a dog bite resulting in total amputation of the upper lip and adjacent ala nasi. The labial artery and three veins, with vessel diameters ranging from 0.3 to 0.5 mm were successfully anastomosed

XIV. Replantation Service

All amputation cases are acute emergencies and it is necessary to be able to perform operations around the clock. In addition, it is necessary to be able to perform immediate revisionary surgery following thromboses. Such demands can only be met by an organised replantation service which is always available. Furthermore, an operating theatre with its personnel must be available and in immediate readiness. The replantation surgeon, in addition to being trained in microsurgery and hand surgery, should have at his command the basic concepts of plastic surgery and traumatology. The successful replantation service is confined to a large unit since, to teach and train microsurgery, close collaboration is essential with the experimental surgery department, and postoperative monitoring and management require trained ward personnel, physiotherapists and occupational therapists. To enable treatment to become routine and to achieve consistent results, a minimum number of cases is required. According to the personal experience of the authors, at least one replantation should be performed every second week.

B. Tissue Transplantation with Microvascular Anastomosis

I. Development of Tissue Transplantation Using Microvascular Anastomosis

Soft tissue defects which result in an exposure of bones, tendons or even foreign material, or cases where a tough covering is necessary, were treated until now by pedicled flaps. This was achieved by using local tissue, in the form of transposition or rotation flaps, or at a distance by using a tubed pedicle. Particularly on the extremities, a local tissue transfer is usually not possible and one must fall back on distant flap surgery. The classical example is the so-called "cross-leg flap", where a flap from the uninjured leg is transferred to the defect on the other lower extremity. Several operations are necessary with intervening periods of several weeks; furthermore, these operations require fixation of the joints. This multiple procedure is very time-consuming for both patient and surgeon, as well as being cumbersome. In 1972, McGregor and Jackson developed the so-called groin flap as an "axial pattern flap". This is a flap which, in contrast to the conventional "random pattern flap" possesses its own individual central vascular system. In the groin, the flap is supplied by the superficial circumflex iliac artery and accompanying veins. Based on anatomical knowledge, the development of microsurgery led to the possibility of transplanting such a flap with its vessels as a free transplant, placing it directly on the defect and anastomosing the appropriate arteries and veins. As early as 1963, Goldwyn et al. experimenting on the dog, imitated these flaps by creating island flaps as they were first called; the flaps were isolated on a vessel strem prior to transfer. In 1965, Krizek et al. carried out experimental flap transplantation. Further laboratory reports came from Strauch and Murray (1967) and McLean and Buncke (1972), who performed transplantations of the omentum in dogs. O'Brien and Shanmugan (1973) reported 27 groin flap transplantations in the rabbit and Daniel and Williams (1973a) reported 15 similar operations in the pig. The first clinical successful transplantation using the groin flap and microvascular anastomosis was reported by Daniel and Taylor in 1973. Previously, in September 1972, Harii in Tokyo had performed a free scalp flap from the contra-lateral temporal region using microvascular anastomosis. Further individual case reports appeared in the literature – O'Brien et al. 1973; Harii (1975; Rigg (1975); Fujino et al. (1975); Biemer and Duspiva (1976a). Experiences following a series of cases were published by O'Brien et al. (1974), Harii et al. (1974, 1975), Ikuta et al. (1975) and Biemer and Duspiva (1977a).

II. Definitions and Nomenclature

The initial publications concerning free tissue transplantation using microvascular anastomosis appeared mostly in the English literature. The term 'flap' has consisently been used in plastic surgery solely to denote pedicle tissue transfer. A free transplant has been termed a 'transplantation' and is further defined by naming the nature of the transplanted tissue.[1] The logical conclusion is to refer to free flap surgery as a 'transplantation of skin and subcuteous tissue' (Biemer and Duspiva 1977a), but in the last few years, the term "free flap" has been adopted world-wide. Since any tissue can be freely transplanted with vascular anastomosis, the generic term "free tissue transplant" or "free tissue transplantation" has been adopted, with or without the addition of "microvascular anastomoses".

Further definition is necessary according to tissue type – e.g., flap transplantation (skin and subcutaneous tissue), muscle transplantation, combined muscle and skin flap transplantation (musculocutaneous flaps) or toe transplantation, etc. The addition of the term "with microvascular anastomosis" is advisable for clarification, since many tissues, such as bone, can also be transplanted without vascular anastomosis. The addition of the term "free" is superfluous when considering the precise definition of the term "transplantation".

1 According to Schmidt-Tintemann (1970)

III. Indications for Free Tissue Transplantation

In principle, the indications are the same as those for pedicle flap surgery, but there are wider indications because of the considerable advantages of this type of procedure when compared to pedicled flaps:

a) A single operation significantly reduces the length of treatment.
b) No immobilisation is required.
c) The additional possibility of innervation (e.g., dorsalis pedis flaps).
d) Less conspicuous donor sites.
e) Better healing since the vascular supply is largely independent from the surrounding tissue.

The main restriction lies in the problems associated with microvascular surgery. In order to be able to use the technique, an additional training is necessary. A rate of thrombosis is always to be considered in microvascular surgery. On the other hand, however, there is likewise a complication rate in pedicle flap surgery, which is quoted at 20% by Stranc et al. (1975). The thrombosis rate, however, is significantly altered by technique and is largely dependent on the individual experience and personal ability of the surgeon in the field of microvascular surgery; this must be taken into account when considering the indications. Basically, flap transplantation will achieve more or less the same result as that obtained using conventional pedicle surgery (see resensitisation by inclusion of a nerve in the transplantation). Therefore in the present day clinical situation, treatment using conventional plastic surgery techniques is always considered first, and the decision for transplantation using vascular anastomosis takes second place. Furthermore, it must be clearly explained to the patient, alongside other possibilities which encompass conventional techniques. Ideal situations exist for free tissue transplantation in traumatic defects of the extremities and in the head and neck region, since inflammatory changes in the vessels are less important and donor vessels are easily isolated and constant in these regions. On the other hand, in chronic ulcers, the severe inflammatory changes of the surrounding tissue must be taken into account. The vessels are difficult to isolate and expose, and their walls are so altered that they are particularly vulnerable and often suffer a separation of the intima from the media. In the authors' experience, the presence of infection is particularly unfavourable – e.g., chronic osteomyelitis – and an infection in the vicinity of the anastomosis leads inevitably to thrombosis. Despite the report from Finseth et al. (1975) regarding two failures using free flap transplantation in the mouth, subsequently Acland in November 1977 was able to demonstrate successful intraoral use. These cases followed excision of tumour in the oral cavity and used free groin flaps for reconstruction. Further indications, in regions where there are no feeding vessels for anastomosis, can be seen in the transfer of distant vessels such as the gastroepiploic vessels from the abdominal cavity for anastomosis in the upper abdominal and thoracic regions (Harii and Ohmori 1973). Relatively clear indications can be seen in transplantation of toes for replacement of the thumb or fingers, in muscle transplantation and in bone transplantation with vascular anastomosis. It is now possible to solve problems, which were either impossible, using conventional techniques, or risked an increased rate of failure.

IV. Preparations for Tissue Transplantation

Precise preparation and planning of the operation is crucial and often determines a successful outcome. Examination and general investigation may show up absolute contraindications for tissue transplantation: e.g. angiopathies, areas of occlusion in the vessels of the legs, and other conditions which contraindicate a long anaesthetic, etc. In some cases, it is possible to localise the arteries in both the recipient and donor areas simply by palpation, and frequently superficial veins can also be seen. In many cases, however, this is not possible and the state of the vessels is unclear. This is particularly true in cases where there have been preceding operations or where there has been additional injury in the donor or recipient areas. In such situations a Doppler investigation can be useful, particularly in the extremities and in the head and neck area. Both the presence of vessels and their capacity and flow can be determined. Frequently, however, final clarification has to rely on angiography. To allow the possible intimal damage resulting from this investigation to settle, the operation should be delayed for several weeks following angiography. Whether angiography is necessary must be decided in each case, since general angiographic investigation is not only unnecessary, but is inadvisable because of the exposure to radiation. In addition to chest x-ray, ECG, full blood count and serum analysis, a clotting and coagulant screen should be performed. The blood group must be determined and two units cross-matched for the operation. The condition of the patient to undergo prolonged anaesthesia in the region of 6–8 hours, must be considered by the internist or the anaesthetist. Because of the length of such operations, the patient must be placed on a well padded table, since decubitus ulcers after such operations have already been described. Furthermore, cooling of the patient, due to exposure, must be prevented to avoid centralisation of the circulation with vasoconstriction and vessel spasm. To facilitate more precise supervision of the patient, a safe and effective central venous line is inserted into the vena cava.

V. Operating Technique

1. General Operative Plan

Despite pre-operative investigation, which has been mentioned previously, the final decision as to whether a free flap is possible can only be made following exposure of the vessels of the donor and recipient areas. For this reason, an alternative solution such as a cross-leg flap should always be discussed and agreed with the patient, so that, under anaesthesia, the first stage can be performed. Equally important is an exact operating plan which will allow the surgeon to precisely explore the vessel situation and enable him to make the final decision without inflicting further damage to the patient (Biemer and Duspiva 1977).

1. Preparation of the donor vessels in the defect area.
2. Preparation of the vessel pedicle in the flap, followed by raising of the flap.
3. Precise marking of the vessel ends, with clear differentiation between arteries and veins.
4. Tacking sutures to fix the flap to the defect area.
5. Microvascular anastomosis – first arterial, then venous.
6. Final suturing of the flap in position and closure of the donor defect.

Exposure of the vessels is performed with the greatest of care under loupe magnification. The extent of exposure of the vessels in the defect must be sufficient, firstly to ensure that the anastomosis can be performed in an area of normal tissue, and secondly to allow a certain variability with regard to siting the anastomosis. In the majority of cases where an end-to-end anastomosis is planned, the vessels of the recipient area are only transected when the transplanted tissue has been gently fixed to the defect. Only then, can the optimal position of the anastomosis be determined and this is also true for end-to-side anastomosis. The planning of the free flap with regard to size and shape can be simplified by using a template. A piece of sterile paper or foil is used to match the defect exactly and the position of the anastomosis can be drawn in. This allows the raising of the flap to be varied so that the vessel pedicle comes to lie exactly in the appropriate position for anastomosis following transplantation (see Fig. 101). Ideal conditions with maximum exposure are essential in order to perform the anastomosis. If necessary, the operating field should be extended and the vessels mobilised over a greater length, or the position of the patient altered. As for microvascular surgery in general, this maximum exposure is essential. The position of the anastomosis must be chosen, so that after the final suturing of the tissue transplant, there are no bends in the vessels and the suture site is well covered. An end-to-end anastomosis is attempted because of the alleged greater safety; calibre differences are accommodated by the insertion of vein grafts (see Chapter "Vein Grafts"). In 1975 Ikuta reported a series of successful cases using end-to-side anastomosis. This has the advantage that the feeding vessel is preserved (see Fig. 103) and this can be of great importance in the extremities. Godina (1979) reported a series of 64 free latissimus dorsi flaps which were all anastomosed in an end-to-side fashion. Necrosis occurred in only one of these cases and as a result of this success, he recommended end-to-side anastomosis. The most suitable vessel for anastomosis is a side-branch which corresponds to the diameter of the flap vessels. Thus the main vessel is retained and, in the majority of cases, a suitable vessel-diameter found for anastomosis (see Fig. 103). Following release of the arterial anastomosis, there is always a relatively fast venous reflux with hyperaemia of the free flap. According to the situation, one or two vein anastomoses can then be performed. The anastomosis of more than two veins appears to the authors to be inadvisable since, such anastomoses will result in a reduction of the flow per vein. The best prophylaxis against venous thrombosis is to obtain as high a flow rate as possible. All veins which are not anastomosed must be ligated exactly to prevent haematoma formation under the flap. For the same reason, the area of the anstomosis should be drained (without drainage the anastomosis may become impaired). In cases where the awaited reflux does not occur and there is no evidence of bleeding from the flap, calm should be preserved and a systematic examination performed:

1. Is the artery anastomosed to artery or has an arterio-venous connection been performed?
2. Is there evidence of spasm of the vessels?
3. Is the anastomosis itself patent?
4. Is there evidence of angulation in the course of the vessels?
3. Has the correct vessel been incorporated in the raising of the flap?
6. Is there evidence of centralisation with hypovolaemia and hypotonicity of the patient?

When considering vessel spasm, it is only patience which is required in the majority of cases (see Chap. 1, Part VII/1). When spasm cannot be overcome, then storage of the free flap for several hours is possible in a fridge at 4 °C (Anderl 1977).

2. Medicinal Treatment

The medicinal treatment is similar to that described in replantations.

Intraoperatively:

a) 500 ml molecular weight Dextran[2].
b) 20 mg Dipyridamol i.v. – 4 hourly[3].

Post-operatively:

a) 500 ml low molecular weight Dextran daily for 6 days[2]
b) Dipyridamol – 20 mg i.v., 4 hourly for the first 24 hours then in a dose of 225 mg orally until the sixth day.[4]
c) Acetylsalicylic acid[5] or a mixture preparation of b) and c).[6]

2 Rheomacrodex, Knoll
3 Persantin, Thomae
4 Persantin forte (3 × 1 tablets) Thomae
5 Colfarit, Bayer
6 Asasantin, Thomae

Antibiotic cover commences pre-operatively according to the bacteriology.

3. Post-operative Treatment and Supervision

The area of the free tissue transplant is slightly elevated from the position of heart level. The dressing must allow good visualisation of the free flap, as it is particularly important to watch for disturbances in venous backflow. Supervision is more difficult than after replantation of peripheral parts since it is often more difficult to establish capillary filling. In addition, temperature monitoring, particularly in very thin flaps gives no clear indication of viability. Colour judgment is often very difficult because of the pale colour, particularly the skin in the groin region. Webster (1977) advised monitoring using a photo-electric pulse meter, but the ideal monitor is not yet available. Perhaps the percutaneous PO_2 measurement offers the possibility of a solution in the future (Werber and Biemer 1978). At the slightest suscpicion of thrombosis, the anastomosis should be quickly re-examined.

4. Complications

Problems sometimes occur during the operation as a result of the amount of subcutaneous fatty tissue. Primary thinning of the flap is not possible because of the vessel course and this thinning must be postponed until a later secondary operation.

Sewing of the free flap under too great a tension can be avoided by inserting a split thickness skin graft at the edge of the flap (Biemer and Duspiva 1976).

The real complication, however, is that of thrombosis, and a venous thrombosis can scarcely be overlooked. The flap swells up and becomes bluish to aubergine in colour (see Fig. 104). The temperature falls and clear blisters soon appear. Swift revision of the anastomosis at the first sign or symptom is advised (see Chap. "Thrombectomy").

An arterial thrombosis is often more difficult to determine. Because of the tissue softness, the "empty feeling" which is demonstrated in finger replantations following arterial thrombosis cannot be determined (see Fig. 105a). Colour, capillary filling and temperature are difficult to monitor, as has been previously metntioned. Occasionally investigation using the Doppler apparatus may clarify the situation, but the surest method is to produce bleeding by inflicting small cuts on the flap edge. Arterial thrombosis is a further absolute indication for swift revision. Total necrosis of the entire transplant always follows an arterial thrombosis, whereas frequently a portion of subcutaneous fatty tissue is retained following venous thrombosis. In this situation a secondary split skin graft is possible (Ohmori 1977; Biemer and Duspiva 1977a) (see Fig. 105f).

Until now it has been impossible to monitor the patency of deep muscle or bone transplantation post-operatively. In such cases the success is determined by the clinical course and by later angiography or scintigraphy.

Fig. 101. A pattern of the defect helps the planning of the free flap. The site of proposed vessel anastomosis is also marked so that the free flap can be raised more exactly, paying attention to size and position of the vessel pedicle

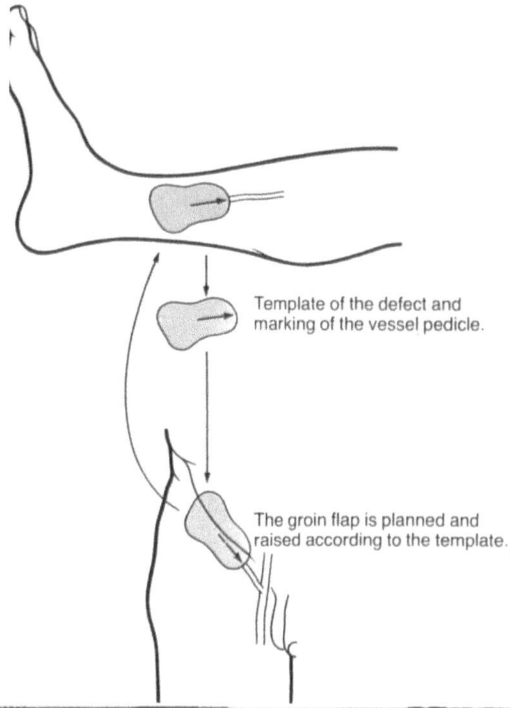

101

Fig. 102 a–d. A chronic ulcer, overlying the heel in a 48 year old woman, had persisted for 2 years following a road traffic accident. Elevation of the groin flap revealed a common origin of the s.e.a. and s.c.i.a. An end-to-side anastomosis with the anterior tibial artery was performed and two end-to-end anastomoses of the accompanying veins

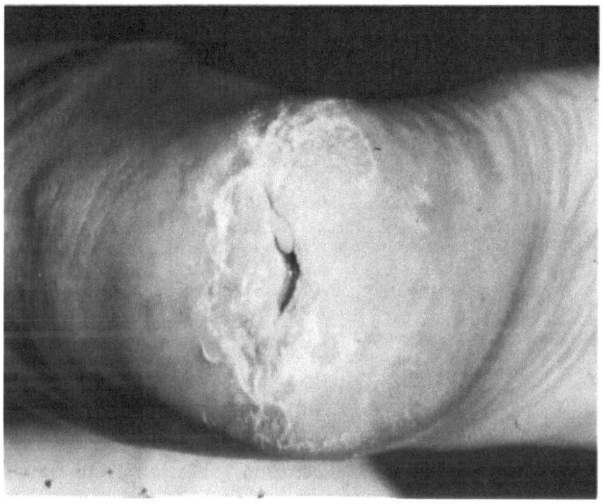

102a

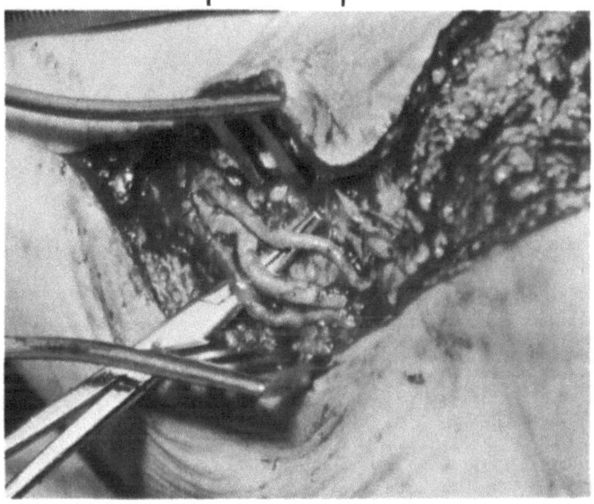

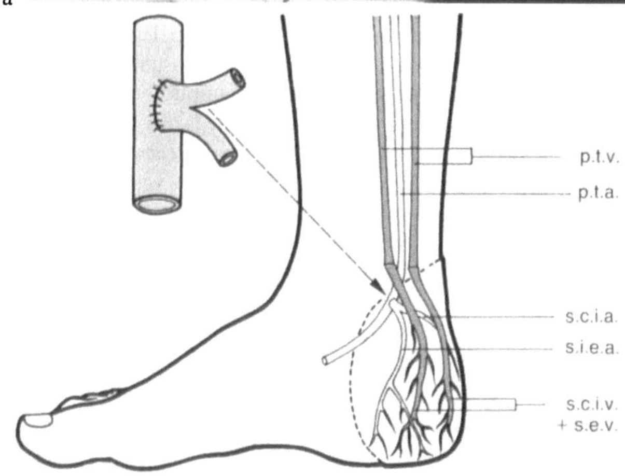

p.t.v. = Posterior tibial vein
p.t.a. = Posterior tibial artery
s.c.i.a. = Superficial circumflex iliac artery
s.i.e.a. = Superficial inferior epigastric artery
End-to-side anastomosis
s.c.i.v. + s.e.v. = Superficial circumflex iliac vein and Superficial epigastric vein

c

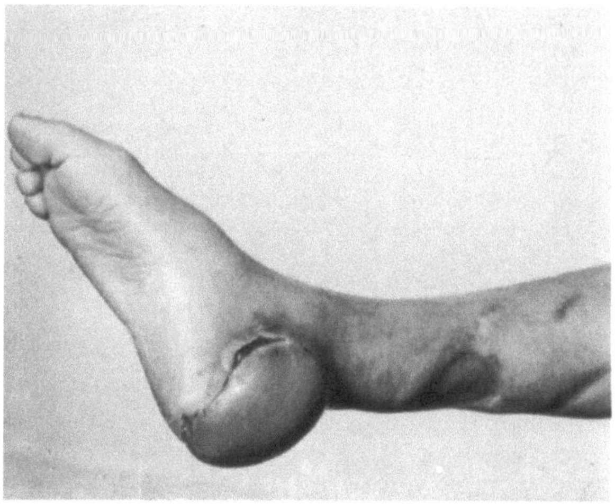

d

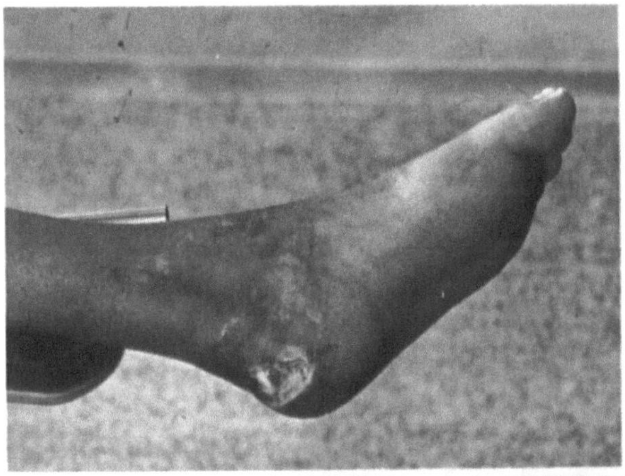

a

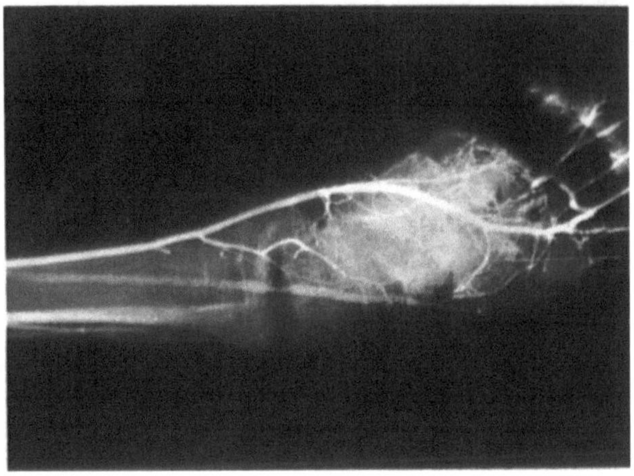

b

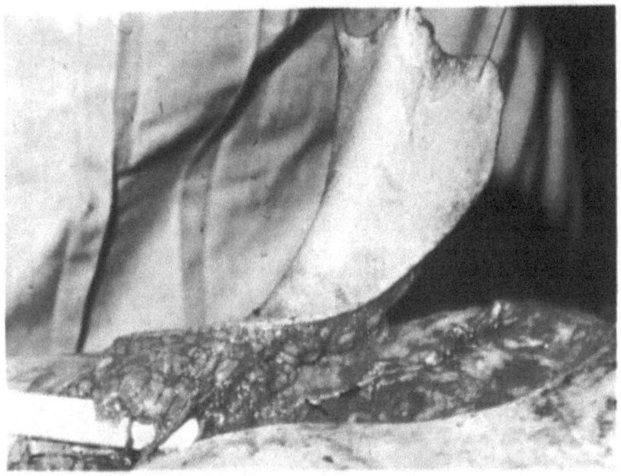

c

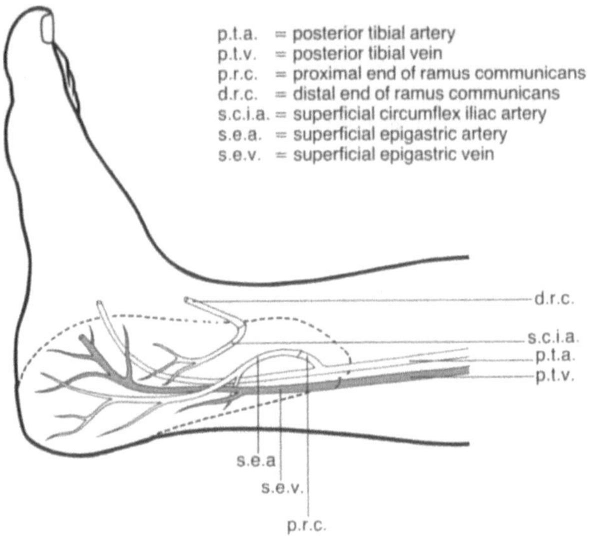

d

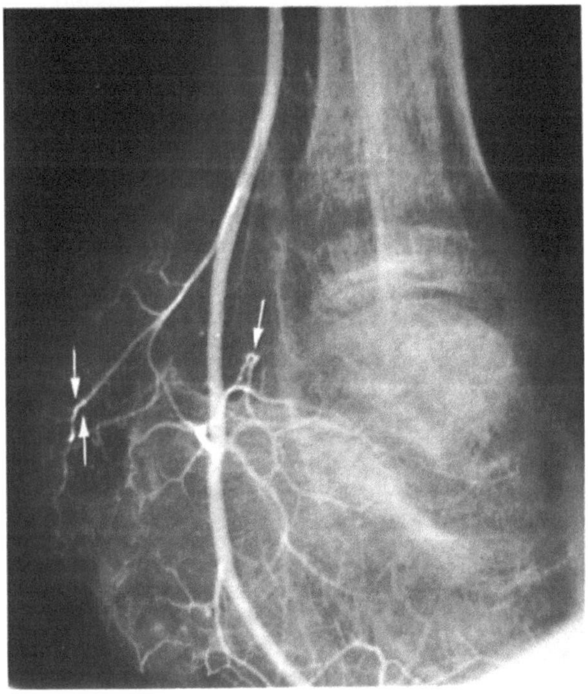

e

Fig. 103 a–g. Chronic ulceration following a compound calcaneal fracture in a 21 year old man. Because of extensive accompanying injury of the lower leg, angiography was performed to determine the vascular pattern. It demonstrated that the foot was supplied only by the posterior tibial artery and therefore the larger side branch was chosen for arterial anastomosis (*arrow*). **c–e** A 10×12 cm groin flap was raised and the vessel pedicle, including the s.e.a. and s.c.i.a. and veins can be seen. The planned anastomosis is shown in the diagram. The larger vessel, the s.e.a., was anastomosed to the proximal end of the ramus communicans and the smaller vessel, the s.c.i.a., was anastomosed to the distal end, since good reflux was demonstrated here.
The post operative angiography shows the sites of the anastomoses (*arrows*)

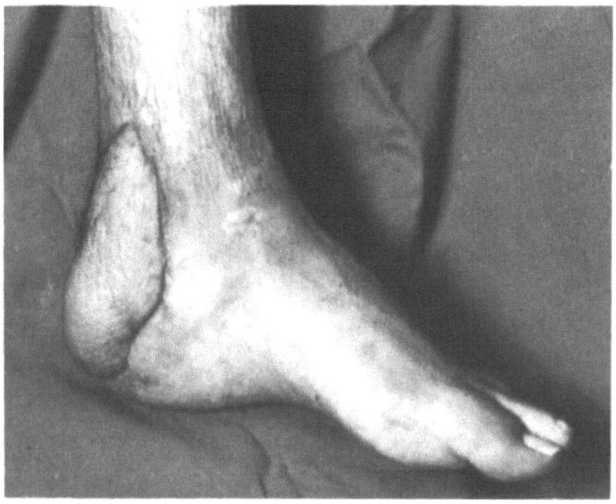

f

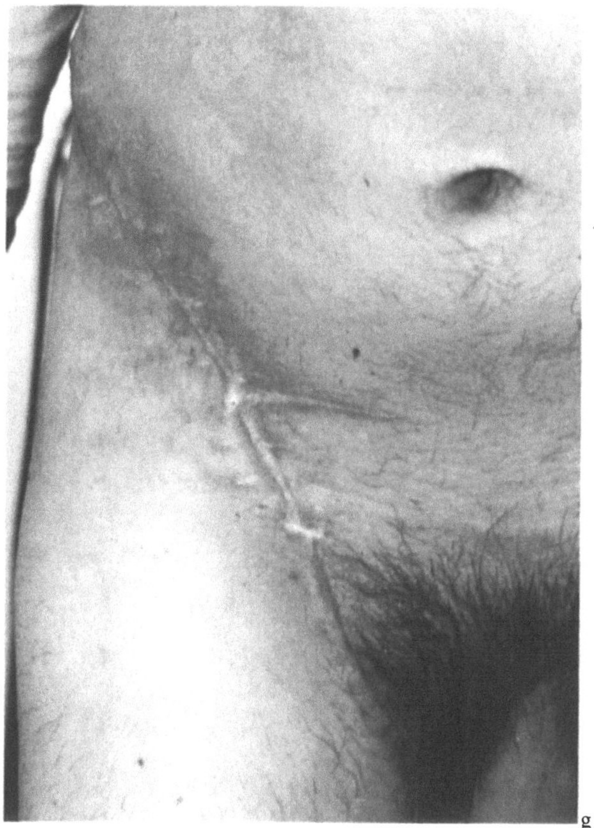

g

f, g Appearance of the free flap at four months postoperatively. The donor site in the groin leaves a relatively unremarkable scar

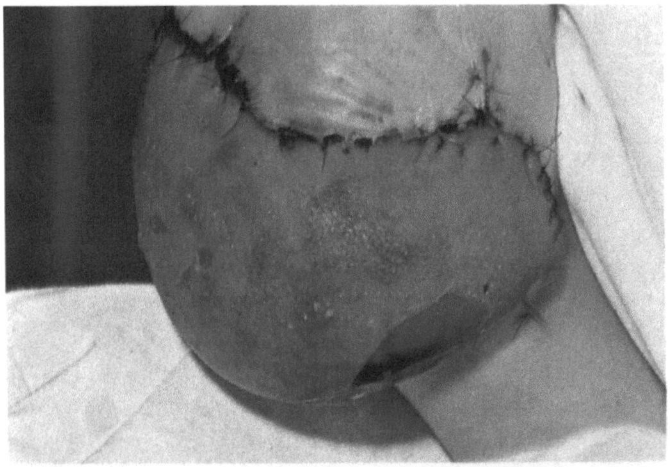

Fig. 104. A fully developed venous thrombosis in a groin flap on the heel. Clearly visible are the swelling and discolouration varying from bluish to aubergine, and blister formation

a

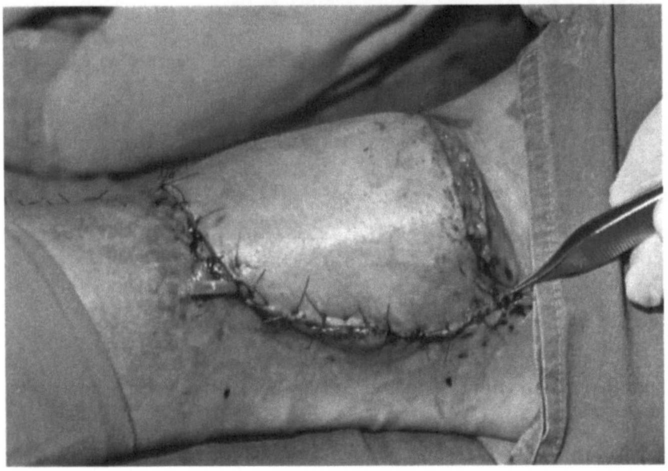

b

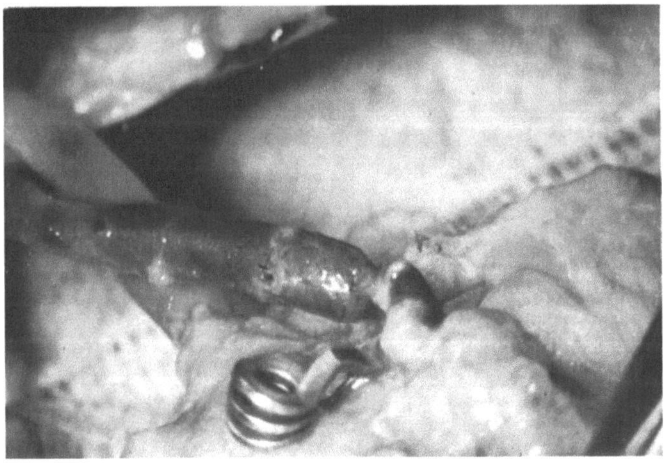

Fig. 105 a. Arterial thrombosis in a free groin flap one day after operation. There is typical corpse-like discolouration of the skin
b–d A fully developed arterial thrombosis in the feeding anterior tibial artery following transplantation of a free groin flap. Thrombectomy, using the finest Fogarty catheter was performed, followed by reanastomosis.
e, f Despite successful thrombectomy, there followed almost complete necrosis of the overlying skin, but some of the fatty tissue was retained so that the defect could subsequently be covered with a split skin graft and the initial goal of treatment was thus achieved

Fig. 105c–f.

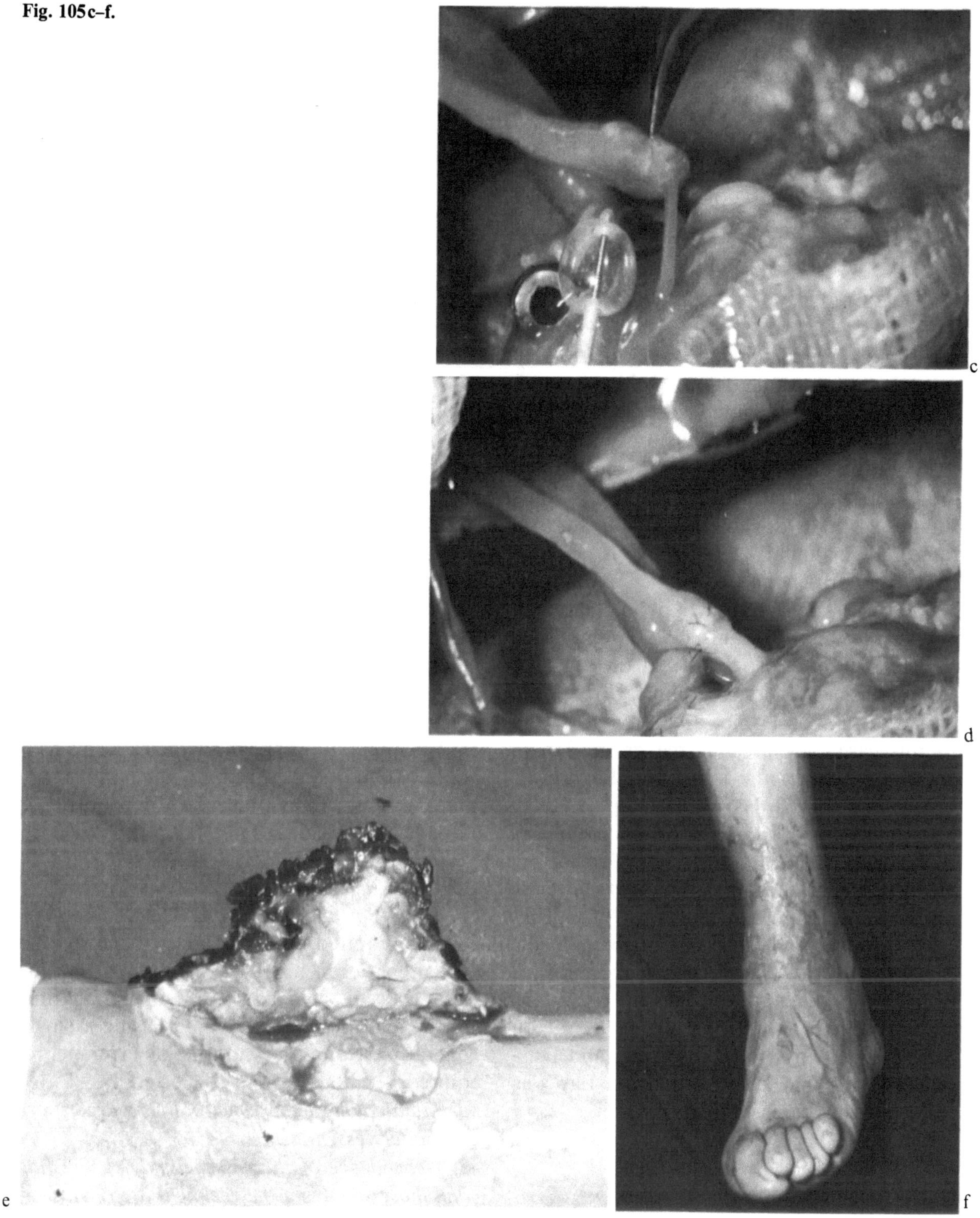

VI. Free Flap Transplantation

1. Development

The first experimental work towards free flap transplantation came from Goldwyn et al. (1963). They transplanted five flaps on the dog, but only a few of these survived for 2–3 days. Strauch and Murray (1967) transplanted groin flaps in the rat with a 61% success rate. Fujino et al. (1972) reported a 58% survival rate in 12 mammary gland flaps in the dog. In 1973, O'Brien and Shanmugan obtained 100% success in 27 groin flaps in the rabbit and Daniel and Williams (1973a) published a successful series of 15 cases in the pig. The first published report of a clinical free groin flap was that of Daniel and Taylor (1973). In this case they used a free groin flap to cover a defect on the lower leg. Previously, in September 1972, Harii and Ohmori (1973) had transplanted a free scalp flap measuring 15 × 3 cm on the temporal vessels. Further single case reports came from O'Brien et al. (1973b), Harii and Ohmori (1975), Rigg (1975), Fujino and Saito (1975), Biemer and Duspiva (1976a). The results of a series of such operations appeared in the literature from O'Brien et al. (1974), Harii et al. (1974), Ikuta et al. (1975) as well as Biemer and Duspiva (1977a). (The authors' first free flap was performed in March 1975.)

2. Advantages and Disadvantages of Free Flap Transplantation

As in every surgical technique, this procedure has advantages and disadvantages.

Advantages:

1. Single stage operation. Whereas pedicle flaps and the creation and migration of tubed pedicle flaps require several operations, with an interval of 3–4 weeks between each stage, this procedure can achieve the same result in a single stage. As a result of this:

2. Shorter hospital stay

3. No fixation of joints. In procedures such as the "cross-leg flap" or the use of the forearm as a carrier for a tube pedicle, the fixation of joints, with all its inherent dangers, is always necessary for several weeks.

4. Aesthetically better donor sites. Free flap transplantations can be taken from less conspicuous areas in the majority of cases.

5. Independence from the vascularity of the defect. The vascular anastomosis of the free flap is independent of the vascularity at the edges of the defect and, in areas of poor vascularity, lead to an overall better vascular supply.

6. Greater variability. As more and more donor regions for free flaps are described, as well as combined transplants such as myocutaneous flaps or osteocutaneous flaps (see appropriate Chapter) with the possibility of additional nerve supply, e.g., the dorsalis pedis free flap, then the most suitable free flap can be chosen according to the requirements, and independent of the site of the defect. This freedom of choice and variability give a great advantage over flaps which are dependent on a pedicle.

Disadvantages:

1. Length of operating time. The subtile techniques required in microvascular surgery and the preparation involved in isolating the fine vessels result in a prolonged operating time in the majority of cases. When using a single operating team, the authors on average required 4–6 hours.

2. Training and experience in microsurgery are absolutely essential.

3. Dependence of the vessel supplying the flap and those supplying the recipient area. This independence makes exact pre-operative planning essential, in order to determine the sites of the vessels by palpation, Doppler investigation or, when necessary, angiography.

Table 10. Free flap transfer

Donor region	Arterial supply	Nerve	Donor defect	Special advantages and uses
Groin flaps	Superficial circumflex iliac artery. Superficial epigastric artery	No	Direct closure	Relatively constant vessels, variable size and form. Is only restricted by the thick subcutaneous fatty layer
Modification of the groin flap	Deep circumflex iliac artery	No	Direct closure	More constant and larger vessels, significantly longer vessel pedicle, especially suited for inclusion of iliac crest bone
Delto-pectoral flaps	Perforating branches of the second intercostal artery	No	Skin graft	Restricted size. Thin subcutaneous tissue. Use is restricted because of the conspicuous donor defect
Axillary flaps	Cutaneous branches of the subscapular artery and throaco-dorsal artery	No	Direct closure	Long vessel pedicle. Because of the variation in vascularity, it is often necessary to include a part of the latissimus dorsi muscle as a musculocutaneous flap
Dorsalis pedis flap	Dorsalis pedis artery	Yes	Skin graft	This flap is particularly suited for hand surgery and to replace the sole of the foot, because of the thin subcutaneous layer and the possibility of anastomosing a sensory nerve which runs in an axial fashion
Modification of the dorsalis pedis flap: flap comprising 1st web space	Dorsalis pedis artery	Yes	Skin graft	Particularly useful in hand surgery to reconstruct interdigital defects
Large toe pulp flap	Dorsalis pedis artery	Yes	Skin graft	This flap is useful as a small island flap, particularly for covering finger-tip defects to regain sensitivity
Temporal flap: scalp flap and forehead flap	Superficial temporal artery with its temporal and ventral branch	No	Most often direct closure by small flaps	When raised as a hair-bearing scalp flap, it is particularly useful in treating areas of alopecia. As a forehead flap it is particularly suited for defects of the face because of the good skin colour. In this instance the great disadvantage is the conspicuous donor site

3. Special Requirements for Free Flap Transplantation

In the clinical situation, there are special requirements for a "free flap":

1. An axial pattern vascularity of both arterial and venous supply.
2. A relatively constant vessel course which is simple to prepare.
3. Variation in the size of the flap should be possible.
4. The subcutaneous fatty layer should be as thin as possible.
5. Axial nerve supply for a nerve anastomosis.
6. Aesthetically and functionally satisfactory donor defect.

An increasing number of donor areas in the human body have been investigated and tested in a clinical situation; all these flaps fulfilled the above requirements in differing ways (see Table 10).

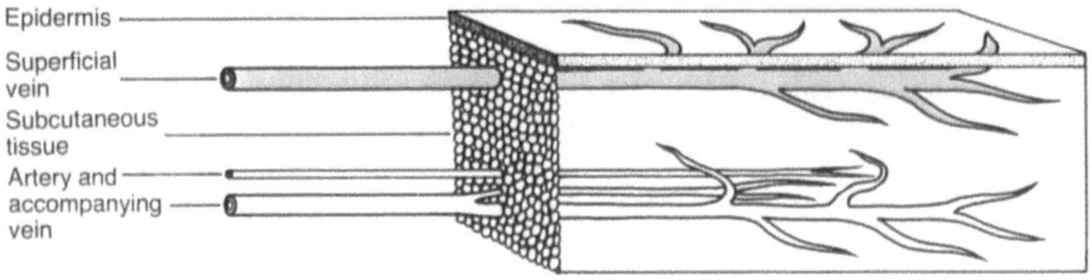

Fig. 106. Diagramatic presentation of a free groin flap

4. Donor Sites

Pedicle flap surgery led to the development of so-called "axial pattern flaps" such as the "groin flap" (McGregor & Jackson 1972), the "delto-pectoral flap" (Bakamjian 1963), the flap from the dorsum of the foot (McGraw and Furlow 1975). In addition, many further donor areas were investigated. These donor areas are presented in the following section, and their uses and advantages are outlined.

a) Groin Flaps (fat flaps, iliac flaps)

The groin flap is supplied by the superficial circumflex iliac artery (s.c.i.a.). A further possible flap can be based on the superficial epigastric artery (s.e.a.) which likewise is a branch of the femoral artery inferior to the inguinal ligament (see Fig. 107a). Each of these two vessels supplies a collective area in the groin (Biemer and Duspiva 1976a). An exact demarcation of the area supplied by each vessel has, until now, not been possible with any investigative technique. The area of the free flap or pure "axial pattern flap" can be extended by incorporating a "random pattern flap". Thus, very large flaps of 28 × 18 cm (Harii 1975a, b), and 20 × 22 cm (Biemer and Duspiva 1976a), can be transplanted, and complete healing achieved by anastomosing only one of these two arteries. The line joining the anterior superior iliac spine and the pubic tubercle acts as a guide to determine the extent of the groin flap. The position of the superficial circumflex iliac artery can be marked over the palpable femoral artery at a distance of two fingerbreadths in men, and one thumb breadth in women, distal to the previously described line (Reimann and Fritz 1975). The s.c.i.a. nearly always passes deep to the fascia lata initially, and gives off a muscular branch to the sartorius before passing into the subcutaneous fat. The vessel pedicle is usually only 1–2 cm long and rapidly branches out. The superficial epigastric artery (s.e.a.) lies superficial to the fascia, and passes in a more cranial direction. The two vessels – s.c.i.a. and s.e.a. – are subject to considerable variation (see Fig. 107). Both arteries are accompanied by veins, but the formation of these veins is extremely variable.
The superficial veins are usually more appropriate for venous anastomosis: they lie close under the skin and follow approximately the same path as the deep arterial supply. These veins, therefore, should be preserved during the lifting of the flap. There is no axial nerve

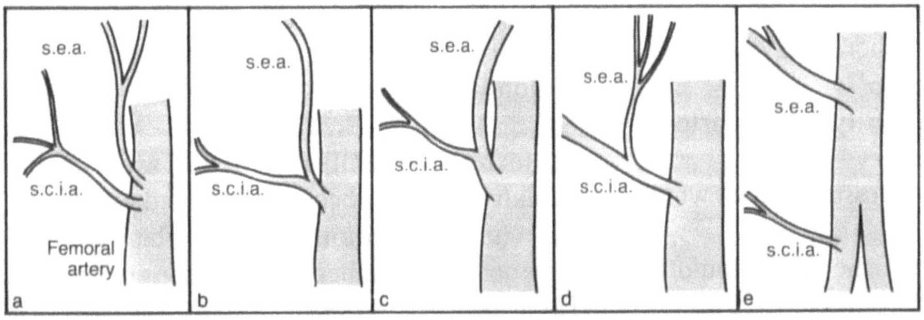

Fig. 107 a–e. Variations in origin of the superficial epigastric artery (s.e.a.) and the superficial circumflex iliac artery (s.c.i.a.). The most common situation by far is shown in Fig. 107a

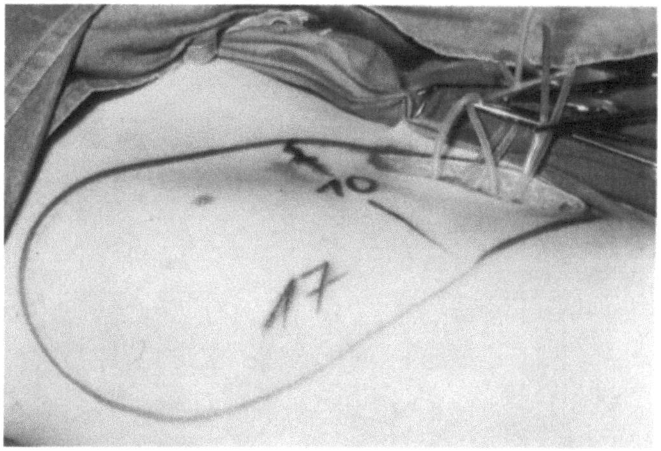

Fig. 108. Raising a groin flap commences with a 5 cm long incision overlying the palpable femoral artery. The vessels are isolated and controlled using soft plastic tubes

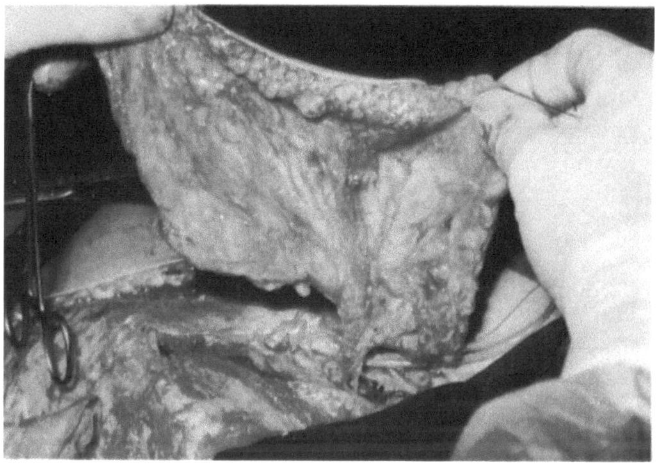

Fig. 109. A groin flap which has been raised to show the superficial circumflex vascular pedicle

in this region in humans since the groin is supplied by several sensory skin branches.

Raising the groin flap commences with a perpendicular incision over the femoral artery, extending for about 5 cm. This exposes the superficial veins (see Fig. 108). The origins of the s.c.i.a. and s.e.a. are prepared, and the area of skin, appropriate to the course and direction of the vessels and the pattern of the flap, is finally determined. In large flaps both arteries can be included and, where possible, both arteries can be anastomosed (see Fig. 103). If it is possible to perform only one single anastomosis, then the larger vessel is chosen and the shape of the flap is moved more into the area supplied by that vessel (see Fig. 110). When both vessels are included, a kind of bilobed flap can be created (Godina 1978).

The flap is raised from a lateral to a medial direction, just superficial to the fascia. The point where the s.c.i.a. pierces the fascia must be carefully sought. The fascia lata from this point to the medial extremity is taken with the flap. Thinning of the flap at its edge is possibly without danger, but in the area of the vessel pedicle, however, the full thickness of subcutaneous fat must be raised with the flap for anatomical reasons. When the flap is isolated on its vessel pedicle, the vascularity must be checked. Because of the very short vessel pedicle, it is extremely important to mark the vessels precisely and safely, since finding them again in the fatty tissue is extremely difficult (Biemer and Duspiva 1976a). Even in very large flaps, the groin defect can almost always be closed, particularly following mobilisation of the abdominal skin. The groin flap until now has proved the most suitable and most versatile free flap. It is the flap which is used most often world-wide, because of its variable size, its relatively large and con-

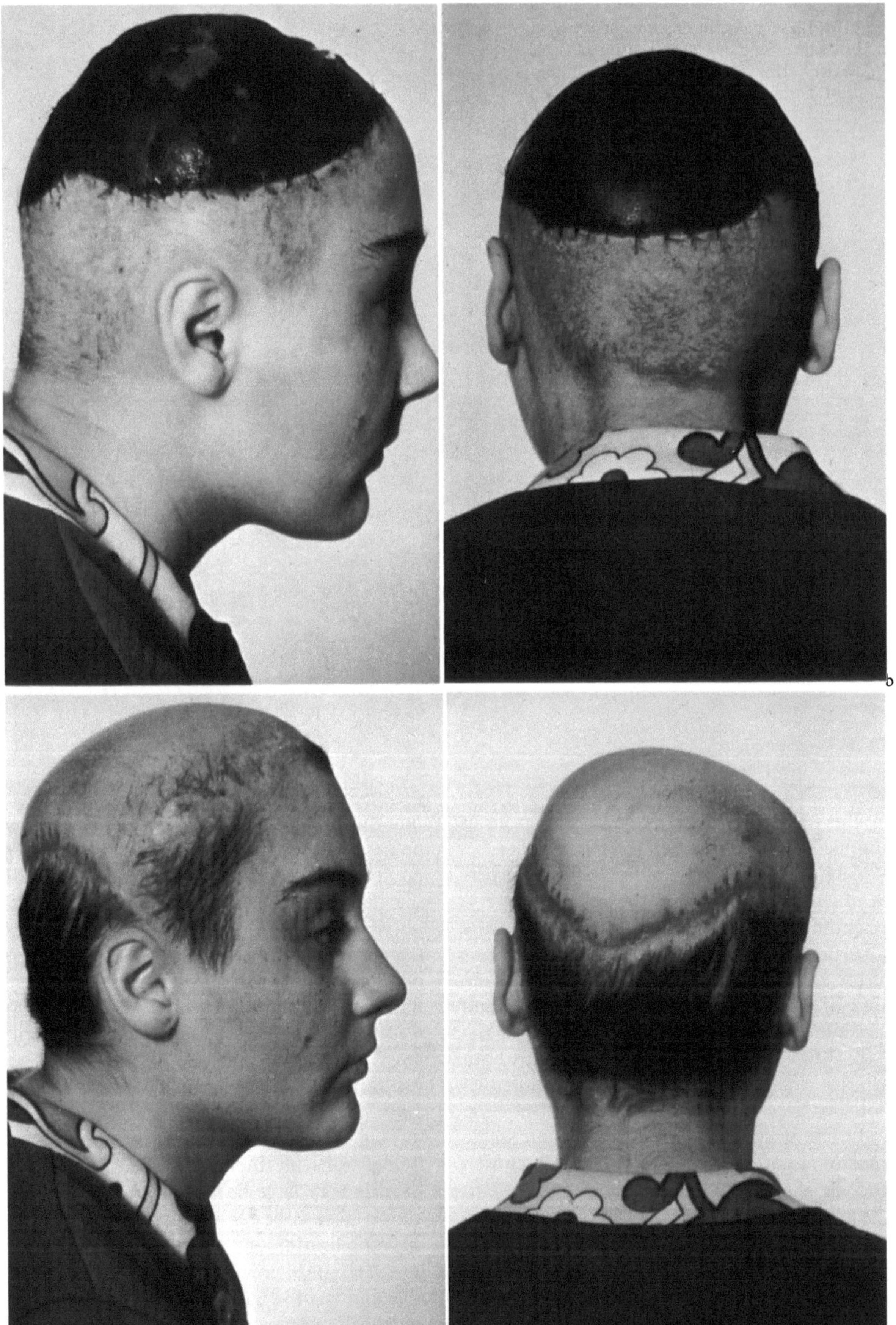

a b c d

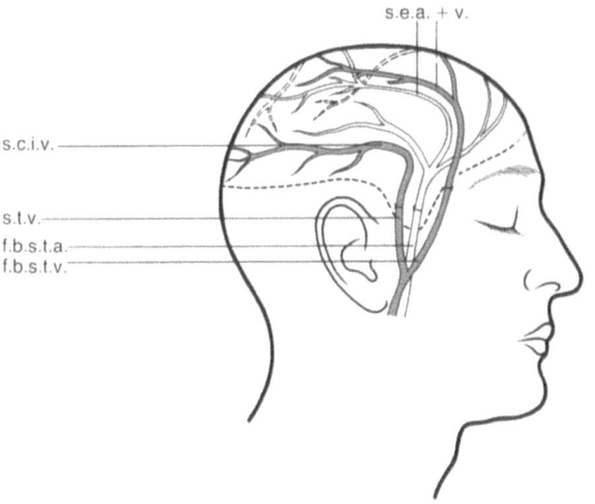

f.b.s.t.a. = frontal branch superficial temporal artery
s.t.v. = superficial temporal vein
f.b.s.t.v. = frontal branch superficial temporal vein
s.e.a. + v. = superficial epigastric artery + vein
e s.c.i.v. = superficial circumflex iliac vein

Fig. 110. a, b Total necrosis of the scalp following an attempted replantation without vascular anastomosis. The 16 year old girl had sustained a total scalping injury from a paper machine. **c–e** The skull was covered with a 20 × 22 cm groin flap with anastomosis as shown in the diagramatic plan

stant vessels and, above all, because of the inconspicuous donor defect. Functional disadvantages lie in the thick subcutaneous fatty layer and in the absence of a usable sensory nerve.

An alternative is found in the so-called "iliac flap" (Acland 1977). Here, the main branches of the superficial circumflex iliac artery and vein are dissected out for a greater length, and the flap is raised in the area of the anterior superior iliac spine. This achieves a longer vessel pedicle as well as a significantly thinner flap, but the size and variability are restrictive. The groin flap can be used as a free fat transplant with vascular anastomosis, following removal of the epidermis (Anderl 1977a, b). Taylor (1979) described a groin flap based on the more constant and significantly larger deep circumflex iliac artery. It originates from the femoral artery, about 1–2 cm above the inguinal ligament, and is accompanied by a large vein. The vessels pass on the inner side of the pelvis over, or in, the iliopsoas muscle. It supplies the skin over, and lateral to, the iliac crest, through perforating branches; it furthermore provides vascularisation of the iliac crest bone (see Chap. "Combined bone flap transplantation").

b) Dorsalis Pedis Flaps (interdigital fold flap, toe pulp flap)

Distal to the extensor retinaculum, the anterior tibial artery becomes the dorsalis pedis ar-

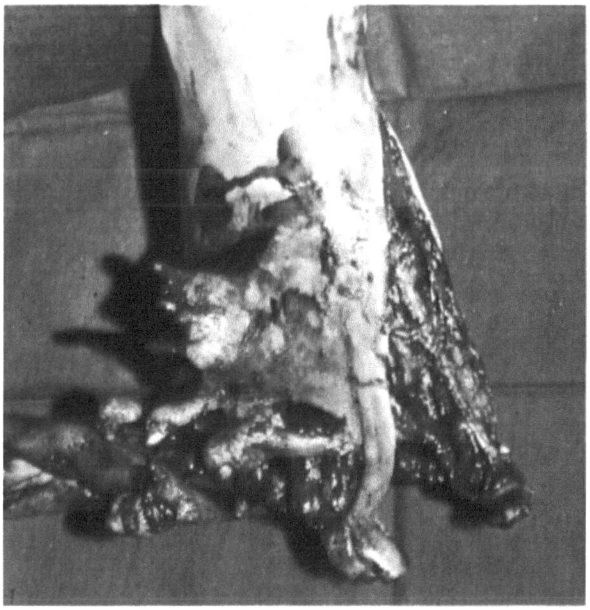
a

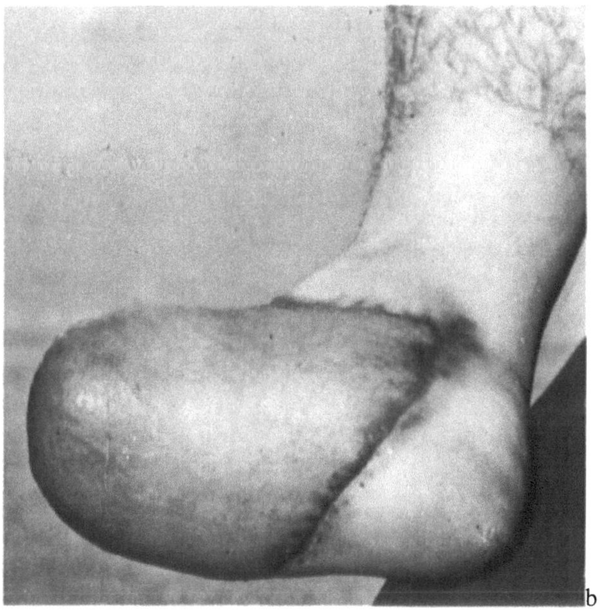
b

Fig. 111 a, b. 28 year old railway man who sustained a crushing amputation of the right forefoot following an injury with a moving locomotive. The raw area was temporarily covered with a skin graft and subsequently the forefoot stump was covered 'mocasin' fashion by a large groin flap. An end-to-end arterial anastomosis using the posterior tibial artery was performed

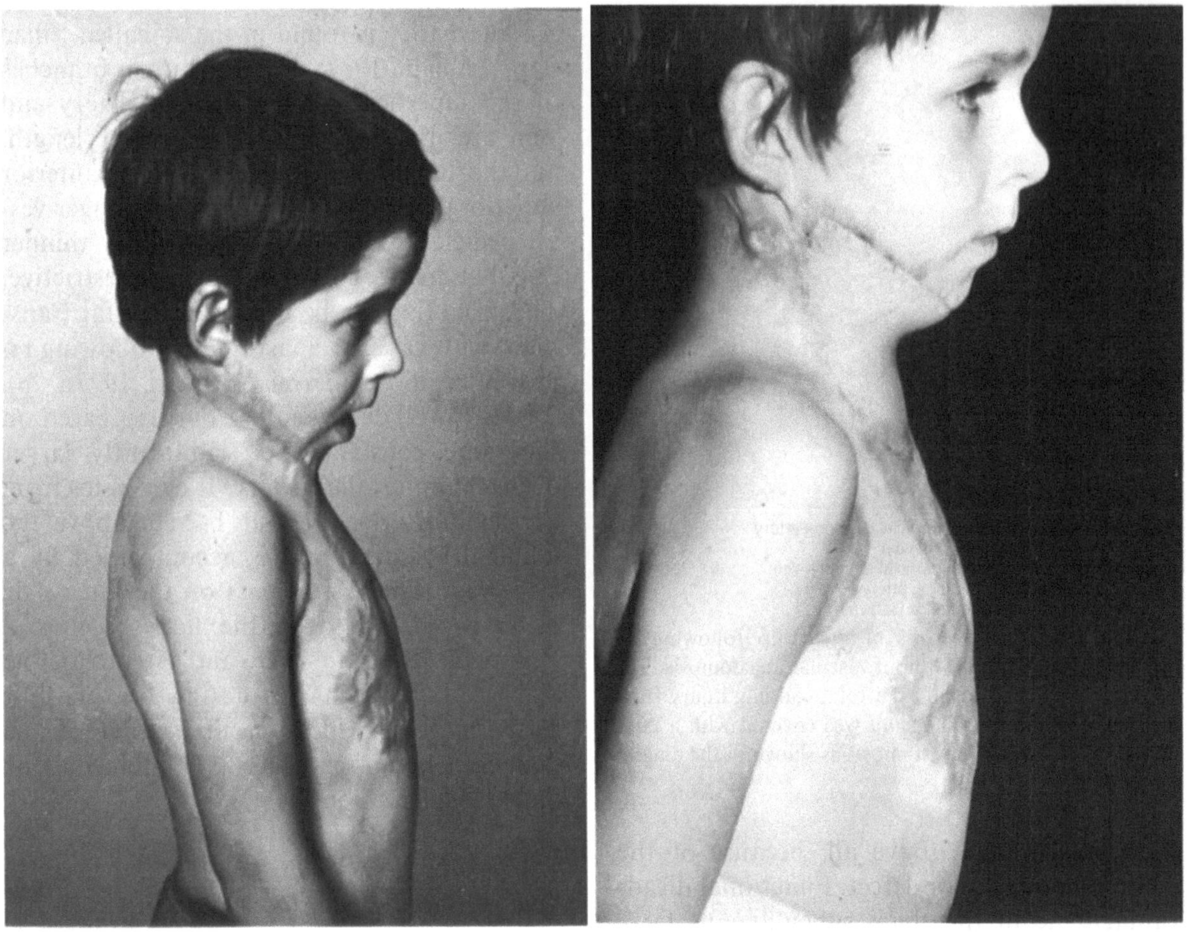

a b

Fig. 112 a, b. Neck contracture in an 8 year old boy following a third degree burning injury. The chin was originally retracted onto the sternum and restoration of neck contour was obtained using a free groin flap, anastomosed to the left facial artery

tery which runs very superficially on the dorsum of the foot over the tarsus. It gives off a deep plantar branch and passes between the first two metatarsals as the dorsal metatarsal artery and distally supplies the latter side of the great toe and the medial side of the second toe (see Fig. 113). In about 30% of cases, the vessel lies deep in the musculature as it gives off its deep plantar branch. The course of the dorsalis pedis artery is crossed by the tendon of the extensor hallucis brevis. The vessel is accompanied by two veins and the deep branch of the fibular nerve which supplies the large toe and the second toe as well as the first web space. It should be noted that in some cases the dorsalis pedis is absent (v. Lanz and Wachsmuth 1972). Anatomical and clini-

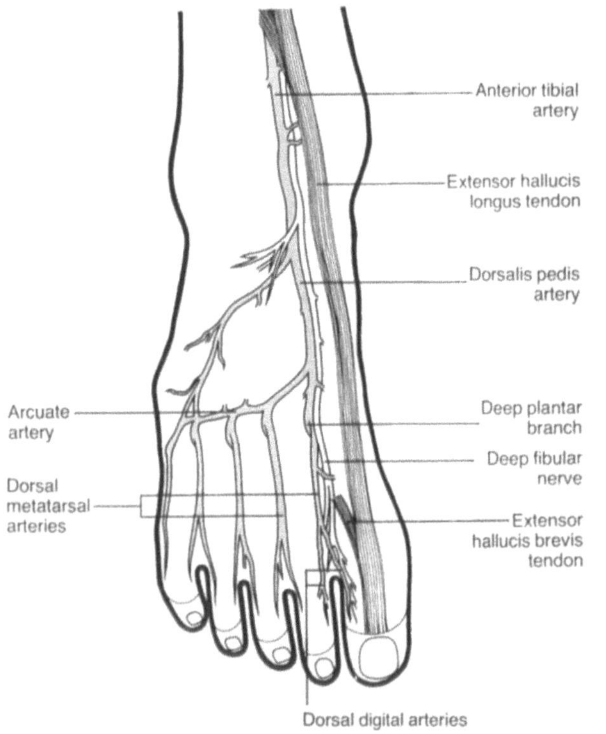

Fig. 113. Diagramatic representation of the anatomy of the dorsum of the foot

cal studies show that the whole skin of the dorsum of the foot, including the first two toes, is supplied by the dorsalis pedis artery. The arcuate artery, which is a branch of the dorsalis pedis artery, collectively supplies the remaining toes of the foot and also gives branches to the metatarsal bones. Because of the thin subcutaneous fat, even in adipose patients, and because of the axial nerve supply, this flap is ideal for hand surgery (see Figs. 114 and 115). The disadvantage of the flap is the necessity to cover the defect with a split skin graft. Careful retention of the paratenon covering the bare tendon is essential for graft-take; particularly in cases where the first web space is taken, subsequent split skin grafting can lead to ulceration. However, according to the authors' experience, this can be overcome using a technique of 'over-grafting'. The size of the flap is determined by the dorsum of the foot. The vessels are large and easily exposed. In addition to the accompanying veins, there are countless veins in the dorsum of the foot and particularly the long saphenous vein is available for venous anastomosis.

When the entire dorsum of the foot is raised as a sensitive flap, the terminal branch of the superficial peroneal nerve, which lies close under the skin, must be included in the flap (see Fig. 116e) ('Anatomy of the Dorsum of the Foot and Exposure of Vessels', see Chap. 'Toe Transplantation').

The course of the artery and vein should be marked before raising the flap. The dorsalis pedis artery with its accompanying veins, as well as the accompanying deep peroneal nerve, are exposed and the flap then raised proximally and from both sides. Variations of this flap use only the distal portion, which encompasses the web space, or a small island flap from the fibular side of the large toe. This latter flap has been termed the 'toe pulp flap' (see Fig. 116).

c) Delto-Pectoral Flap

The free delto-pectoral flap is taken from the area described by Bakamjian in 1963. The flap is supplied by perforating branches of the first and second intercostal arteries. The larger supply is usually from the second intercostal artery and it is this vessel which is most suitable for anastomosis (see Fig. 117). The vessel pedicle is usually very short and the diameter of the artery varies from 0.8 to 1.2 mm (Harii et al. 1974). The flap is raised laterally in a plane superficial to the fascia covering the deltoid muscle.

Medial to the cephalic vein, the fascia of the pectoralis major muscle should be included with the flap (Harrii et al. 1974). The subcutaneous fat is usually thinner than that of the groin flap and furthermore the skin colouring is more suitable for covering defects on the face. The use is often limited in men because of the degree of hair growth on the chest. The main disadvantages are a very noticeable donor defect, which must be covered with split thickness skin grafts, and the very small calibre of vessels: therefore today it is almost never used in clinical practice.

d) Temporal Flaps

The so-called forehead flap can be raised including the frontal branch of the superficial temporal artery and pedicled on the branches of this lateral artery (see Fig. 118). Because of the great variability of the vessels and particularly because of the disfiguring donor defect, this flap has extremely few indications in clinical practice. Of greater significance is the hair-bearing flap pedicled on the parietal branch of the superficial temporal artery. This can be used, for example, to cover an area of traumatic alopecia on the opposite side (Harii et al. 1974; Baudet et al. 1974).

e) Axillary Flaps

Free axillary flaps have been described by Boeck (1976) and Baudet et al. (1976). They are pedicled on the cutaneous branches of the thoraco-dorsal or lateral thoracic vessels (see Fig. 119). Part of the latissimus dorsi muscle can be raised as a musculocutaneous flap (see Chap. 'Musculo-cutaneous Flaps'), carried on the main trunk of the thoraco-dorsal vessels. Disadvantages of this donor region are the

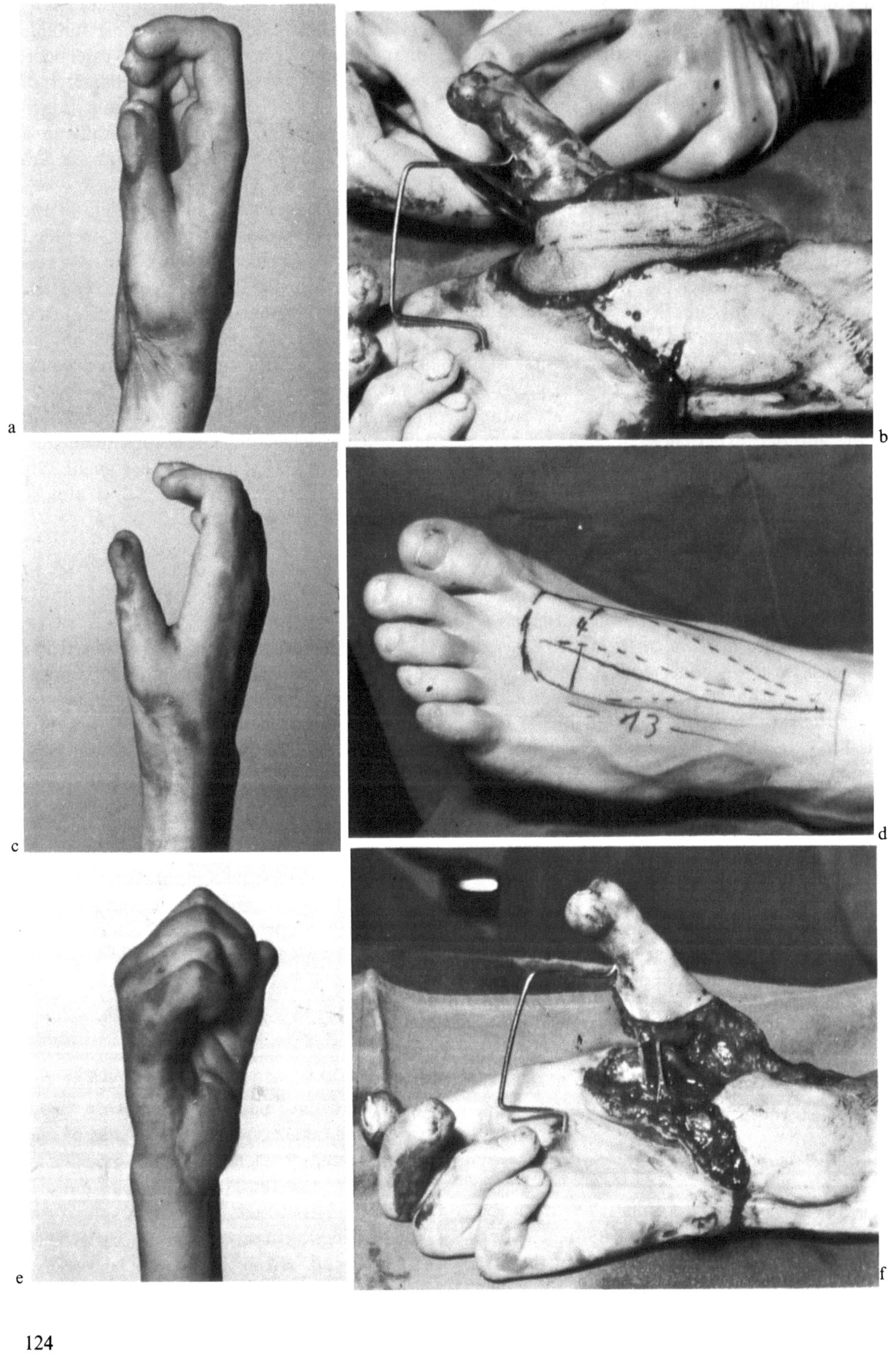
a
b
c
4
13
d
e
f

a b c d

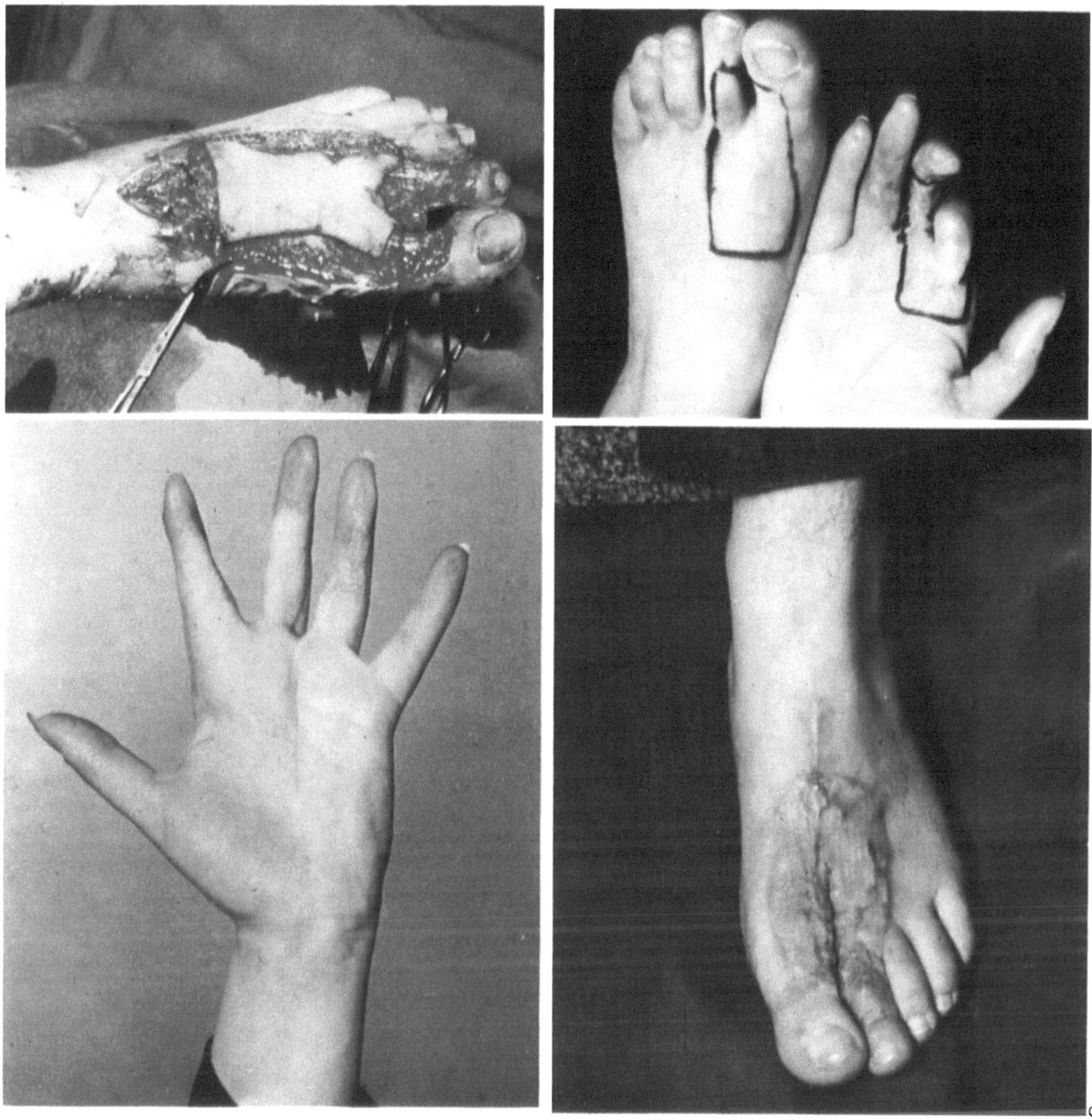

Fig. 115 a, b. Marking of a dorsalis pedis free flap to release a flexion contracture of the index and middle fingers following a third degree burning injury sustained in a press machine. **c, d** The appearance following one thinning procedure of the flap and deepening of the second web space. A digital artery was used for the arterial anastomosis and a vein graft was required to anastomose the vein to the dorsum of the hand. The deep fibular nerve was anastomosed to a digital nerve and the donor defect covered with a split thickness skin graft.

Fig. 114. a. The condition of the hand in an 18 year old man following a severe combined hand injury. There is fixed contraction of the hand with a flexion contracture of all the long fingers and an adduction contracture of the thumb. **b–d** Release of the contracted muscles allows the thumb to be abducted and the resultant soft tissue defect is covered using a 4 × 13 cm free dorsalis pedis flap. The artery is anastomosed to the radial artery and the superior fibular nerve is anastomosed to branches of the radial nerve. **e, f** Functional result following complete healing of the flap and subsequent tenolysis of the long fingers

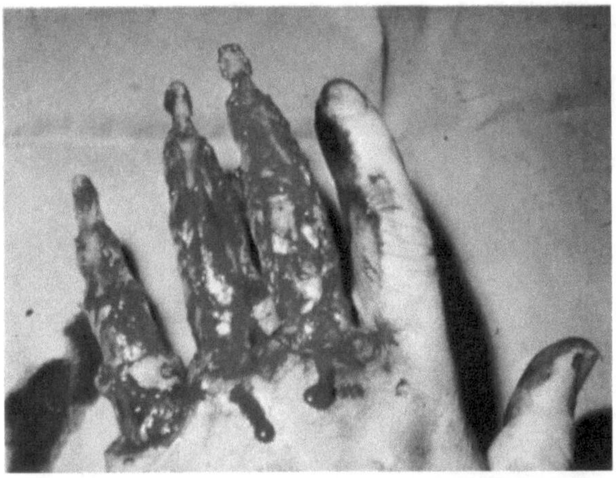

a

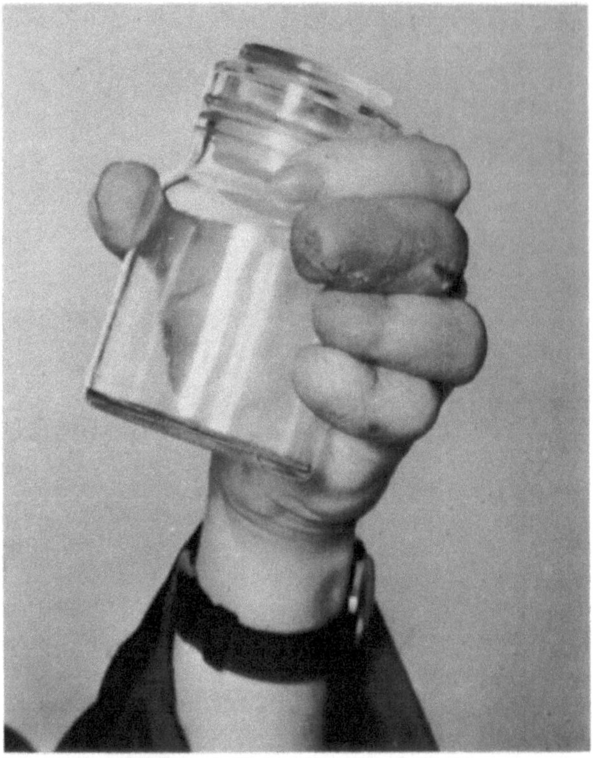

b

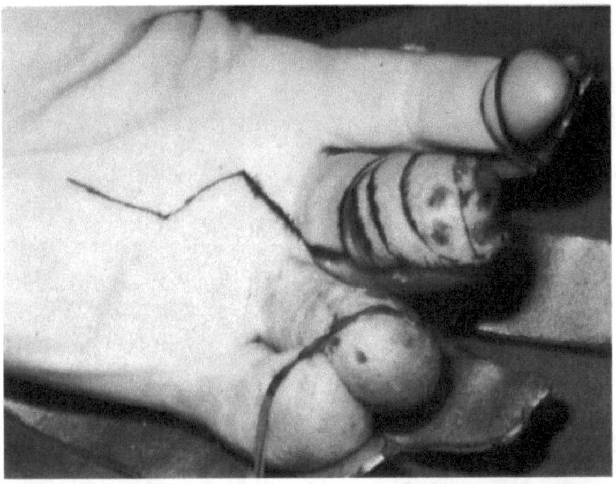

c

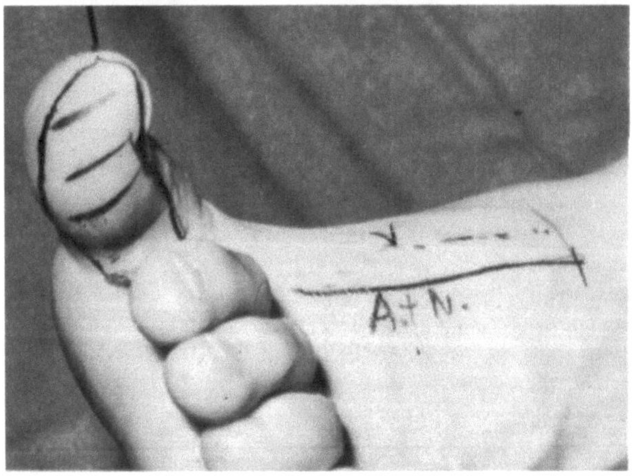

d

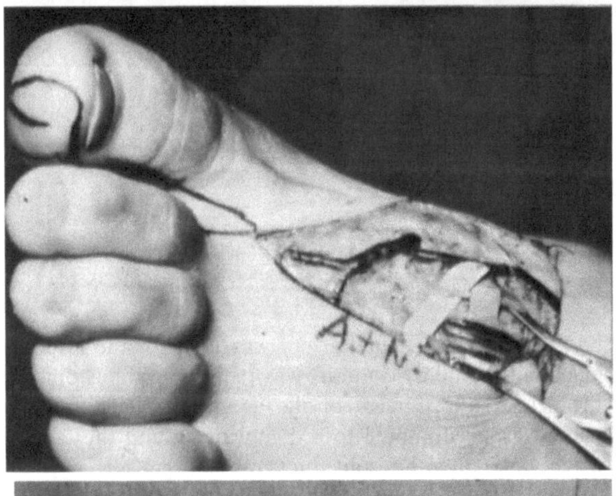

e

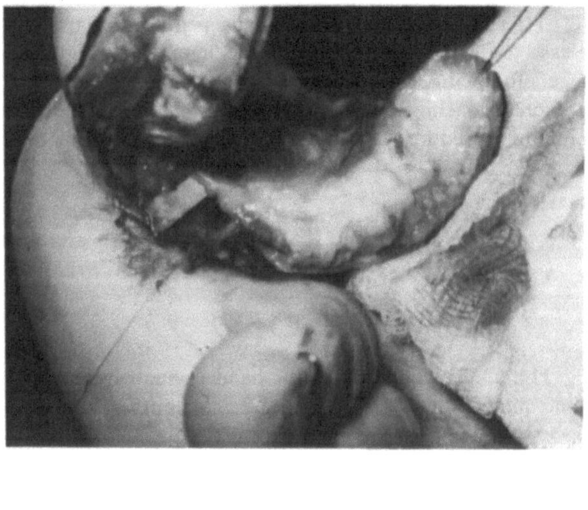

f

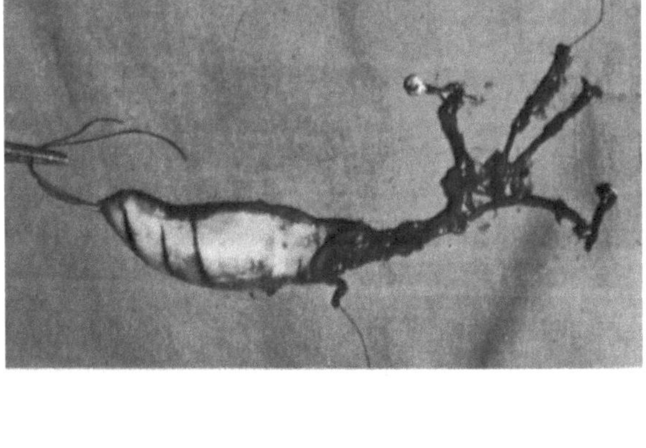

g

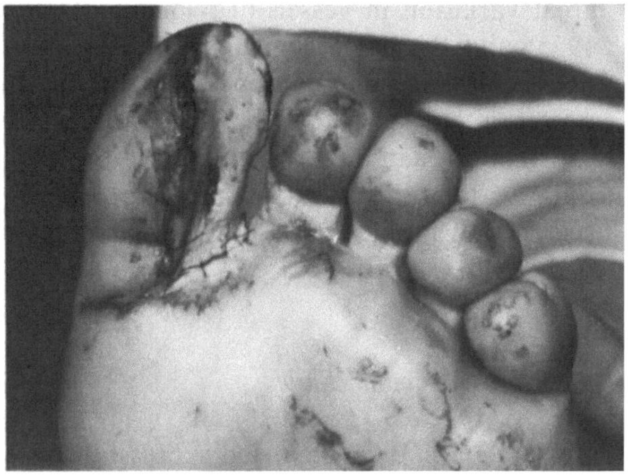

h

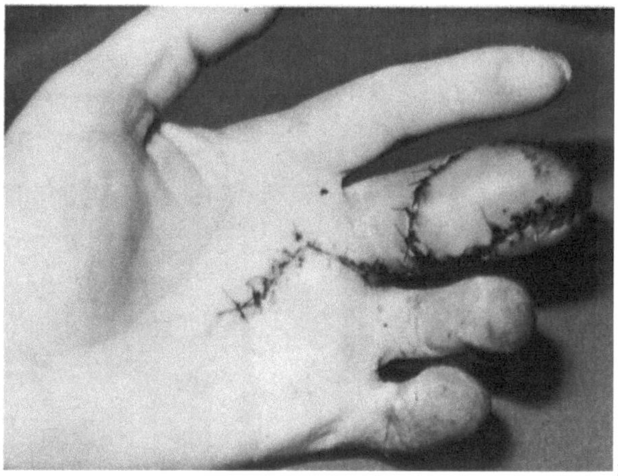

i

◀ **Fig. 116. a–c** Degloving injury of the middle, ring and little fingers in a 35 year old man, the result of an accident involving a roller. The defect was covered using a pedicled groin flap with subsequent separation and thinning. Although quite good function of the fingers was obtained, this was strongly impaired by the lack of sensitivity, which, particularly in the middle finger, led to episodes of inflammation and ulceration. **d, e** The volar aspect of the proximal and distal joints of the middle finger were covered with a toe pulp flap from the fibular side of the large toe. The course of the dorsalis pedis artery and the superficial veins are marked. **f** The dorsalis pedis artery and its two accompanying veins, together with the deep branch of the fibular nerve, which runs medially, are prepared. Further veins draining into the dorsal venous arch are also prepared. The superficial branch of the fibular nerve is exposed and divided. **g, h** The toe pulp flap is raised, together with a small arterial branch of the dorsal digital artery which supplies the flap. The plantar digital nerve from the plantar fibular nerve, which innervates the plantar surface of the flap, is marked with a suture. Together with the deep fibular nerve, which supplies the dorsal part of the flap, it is anastomosed onto a digital nerve. All structures are carefully marked on the completely raised free flap, using different clips for the vessels, and sutures for the nerves. **i** The donor defect is covered with a small split thickness skin graft. The free flap healed satisfactorily and nine months following operation, a 2 point discrimination of 21 mm was achieved, the same as that on the remaining large toe

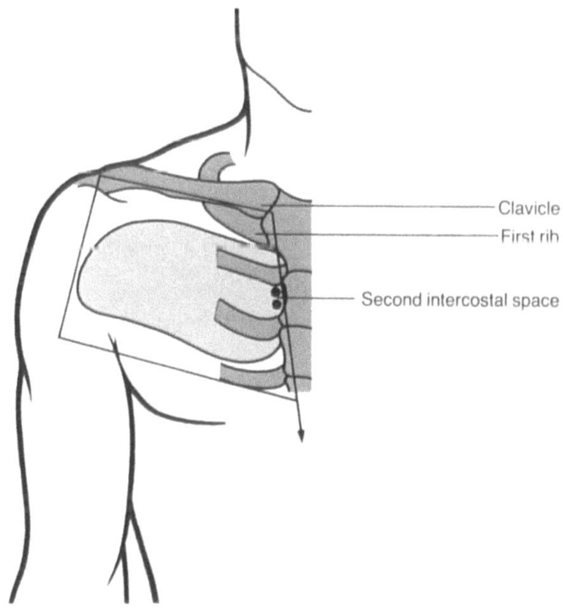

Fig. 117. Diagramatic representation of the delto-pectoral flap

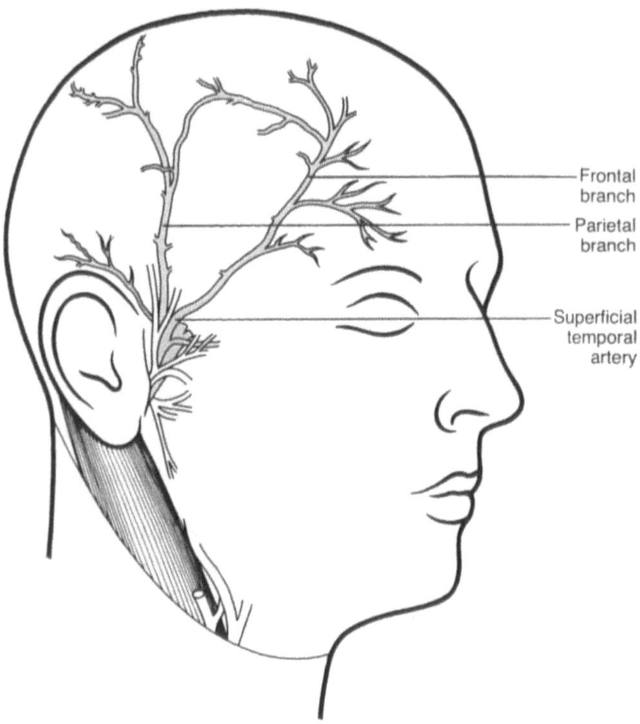

Fig. 118. Diagram showing the course of the superficial temporal artery

great variation in vessels (Taylor and Daniel 1975) and the extent of subcutaneous fat in obese patients. In addition, the scar on the posterolateral aspect of the chest wall is less satisfactory than the scar achieved in the groin flap. On the other hand, Baudet et al. emphasise the advantage of the long and large vessel pedicle.

f) Retro-Auricular Flaps

Fujino et al. (1975) reported successful use of the so-called retro-auricular flap to cover a defect on the nasal bridge. The flap is supplied by the posterior auricular artery with accompanying veins and the resulting defect covered with split thickness skin graft. The size of the flap is, of course, limited by the adjoining head hair.

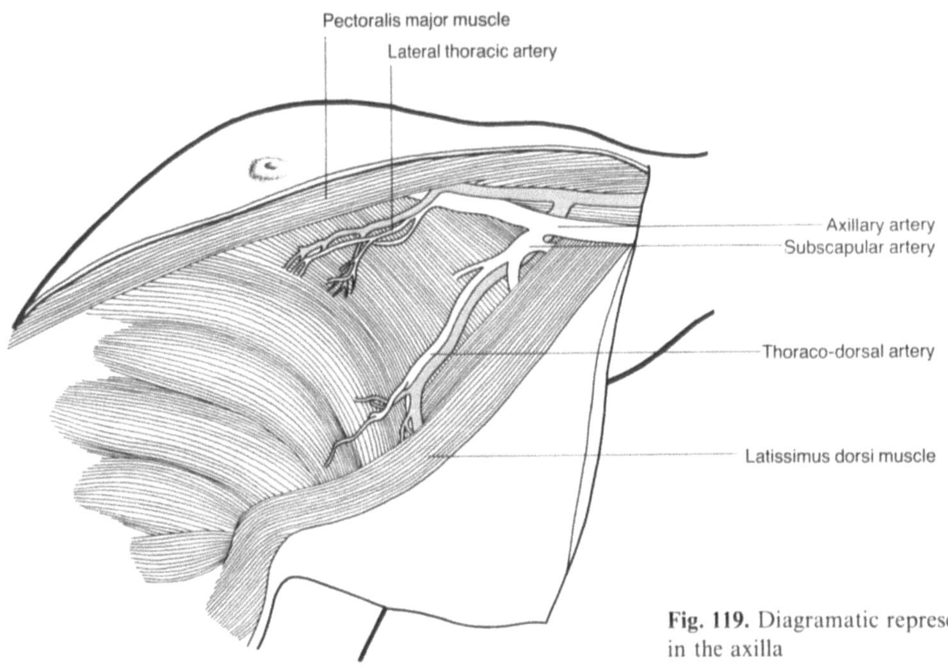

Fig. 119. Diagramatic representation of important vessels in the axilla

VII. Combined Skin and Muscle Flap Transplantation

(musculo-cutaneous flaps)

The principle of musculo-cutaneous flaps depends on the overlying skin being supplied by delicate perforating branches of vessels which supply the muscle (see Fig. 120). Advantages for the use of this combined flap are as follows: It expands the possible donor site into areas in which no subcutaneous axial vessel pattern can be found. It increases the possibility of a thick and well padded flap. In the majority of cases, the vessels are large, since they provide nourishment for the muscle. By performing simultaneous nerve anastomosis, the muscle can subsequently be utilised functionally. Musculo-cutaneous flaps illustrate the progression towards using larger central vessels, leaving the small delicate superficial cutaneous vessels, thus simplifying the anastomosis and making it safer. A similar example can be seen in toe transplantation where the larger dorsalis pedis artery is used instead of the delicate plantar digital vessels. According to the tissue required, the whole of the overlying skin, or only part of the skin, can be raised as an island myocutaneous flap.

a) Gracilis Flaps

The skin on the inner surface of the thigh overlying the gracilis muscle can be raised with the muscle as a musculo-cutaneous flap (Harii et al. 1976a). The main pedicle supplying the muscle arises, in the majority of cases, directly from the profunda femoris artery or from the medial femoral circumflex artery, and enters the muscle in its cranial third. According to Harii, the outer diameter of the artery varies from 1.2 to 1.8 mm and the accompanying veins from 1.5 to 2.2 mm. The nerve supply to the muscle is a branch of the obturator nerve which passes into the muscle proximal to the arteries (see Chap. 'Muscle Transplantation') (see Fig. 122). The donor defect can be closed directly in the majority of cases.
In the presence of fully functioning adductors of the leg there is no functional loss following removal of the gracilis muscle (Harii 1976).

b) Latissimus-Dorsi Flaps

A latissimus dorsi flap has approximately the same scope as the axillary flap (see Section – 'Axillary Flaps'). Small- to medium-sized flaps allow the defect to be closed directly. The feeding vessels are the thoraco-dorsal vessels (see Fig. 119) and these large vessels are usually over 2 mm in diameter: they are situated on the anterior palpable edge of the latissimus dorsi muscle and are relatively easy to find. The vessels can be dissected out of a portion of a muscle so that a 10 to 15 cm long vessel pedicle can be formed if required. In well developed muscular patients, the flap is frequently very thick, particularly in the cranial portion. Atrophy of the muscle, following denervation, can spontaneously resolve this problem. Godina in 1979 reported 64 such flaps and, in this series, only one case suffered necrosis.

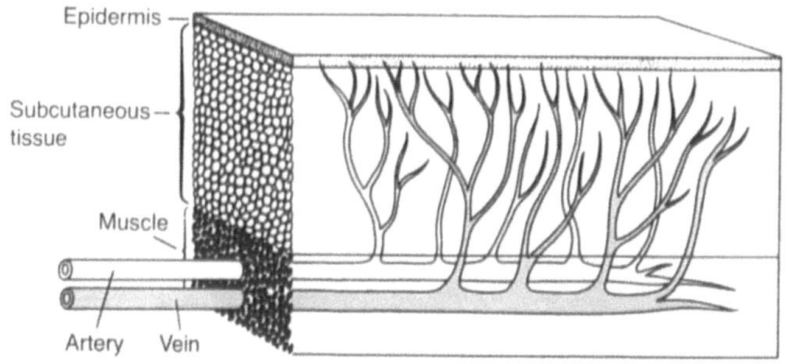

Fig. 120. Diagramatic plan of the musculo-cutaneous flap

VIII. Combined Skin Flap with Bone Transplantation

(osteo-cutaneous flaps)

Analogous to the situation of musculo-cutaneous flaps, it is also possible to transplant skin with underlying bone, where the feeding vessels give branches to both tissues. Until now, three such transplants have been examined.

1. Rib and chest wall.
2. Second metatarsal, with the dorsalis-pedis flap.
3. Iliac crest with the groin flap.

The rib chest wall flap is supplied by the intercostal vessels (see Chap. 'Bone transplantation'). Buncke et al. in 1977, reported one example where this combined flap was used to bridge a tibia and cover a soft tissue defect. Ohmori (1977) described a case in which a combined flap comprising the dorsalis pedis with underlying second metatarsal was used for the total reconstruction of a nose. The feeding vessel, i.e. the dorsalis pedis artery, was dissected free proximally to obtain lengthening, and was raised as the anterior tibial artery, so that the anastomosis could be performed onto the temporal vessels at a long distance with a long vessel pedicle. The authors have used a similar transplant to replace a traumatically lost first metacarpal and overlying skin. By including the long extensor tendon of the second toe and the short extensor tendon of the large toe, the abductor tendons of the thumb, as well as the long extensor tendon of the thumb, could also be reconstructed. A similar combined flap can be achieved by inclusion of the anterior iliac spine, or alternatively a portion of iliac crest, together with a groin flap. Taylor (1979) demonstrated a more certain and safe arterialisation using the deep circumflex iliac artery (see Chap. 'Groin flaps').

Indications for such combined bone/skin flaps exist where there are bone defects of the extremities and particularly of the face, with additional lack of soft tissue covering.

IX. Bone Transplantation

As early as 1918, Blair described the transfer of live bone on a pedicle: here, either muscle or skin may be used as feeding pedicle. Strauch et al. (1971) isolated a rib using the vessel pedicle of the internal mammary artery and used it to reconstruct the lower jaw in a dog. McCulloch and Fredrickson (1973) divided this vessel pedicle and re-anastomosed the vessels using microvascular surgical techniques.

Tschopp (1976), in addition to vessel anastomosis, also anastomosed the intercostal nerve which supplied the transplanted intercostal muscles. Bos reported the use of free fibula grafts in the legs of dogs in 1977. He showed that, by maintaining a patent anastomosis, bone could be retained in its fully live state, whereas loss of its vascular connection led to almost total bone resorbtion. Taylor et al. (1975) first described clinical examples using free fibular grafts. In one case, the graft had to be removed because of infection, but the second case healed satisfactorily. O'Brien (1977) transplanted the fibula to reconstruct a defect in the vertebral canal of a patient.

In free rib transplantation, the intercostal vessels are raised with the flap. The problem here lies on the venous side, since the intercostal veins are often poorly developed. On the other hand, the intercostal nerve can be used, e.g., as a graft, in cases where there is simultaneous nerve destruction. A disadvantage lies in the necessary thoracotomy which, particularly when the pleural cavity is opened, can be particularly stressful for the patient. The more suitable ribs are the 5th and 6th, and the amount of rib removed varies according to the clinical requirements, particularly with regard to the curve of the rib. Basically, however, the rib should be removed as far dorsal as possible. Here, the vessels are not only larger, but, because of the greater amount of muscle, the danger of subsequent chest wall herniation is reduced (see Fig. 121).

The main indication for rib transplantation is in reconstruction of the mandible. By including the pleura or, alternatively, the chest wall, a three layer reconstruction of the mandible can be performed in a single stage.

The fibula transplant is particularly suited to bridge long, regular bone defects. When elevating the bone, a tuft of muscle approximately 1 cm thick must be retained on the bone in order to ensure the periosteal blood supply; the feeding vessel, with a portion of artery, is also raised. It is important that the proximal head of the fibula, as well as the distal third, is preserved, to retain stability of the knee and ankle joints (Taylor et al. 1975). In addition to these two bone transplants, combined skin/bone flaps such as the iliac crest with the groin flap or the second metatarsal with the dorsalis pedis flap, can be raised and transplanted (see Chap. 'Combined skin/bone flaps').

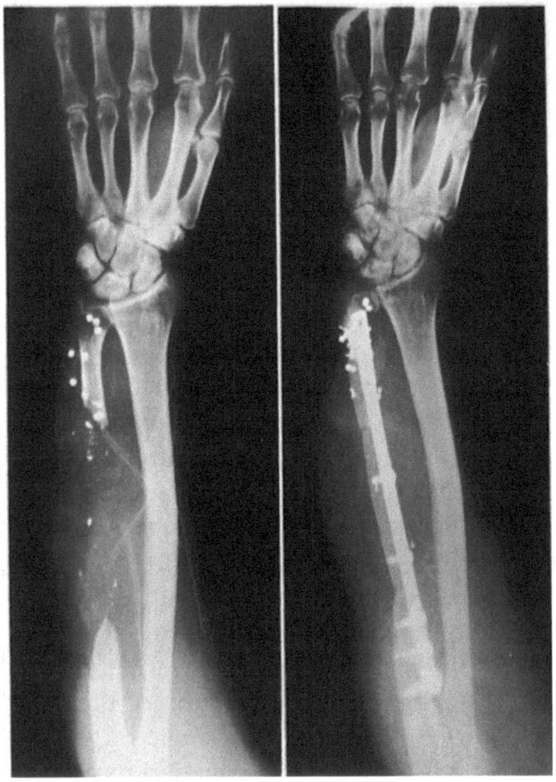

a b

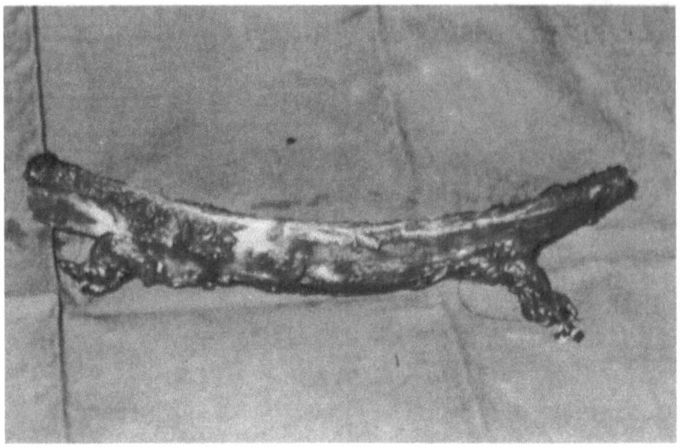

c

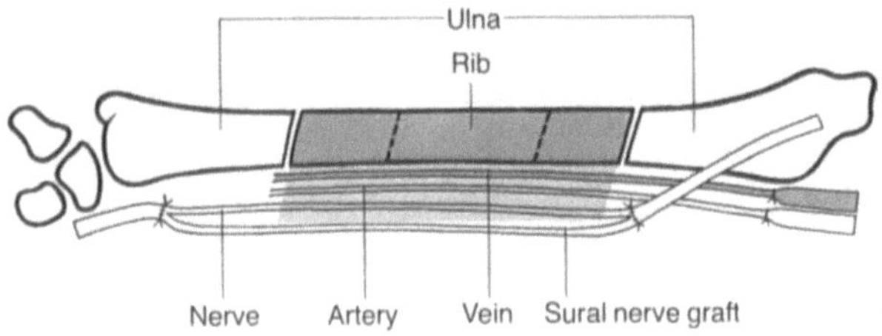

d

Fig. 121. a, b 38 year old man who was involved in a hunting accident resulting in the loss of 12 cm of the ulna and ulnar nerve. The soft tissue loss was replaced using a pedicle flap from the lower abdomen. The bone defect was replaced using a 13 cm long free rib graft with anastomosis of the intercostal artery to the stump of the ulnar artery. A 15 cm gap in the ulnar nerve was repaired using the intercostal nerve and two sural nerve grafts. Thirteen months following surgery there were signs of reinnervation. **c–e** The free rib graft was taken from the 5th rib on the right side. The vessels and nerves are marked, and by means of subperiosteal crack fractures, the rib was straightened and extended so that it could be inserted using a long osteo-synthetic plate. Because of the short distal ulnar fragment, it was necessary to use additional fixation

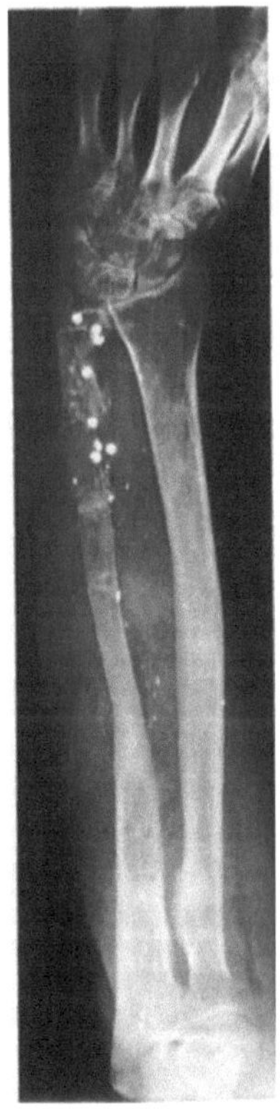

e

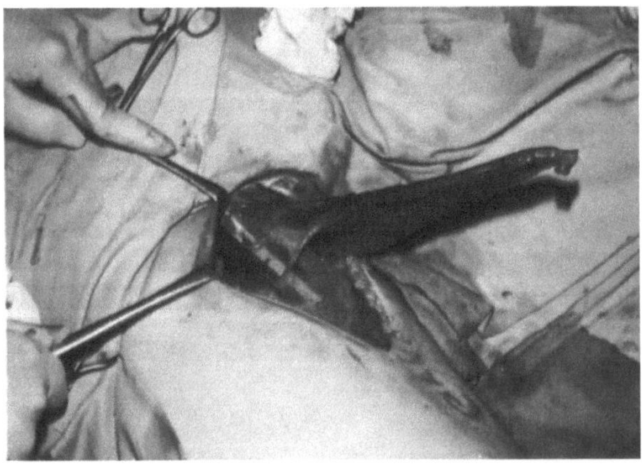

Fig. 122. The gracilis muscle is raised. The nerve lies cranially, whereas the vessel bundle lies more caudally

X. Muscle Transplantation

In 1970 Tamai et al. described the successful transplantation of the rectus femoris muscle in dogs. Harii et al. (1975) first reported the clinical use of muscle transplantation with vascular anastomosis, using the gracilis muscle to reconstruct an established facial paralysis. The upper third of the gracilis muscle can be exposed through an incision approximately 10 cm in length on the inner surface of the thigh. The motor branch supplying the muscle is derived from the obturator nerve and passes cranial to the vessel pedicle into the muscle. The vascular branch of the pedicle, branches of the profunda femoris artery, and accompanying veins, lie somewhat distal to the nerve (see Fig. 122). A third incision, a hand's breadth above the knee joint, exposes the distal portion of the muscle, allowing the muscle to be totally removed. The muscle is transplanted to the head and fixed in its cranial part to the temporalis fascia.

Vascular anastomosis is performed to the temporal vessel and nerve anastomosis uses either a motor branch of the trigeminal nerve (Harii 1976), or a cross facial nerve graft from the opposite healthy facial nerve, inserted six months previously (Anderl 1973).

The gracilis muscle is placed in a pocket under the cheek skin and brought out through an incision in the naso-labial fold. The distal end of the muscle is split and passed around the upper and lower lip prior to fixation. The large muscle atrophies to some degree initially until reinnervation is established. The skin overlying the gracilis muscle can be included as a combined musculo-cutaneous flap (see Chap. 'Musculo-cutaneous flap').

In 1973, at the No. VI People's Hospital, Shanghai, the lateral half of the pectoralis major muscle was used to reconstruct the destroyed flexor musculature on a patient's forearm (No. VI People's Hospital, 1976). The muscle was raised on the lateral thoracic vessels and included the lateral pectoral nerve; as a result of this operation, active flexion of the long fingers was achieved.

XI. Transplantation of the Omentum

Until recently the omentum, maintained on a pedicle, was used by many authors for covering large soft tissue defects. McLean and Buncke (1972), performed a free transplant of omentum with vessel anastomosis to cover a defect on the skull. The omentum was subsequently covered with split thickness skin grafts. Similarly, Harii (1975) and Ikuta (1975) have used omentum with vascular anastomosis for similar cases.

The indication for the use of free transplantation of the omentum is particularly strong in large soft tissue defects which, either because of their size or because of their depth, cannot be covered or filled by other flaps. In these cases the omentum is subsequently covered with split thickness skin grafts.

XII. Toe Transplantation

In 1897, Nicoladoni described a technique for reconstructing the thumb using a toe, but it was necessary to fix the hand to the foot for 3 weeks.

For this reason, the procedure was only used in special cases.

In 1900 Eiselsberg reported a case of reconstructing the index finger using a pedicled second toe transplant.

The preference for thumb reconstruction then moved to the long fingers i.e. pollicization. Buncke et al. (1966), first achieved successful free transplantation of the large and second toes in rhesus monkeys, using vascular anastomosis. The first successful clinical case of large toe transplantation for reconstructing the thumb was published by Cobbett in 1969a). He transplanted the large toe to the thumb with anastomosis of the plantar arteries of the toe. The venous anastomosis was performed on the dorsum of the hand.

Buncke et al. (1973) anastomosed the first dorsal metatarsal artery when using the large toe to reconstruct a thumb. In both these cases, as well as later operations, there were reported post-operative difficulties with regard to the anastomosis. O'Brien et al. in 1975, reported their experience of a procedure which appeared free from complication. Reconstruction of the thumb and fingers using the second toe was reported in individual case reports by Buncke et al. (1973) and Ohmori and Harii (1975a). In the spring of 1977, the authors reported a case of reconstruction of the thumb using the 2nd toe, which had been performed in October 1976. In these cases, the dorsalis pedis artery or its terminal branch, the first dorsal metatarsal artery, was chosen for the arterial anastomosis.

In reconstruction of the thumb and fingers by toe transplantation, the anatomical similarity in relation to nerves, extensor and flexor tendon apparatus and joints, can be utilised.

Anatomy of the Neurovascular Supply to the Large and Second Toe

In the malleolar region, the tendon of the extensor hallucis longus muscle passes from lateral to medial, over the neurovascular bundle of the tibialis anterior vessels. As this artery passes under the extensor retinaculum distally over the dorsum of the foot, it is termed the dorsalis pedis artery and it gives branches to the medial and lateral aspects of the ankle and three further branches to the lateral border of the foot: the proximal lateral tarsal artery, the distal lateral tarsal artery and, in the region of the tarsal-metatarsal joints, the arcuate artery. From this arcuate artery arise the dorsal metatarsal arteries, which divide at the level of the metatarsal phalangeal joints into the dorsal digital arteries, which in turn divide to supply each side of the neighbouring toe. Proximal to the dorsal metatarsal artery, the arcuate artery gives off a deep plantar trunk, which descends between the first and second metatarsal bones to the sole of the foot (see Fig. 113). Normally, the dorsal metatarsal arteries pass distally over the interossei muscles. In about 30% of cases (v. Lanz and Wachsmuth 1972), the vessels pass under the interossei muscles or, alternatively, into the muscle while passing distally. In such cases, preparation and isolation of the vessels is complicated. The first dorsal metatarsal artery supplies the large toe in the majority of cases and 1–3 smaller dorsal digital vessels to the medial side of the 2nd toe (see Fig. 113). It should be noted that in about 15% of cases, however, the dorsalis pedis artery is not available (v. Lanz and Wachsmuth 1972).

Running parallel and usually lateral to the artery is the deep peroneal nerve, which passes into the first web space and provides sensation to this area. The most proximal skin of the dorsum of the foot is supplied by the superficial peroneal nerve, which passes over the fascia of the dorsum of the foot.

The dorsalis pedis artery is usually accompanied by two veins which communicate with one another (see Fig. 116).

The entire neurovascular bundle is crossed by the tendon of the extensor hallicis brevis muscle on the dorsum of the foot, and in preparation and lifting this muscle must be divided. The superficial plexus of veins in the dorsum of the foot runs laterally predominantly to the short saphenous vein and medially towards the long saphenous vein.

Operative Procedure

Toe transplantation to the hand is best performed using two operating teams: incision is made over the palpable dorsalis pedis artery on the back of the foot for exposure. It is important to first ascertain that the posterior tibial artery will supply the forefoot, following removal of the dorsalis pedis artery. Furthermore, pre-operatively, in addition to the marking of the course of the artery, the appropriate veins draining the toe superficially on the back of the foot should be marked and should be raised with the flap, in case there is difficulty in preparing the venae comitantes.

Preparation and raising of the flap continues with careful haemostasis and division and ligation of all side branches. (Ideal conditions for preparation and lifting of the flap can be achieved as follows: the foot is exsanguinated, a tourniquet applied and subsequently released for a short time until the artery and veins are filled. Thereafter the tourniquet is re-inflated) (see Fig. 116f). In 2nd toe transplantation, particular care must be taken with the delicate dorsal digital artery which supplies it. Depending on the toe to be transplanted and the amount of soft tissue required, a large or small triangular skin flap can be raised (see Fig. 123c). In extreme cases, the toe can be transplanted with a total dorsalis pedis skin flap. Equally, the neighbouring web or, with the second toe, the inner surface of the large toe, can be transplanted when required. On the plantar side following removal of the toe, the resulting scar should never extend as far as the weight-bearing surface of the sole of the foot. The extensor tendons, taken with the transplanted toe, are always initially somewhat longer than required. Depending on the requirements, an osteotomy can be performed on the distal third of the

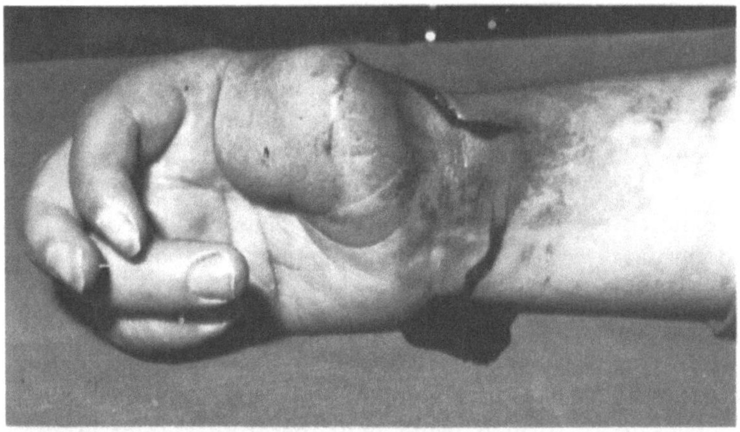

a

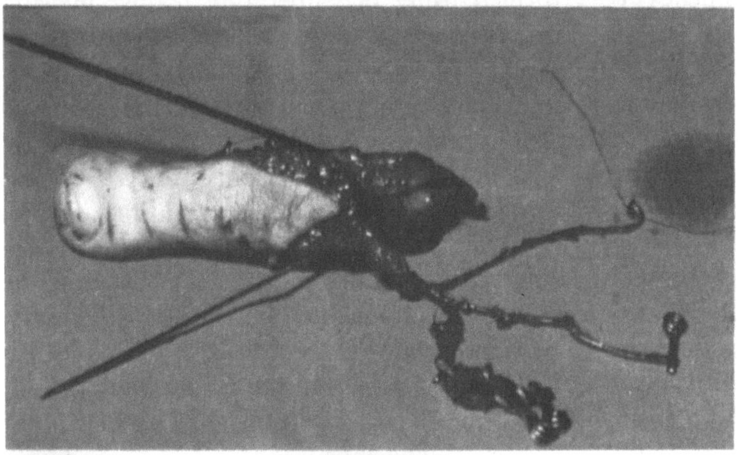

b

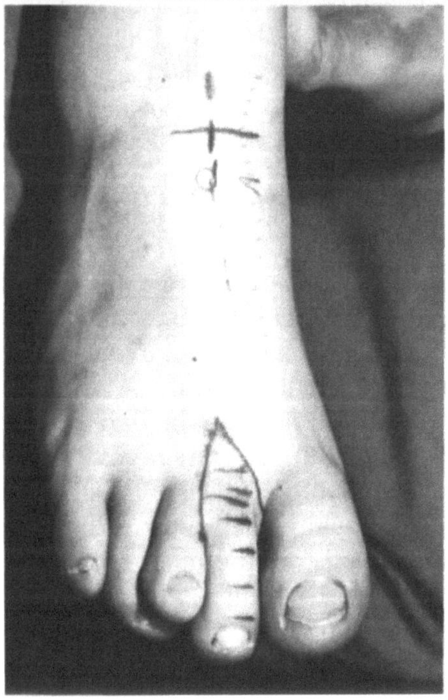

c

Fig. 123 a–c. A 21 year old farmer's wife who sustained total amputation of her right thumb following an accident involving farm machinery. In addition there was limitation of movement of the index and middle fingers. Thumb reconstruction was achieved by means of a second toe transfer

second metatarsal, or the toe divided through the metatarsal phalangeal joint. In the case of the large toe, at least the plantar half of the first metatarsal head must be retained for functional reasons. In 2nd toe transplantation, the head of the second metatarsal is removed to allow the foot to narrow and give a functionally and aesthetically better closure (see Fig. 126g).
Because of the extreme hyperextensibility of the metacarpophalangeal joint of the 2nd toe, it will not function well on flexing the hand. The inclusion of this joint into the transplant achieves lengthening, but flexion function can only occur in the proximal and distal interphalangeal joints.
Two plantar nerves are found on the plantar side of the toe and sufficient length is raised with the transplant. Exposure of the flexor tendons can readily be achieved following the osteotomy, and this avoids opening the sole of the foot. Direct wound closure is performed in layers and achieves a degree of narrowing

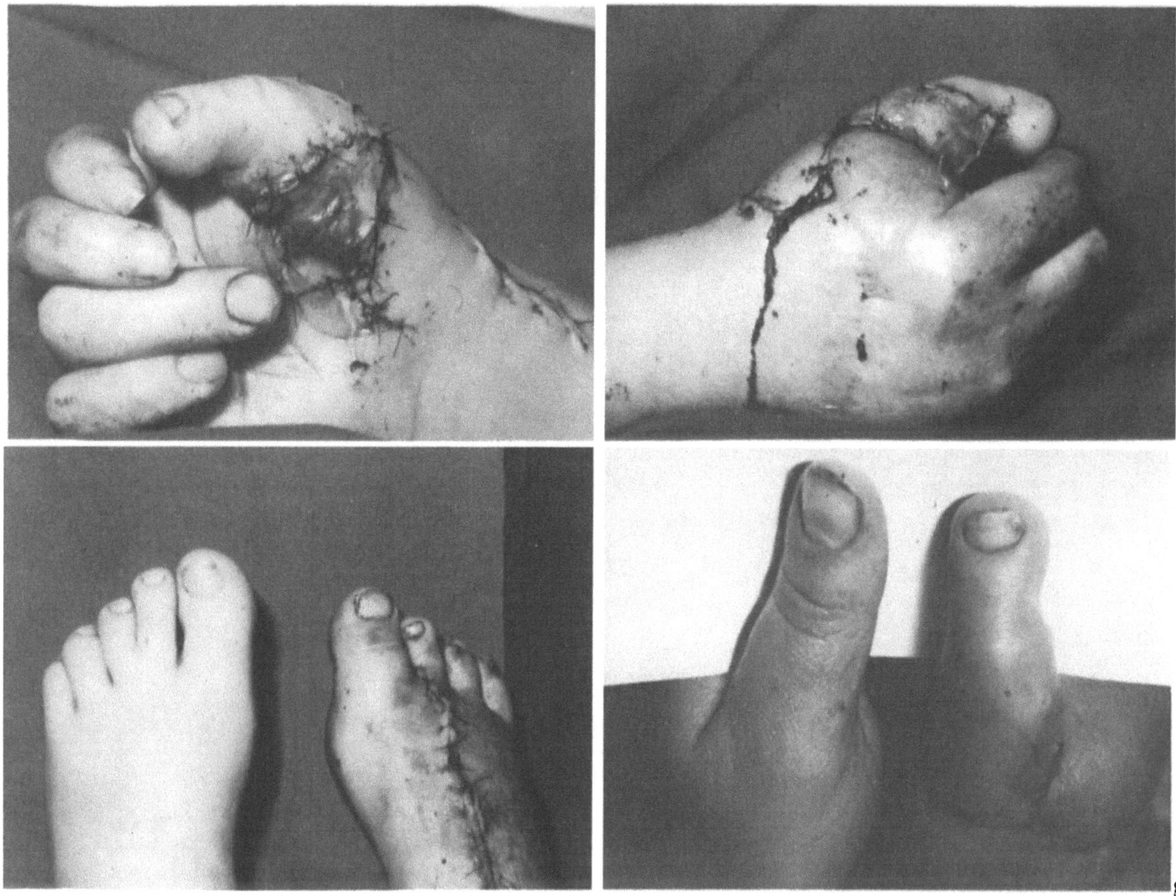

d e f g

Fig. 123d–g. Lack of soft tissue on the stump and the partial syndactyly between the second and third toes, necessitated a sickle-shaped split thickness skin graft at the base of the toe transfer. The toe defect was closed directly, by narrowing the foot. **g** The new "thumb" matches the normal contralateral thumb in overall shape and length

of the foot. The bone in the stump of the thumb is exposed through a fish-mouth incision and is appropriately prepared (see Fig. 124a). The tendons of extensor pollicis longus, flexor pollicis longus and the two volar nerve stumps are exposed and marked. An additional 'S'-shaped incision is made over the trapezium joint and the dorsal aspect of the thumb explored. Here, in the radial fossa, the radial artery, as well as 2–3 veins and a branch of the radial nerve are identified (see Fig. 126e). The 2nd toe is fixed to the thumb stump using two crossed Kirschner wires or screws. Following this, the extensor pollicis longus is sutured to the extensor tendon of the toe.

The arterial anastomosis to the radial artery is performed, followed by 1–2 venous anastomoses as well as a nerve repair using the deep fibular nerve.

The flexor tendon is repaired and likewise two volar or, alternatively, plantar nerves are anastomosed (see Fig. 126e).

In many cases, it is necessary to split-skin graft two lateral crescent-shaped areas at the base of the toe (see Fig. 123). These areas are relatively larger in cases where there is the frequent partial syndactyly between the 2nd and 3rd toes.

In the authors' experience, it may take approximately 1–2 hours until a clear circulation is established or until there is evidence of active hyperaemia in the toe transplant. A possible reason is the likelihood of vessel spasm of the dorsalis pedis artery, resulting from the lengthy preparation of this vessel. The usual medication for free tissue transplantation is administered. When the 2nd toe is used as a finger, the arterial anastomosis is more fa-

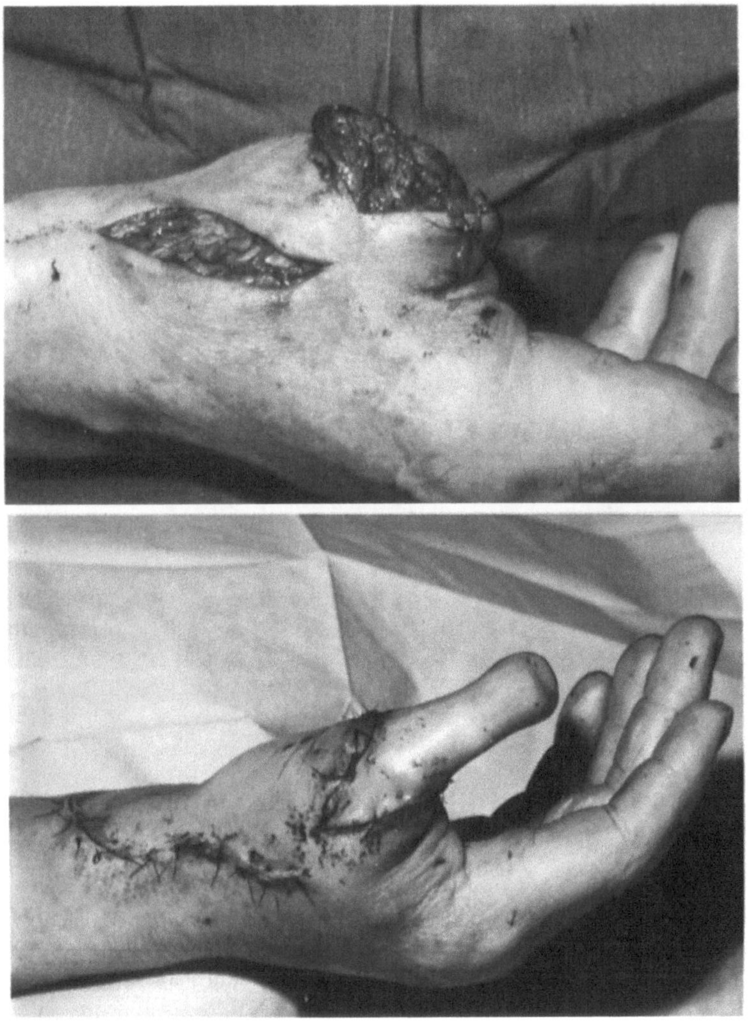

a

b

Fig. 124 a, b. A fish-mouth incision on the thumb stump exposes the bone, the volar nerves and arteries and the long flexor tendon. An S-shaped incision over the anatomical snuff box exposes the radial artery, 1–2 veins, a branch of the radial nerve and the extensor tendon. The triangulated base of the toe transfer matches well into the incision made in the thumb stump

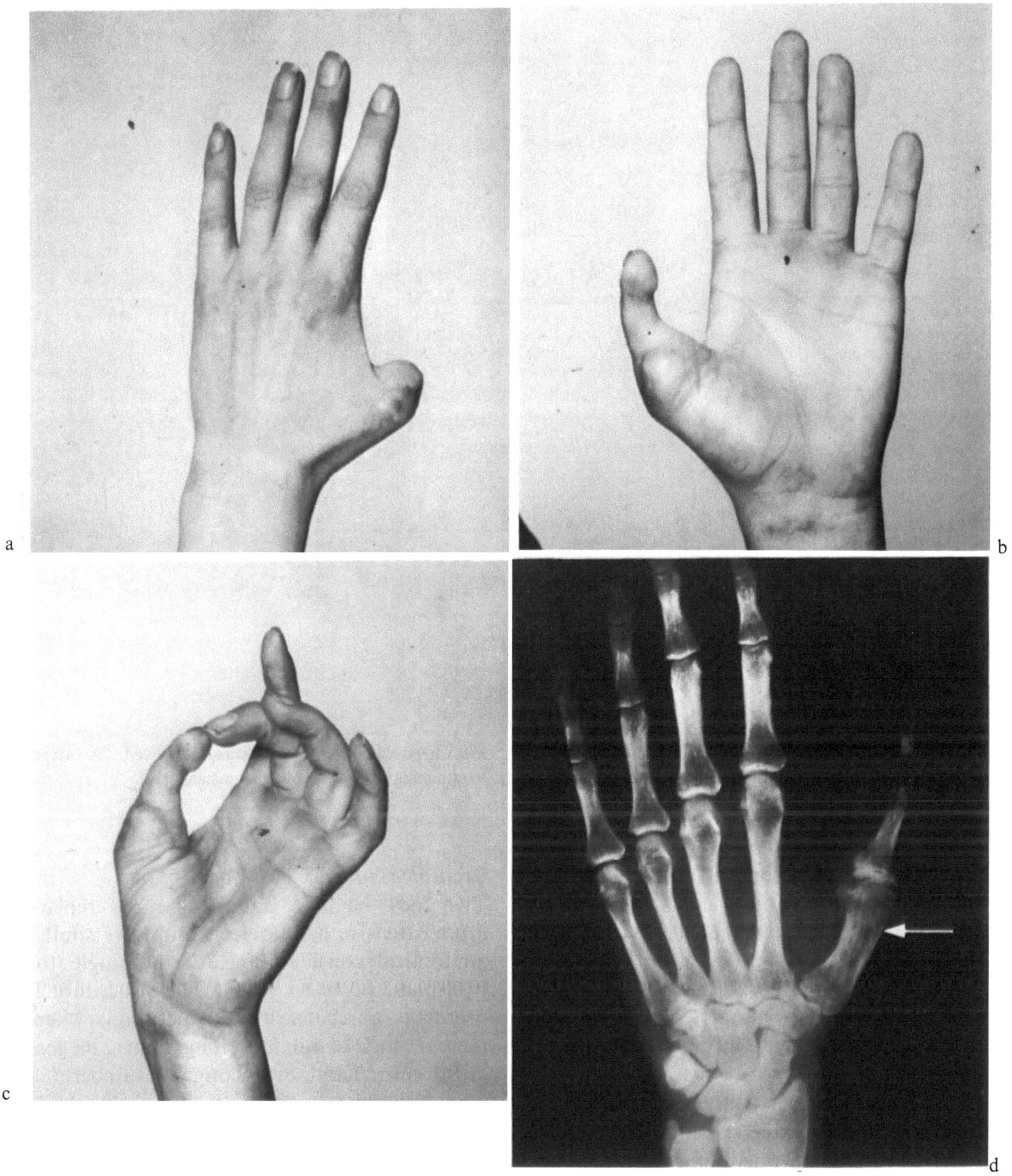
a b c d

Fig. 125 a–d. Loss of the left thumb in a 46 year female concert pianist resulting from a road traffic accident. One year following reconstruction using the second toe, the patient could again give concerts. The x-ray shows good healing of the osteosynthesis site (arrow). The new "thumb" possesses one joint more than the natural extremity

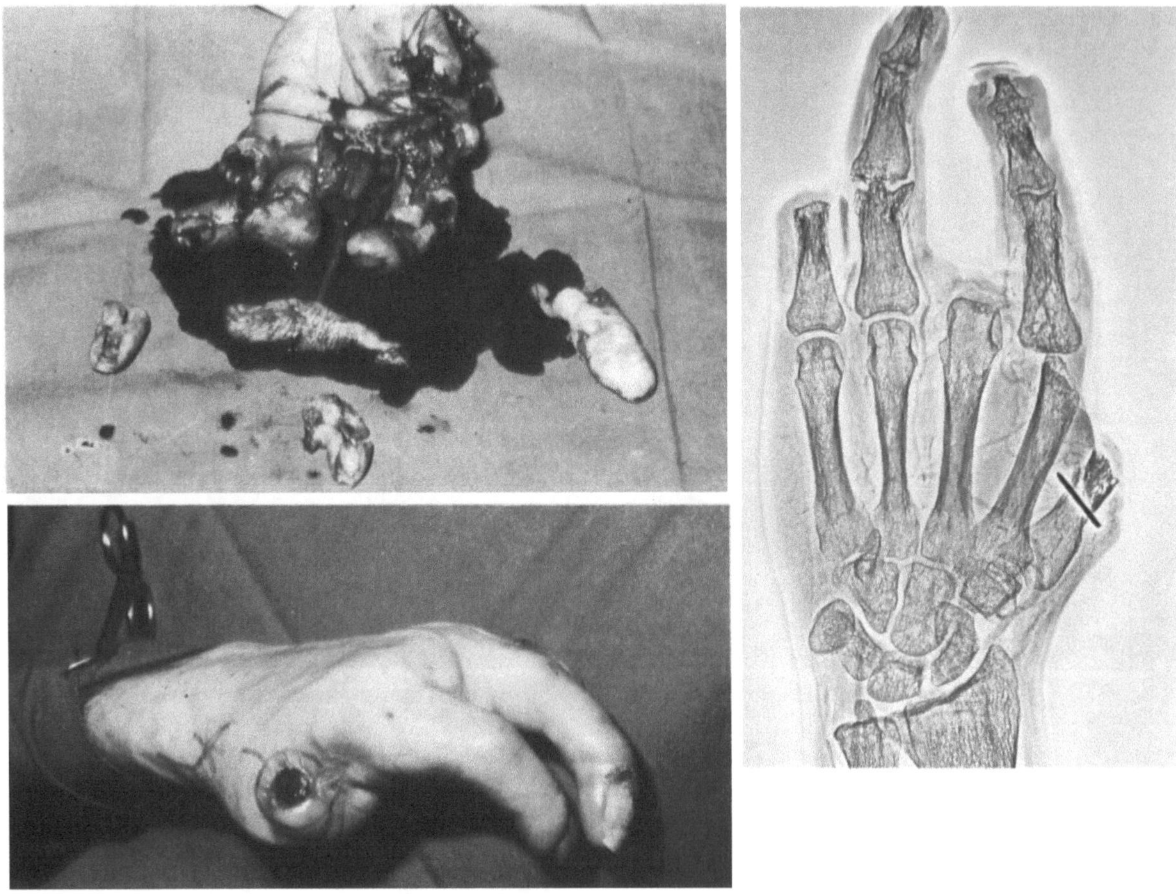

a

b

c

Fig. 126 a–c. Mill cutting injury in the left hand of a 34 year old carpenter. It was only possible to retain a two finger hand by replantation, and the index finger metacarpophalangeal joint was destroyed. A staged lengthening of the thumb was unsuccessful

vourable, using the communal digital artery, and there is an obvious venous anastomosis using the large veins on the back of the hand (see Fig. 127).

In the opinion of the authors, the 2nd toe has the following advantages, when compared to the large toe, for use in thumb reconstruction:

1. It is usually longer than the large toe.
2. It is a more suitable size and shape, compared with the retained thumb of the opposite side, particularly in women.
3. The aesthetic and functional results of the donor defect on the foot are much better than those following removal of the large toe.

Transplantation of Two Toes 'en bloc'

Two toes 'en bloc' can be used to replace more extensive hand defects and have similar anatomical considerations to the single toe transplant (O'Brien 1977). The procedure is useful as a reconstructive operation, where there is loss of all four long digits, or loss of the entire hand, or in congenital finger and hand aplasias.

If necessary, this can be combined with a further transplantation of the large toe or a further transplantation of second toe from the opposite foot to build up a thumb.

Fig. 126 d. A second toe transfer was performed according to the plan shown in the diagram

Fig. 126e–i. The MP joint of the index finger was replaced using a joint prosthesis (St. George prosthesis). The donor defect on the foot is closed directly; two years postoperatively there is no discomfort and the young carpenter wears normal footwear. In addition, he can return to his previous employment

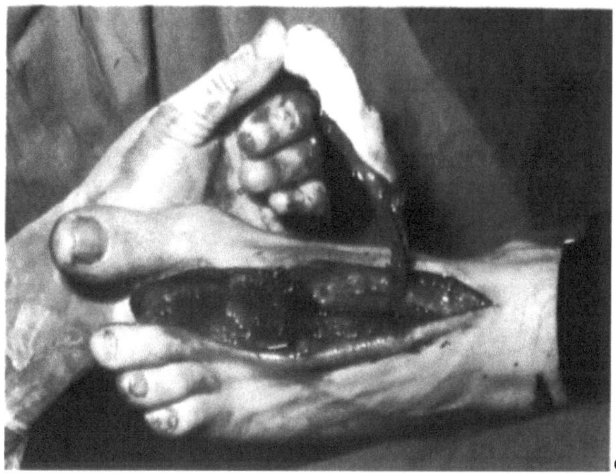

d

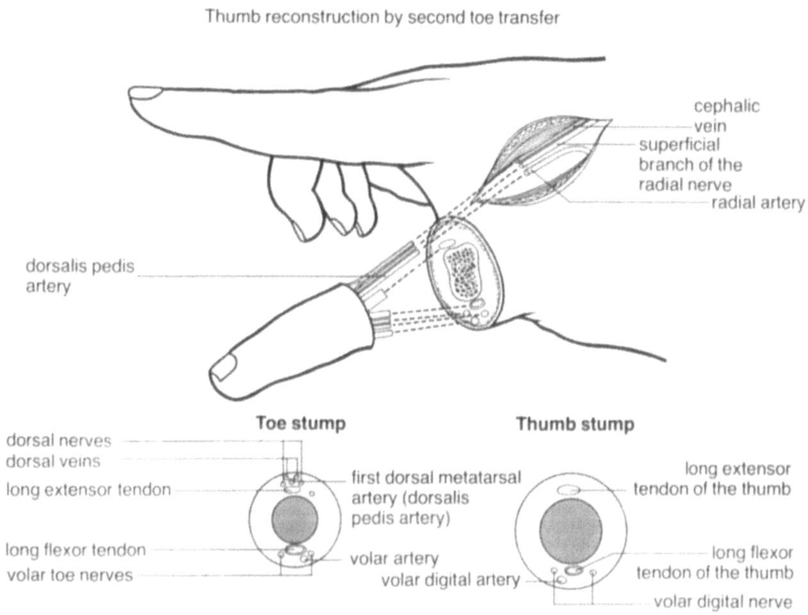

e

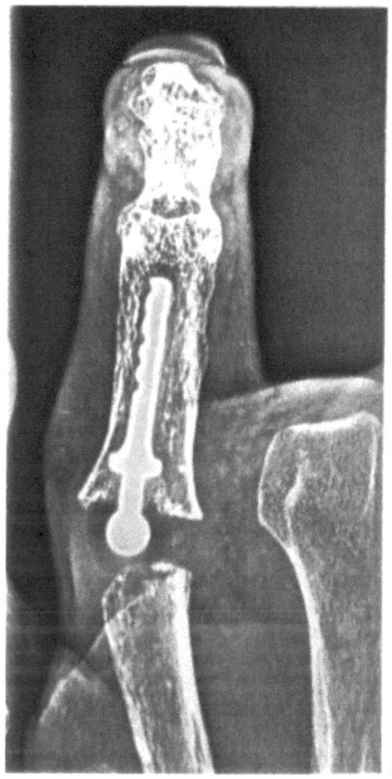

f

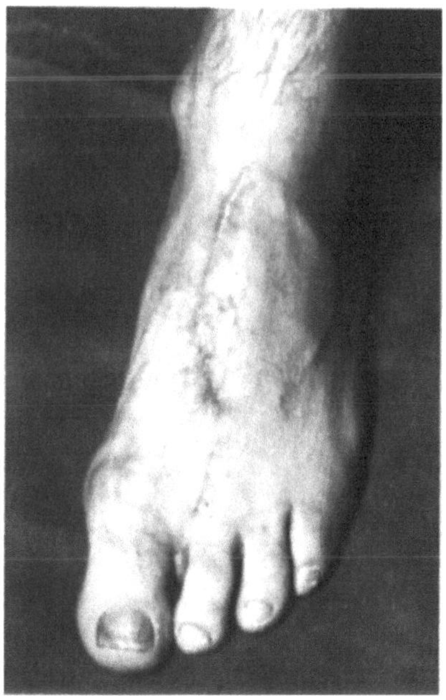

g

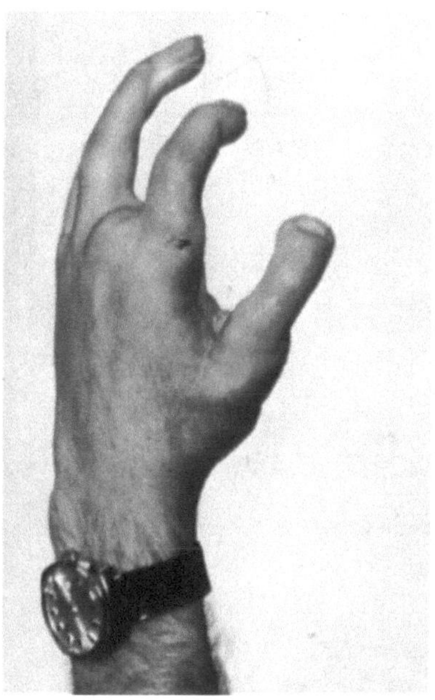

h

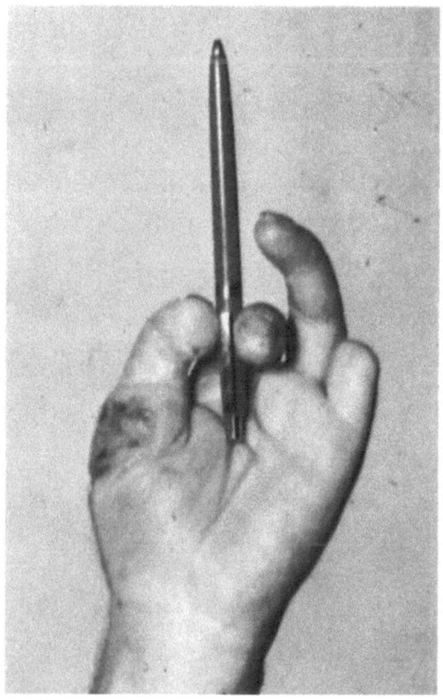

i

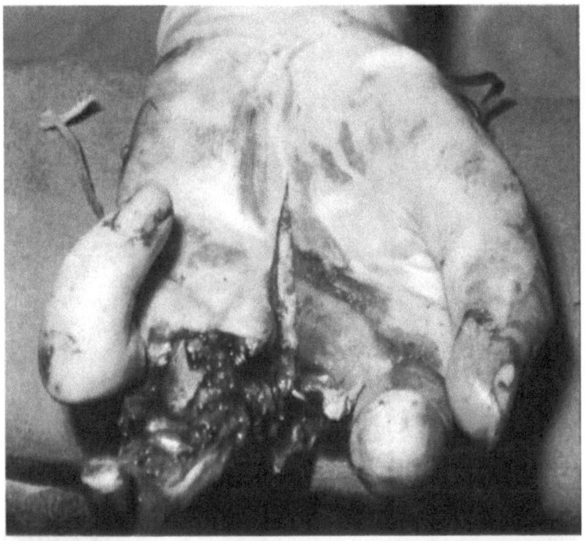

a

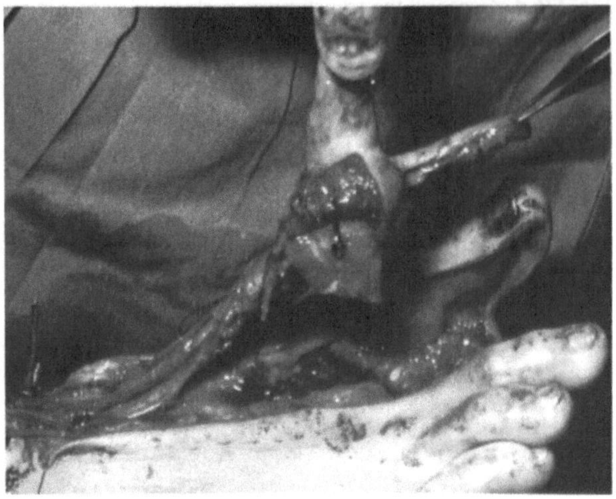

b

Fig. 127. a, b. Nineteen year old farm boy who presented with a stiff index finger stump, absent middle finger, unstable fracture of the proximal phalanx of the ring finger, and complete destruction of the flexor tendon bed and palmar skin, as a result of a previous accident. The small finger showed a fixed flexion deformity and there was no finger capable of opposition with the fully competent thumb. A combined transfer comprising the second toe and fibular side of the large toe was used to replace the middle finger and volar aspect of the ring finger. **c–e** The appearance after six months shows a good pincer grip between the thumb and the new middle finger

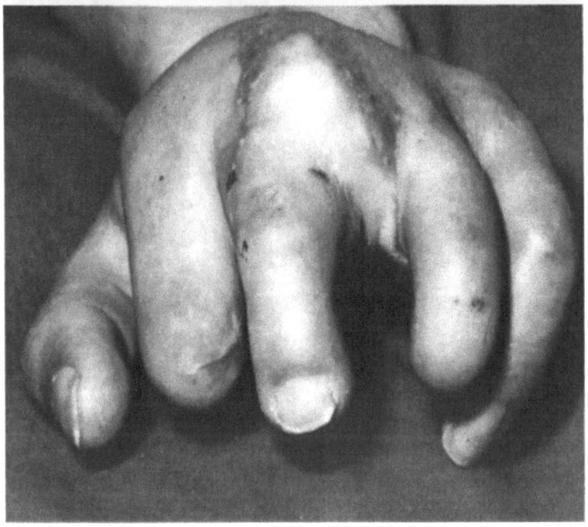

c

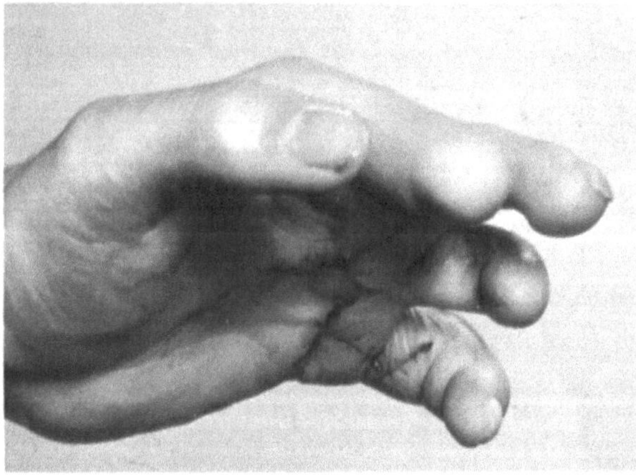

d

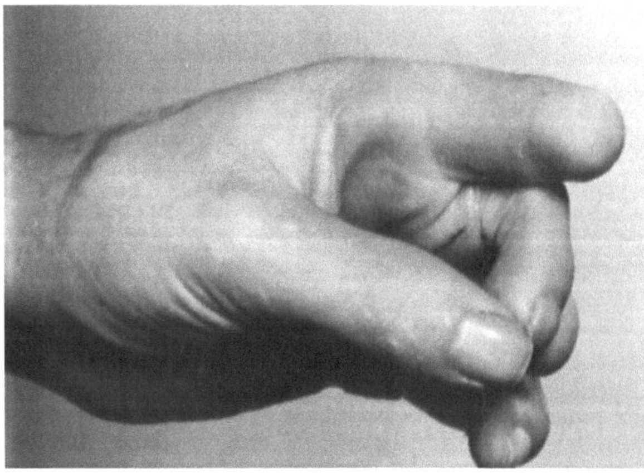

e

References

Acland RD (1972) Prevention of thrombosis in microvascular surgery by use of magnesium sulphate. Br J Plast Surg 29:292

Acland RD (1973) Thrombusformation in microvascular surgery: An experimental study of the effects of surgical trauma. Surgery 73:766

Acland RD (1977) Personal communication

Acland RD, Smith P (1976) Microvascular surgical techniques used to provide skin cover over an ununited tibial fracture. J Bone Joint (Am) Surg 583:471

American replantation mission to China (1973) Replantation surgery in China. Plast Reconstr Surg 52:476

Anderl H (1973) Reconstruction of face through cross face nerve transplantation in facial paralysis. Chir Plastica 2:17

Anderl H (1977a) Freie Fett-Transplantation mit Mikrogefäßanastomosen. 8. Tagung d. Vereinigung Deutscher Plastischer Chirurgen, Erlangen (12.–15. Okt. 1977)

Anderl H (1977b) Mikrochirurgische Transplantation eines Inguinallappens, der 30 Stunden gebankt wurde. Diskussionsbemerkung, 8. Tagung d. Vereinigung Deutscher Plastischer Chirurgen, Erlangen (12.–15. Okt. 1977)

Antia NH, Buch VI (1971) Transfer of an abdominal dermo-fat graft by direct anastomosis of blood vessels. Br J Plast Surg 24:15

Bakamjian V (1963) A technique for primary reconstruction of the palate after radical maxillectomy for cancer. Plast Reconstr Surg 31:103

Baudet J, Lemaire M, Legroux PH, Vidal L, Sargos P, deConnick L, Goumain AJM (1974) Transfer par microanastomoses dùn lambeau de cuir chevelu dans un cas dàlopècie cicatricielle. Ann Chir Plast 19:213

Baudet J, Guimberteau JC, Nascimento E (1976) Successful clinical transfer of two free thoracodorsal axillary flaps. Plast Reconstr Surg 58:680

Berger A, Meissl G, Millesi H, Piza-Katzer H (1976) Replantation amputierter Gewebeteile durch mikrovaskuläre Anastomosen. Vortrag: 17. Tagung d. Österr. Gesellschaft f. Chirurgie, Salzburg, 27.–29. Mai, 1976. Veröffentlicht: Acta Chirurgica Austriaca, Bericht von H Steiner, G Zimmermann, 1976/77

Biemer E (1977a) Replantation von Fingern und Extremitätenteilen. Technik und Ergebnisse. Chirurg 48:353

Biemer E (1977b) II.-Zehentransplantation. Vortrag auf Third Congress of the European Section of the Int. Confederation for Plastic and Reconstructive Surgery. The Hague 22.–27. Mai 1977

Biemer E (1977c) Klassifizierung von totalen und subtotalen Amputationen. Handchirurgie 9:21

Biemer E (1977d) Vein grafts in microvascular surgery. Br J Plast Surg 30:197

Biemer E (1977e) Erstbehandlung bei Amputationsverletzungen. Ther Ggw 116:146

Biemer E (1978) Replantation at the hand by microvascular anastomoses. In: Balas P (ed) Proceedings of the Int. Congress of Cardiovascular Surgery, Athen 11.–15. Juni 1978. Sulocton, Athen, p 441

Biemer E, Duspiva W (1976a) Free microvascular transfer of a groin flap to the skull following scalp avulsion. Chir Plast 3:277

Biemer E, Duspiva W (1976b) Erfolgreiche Replantation eines völlig abgetrennten Daumens. Münch Med Wochenschr 118:711

Biemer E, Duspiva W (1976c) Erfolgreiche Replantation der Mittelhand Münch Med Wochenschr 118:473

Biemer E, Duspiva W (1977a) Freie Verpflanzung von Haut- und Weichteilgewebe mit mikrovaskulären Anastomosen zur Defektdeckung. Münch Med Wochenschr 119:587

Biemer E, Duspiva W (1977b) Komplikationen bei der Replantation abgetrennter Gliedmaßen. Handchirurgie 9:67

Biemer E, Duspiva W (1978) Erfahrungen nach über 272 Replantationen peripherer Extremitätenteilen mit mikrovaskulären Anastomosen. Z Orthop 116:587

Biemer E, Heiss J (1978) Free flap transfer by microvascular anastomoses. In: Balas P (ed) Proceedings of the Int. Congress of Cardiovascular Surgery, 11.–15. Juni 1977, Athen, p 446

Biemer E, Duspiva W, Herndl E, Stock W, Ramatschi P (1977) Replantation an der oberen Extremität durch mikrovaskuläre Anastomosen. Chir Praxis 22:281

Biemer E, Duspiva W, Herndl E, Stock W, Ramatschi P (1977) Early experiences in organising and running a replantation service. Br J Plast Surg 31:9

Blair VP (1918) Surgery and disease of the mouth and jaws. Mosby, St. Louis

Boeckx WD, DeConinck A, Vanderlinden E (1976) Ten free flap transfers. Plast Reconstr Surg 57:707

Bos KE (1977) Bone transplantation revascularized by microvascular anastomoses. Vortrag auf dem Third Congress of the European Section of the Int. Confederation for plastic and reconstructive surgery. Mai 22.–27. 1977, The Hague

Bowen JE, Poole MD (1975) Multiple digital replantations. A case report. Br J Plast Surg 28:8

Buck-Gramcko D (1974) Mikrochirurgie peripherer Gefäße. Experimentelle Untersuchungen und klinische Anwendung. Handchirurgie 6:101

Buck-Gramcko D (1978) Indikation und Technik der Replantation. Langenbecks Arch Chir 347:97

Buncke HJ, Schulz WP (1966) Total ear reimplantation in the rabbit utilizing microminiature vascular anastomoses. Br J Plast Surg 10:15

Buncke HJ, Buncke CM, Schulz WB (1965) Experimental Digital Amputation and Reimplantation. Plast Reconstr Surg 36:62

Buncke HJ, Buncke CM, Schulz WP (1966) Immediate

Nicaladoni procedure in the rhesus monkey, or hallux-to-hand transplantation, utilizing microminiature vascular anastomoses. Br J Plast Surg 19:332

Buncke HJ, McLean DH, George PT, Creech BJ, Chater NL, Commons GW (1973) Thumb replacement: great toe transplantation by Microvascular anastomosis. Br J Plast Surg 26:194

Buncke HJ, Furnas DW, Gordon L, Achauer BM (1977) Free osteocutaneous flap from a rib to the tibia. Plast Reconstr Surg 59:799

Chen CW (1976) Personal communication

Chen YC, Chen CW, Pin CT, Pao YS (1966) Some problems concerning small vessel anastomosis in the reattachment of complete traumatic amputations. Chin Med J 85:79

Chi-Shui-Tan Hospital, Peking (1976) Personal communication

Cobbett JR (1969a) Free digital transfer. Report of a case of transfer of a great toe to replace an amputated thumb. J Bone Joint Surg 51B:677

Cobbett JR (1969b) Small vessel surgery in hand. The Hand 1:57

Cohen BE, May JW, Daly JSF, Young HH (1977) Successful clinical replantation of an amputated penis by microneurovascular repair. Plast Reconstr Surg 59:276

Daniel G, Entin MA, Kahn DS (1971) Autogenous transplantation in the dog of metacarpophalangeal joint with preserved neurovascular bundle. Can J Surg 14:253

Daniel RK, Taylor GI (1973) Distant transfer of an island flap by microvascular anastomoses. Plast Reconstr Surg 52:111 (1973)

Daniel RK, Terzis JK (1977) Reconstructive microsurgery. Little Brown, Boston

Daniel RK, Williams HB (1973a) The free transfer of skin flaps by microvascular anastomoses: An experimental study and a reappraisal. Plast Reconstr Surg 52:16

Daniel RK, Williams HB (1973b) The free transfer of skin flaps by microvascular anastomoses. Plast Reconstr Surg 52:16

Daniel RK, Terzis JK, Schwartz G (1975) Neurovascular free flaps. Plast Reconstr Surg 56:13

Duspiva W, Biemer E (1976a) Technik der Mikrogefäßchirurgie. Med Welt 27:852

Duspiva W, Biemer E (1976b) Tecnicas de cirurgia microvascular. Med Welt 9:46

Duspiva W, Biemer E (1977) Komplikationen bei der freien Gewebeübertragung mit mikrovaskulären Anastomosen. Handchirurgie 9:71

Duspiva W, Biemer E, Herndl E, Stock W, Alberti Irene von (1979) Knochenheilung in der Replantationschirurgie der Hand. Fortschr Med 97:953

Eiselsberg Fr. v. (1900) Ersatz des Zeigefingers durch die zweite Zehe. Arch Klin Chir 61:2

Emmans PR, Harrison MJG, Honour AJ, Mitchell IRH (1965) Effect of pyrimidopyrimidine derivate on thrombus formation in the rabbit. Nature 208:255

Finseth F, Kavarana N, Antia N (1975) Complications of free flap transfers to the mouth region. Plast Reconstr Surg 56:652

First Teaching Hosp. of Chung Shan Med. College (1973) Experience in replantation of severed fingers. Chin Med J 6:71

First Teaching Hosp. of Chung Shan Med. College (1973) Replantation of severed limbs. Chin Med J 6:70

Fujikawa S, O'Brien BMcC (1975) An experimental evaluation of microvenous grafts. Br J Plast Surg 28:244

Fujino T, Harashina T, Mikato A (1972) Autogenous en-bloc transplantation of the mammary gland in dogs using microsurgical technique. Plast Reconstr Surg 50:376

Fujino T, Harashina T, Nakajima T (1975) Free skin flap from the retroauricular region to the nose. Plast Reconstr Surg 57:338

Fujino T, Saito S (1975) Repair of pharyngoesophageal fistula by microvascular transfer of a free skin flap. Plast Reconstr Surg 56:549

Geldmacher J, Brug E (1973) Arbeitsunfall und Handverletzung. Münch Med Wochenschr 115:1212

Godina M (1978) Persönl. Mitteilungen auf Arbeitstreffen über Mikrochirurgie, München, Klinikum rechts d. Isar, April 1978

Godina M (1979) Paper at Fifth International Symposium on Microsurgery. Guarujá, Brasilien, May 21–24

Goldwyn RM, Lamb DL, White WL (1963) An experimental study of large island flaps in dogs. Plast Reconstr Surg 31:528

Harashina T, Nakajima T, Yoshimura Y (1977) A free groin flap reconstruction in progressive facial hemiatrophy. Br J Plast Surg 30(1):14

Harii K (1974) Free deltopectoral skin flaps. Br J Plast Surg 27:231

Harii K (1975) Omentumtransplant. Vortrag auf Third Int. Symposium on Microsurgery. East Grinstead 1975

Harii K, Ohmori S (1973) Use of the gastroepiploic vessels as recipient or donor vessels in the free transfer of composite flaps by microvascular anastomoses. Plast Reconstr Surg 52:541

Harii K, Ohmori K (1975a) Direct transfer of large free groin skin flap to the lower extremity using microvascular anastomoses. Chir Plast 3:1

Harii K, Ohmori K (1975b) Free groin flaps in children. Plast Reconstr Surg 55:588

Harii K, Ohmori K, Ohmori S (1974) Successful clinical transfer of then flaps by microvascular anastomoses. Plast Reconstr Surg 53:259

Harii K, Ohmori K, Torii S, Murakami F, Kasai Y, Schiguchi J, Ohmori S (1975) Free groin skin flaps. Br J Plast Surg 28:225

Harii K, Ohmori K, Schiguchi J (1976a) The free musculocutaneous flap. Plast Reconstr Surg 57:294

Harii K, Ohmori K, Torii S (1976b) Free gracilis muscle transplantation with microvascular anastomoses for treatment of facial paralysis. Plast Reconstr Surg 27:133

Hirsch J (1965) Increased platelets adhesiveness in recurrent venous thrombosis and pulmonary embolism. Br Med J II:797

Höpfner E (1903) Über Gefäßnaht, Gefäßtransplantation und Reimplantation von amputierten Extremitäten. Arch Klin Chir 70:417

Holzmann T, Wriedt-Lübbe I, Kramann B, Biemer E, Blümel G (1973) An experimental study of venous grafts in microvascular surgery. – A functional and micromorphological investigation. Paper at 13th Congress of European Society for Surgical Research, Helsinki, May 21.–24. 1978

Ikuta Y (1975) Autotransplant of omentum to cover large denucation of the scalp. Plast Reconstr Surg 55:490

Ikuta Y (1977) Replantation surgery in upper extremity. Handchirurgie 9:51

Ikuta Y, Kubo T, Tsuge K (1976) Free muscle transplantation by microsurgical technique to treat severe Volkmann's contracture. Plast Reconstr Surg 58:407 (1976)

Ikuta Y, Vatari S, Kowamuna H, Sluma R, Matamaski Y, Mugaski Y, Tsuge K (1975) Free flap transfer by end-to-side-anastomoses. Br J Plast Surg 28:1

Jacobson JH, Suarez EL (1960) Microsurgery in anastomoses of small vessels. Surg Forum 11:243

Kleinert HE, Kasdan ML (1963) Salvage of devascularized upper extremities, including studies on small vessel anastomoses. Clin Orthop 29:29

Kleinert HE, Kasdan ML (1965) Anastomosis of digital vessels. J Ky Med Assoc 63:106

Komatsu S, Taimai S (1968) Successful replantation of a completely cut-off thumb. Plast Reconstr Surg 42:374

Krizek TJ, Tani T, Desprez JD, Kiehn CL (1965) Experimental transplantation of composite grafts by microsurgical vascular anastomoses. Plast Reconstr Surg 36:538

Kutz JE, Hay EL, Kleinert HE (1969) Fate of small vessel repair. J Bone Joint Surg 51a:792

Lanz T, Wachsmuth W (1972) Praktische Anatomie, Bd I, Springer, Berlin Heidelberg New York

Lapchinsky AG (1960) Recent results of experimental transplantation of preserved limbs and kidneys and possible use of this technique in clinical practice. Ann NY Acad Sci 64:539

Leeb DC, Ben-Hur N, Mazzarella L (1977) Reconstruction of the floor of the mouth with a free dorsalis pedis flap. Plast Reconstr Surg 59(3):379

Lendvay PG (1968) Anastomoses of small digital vessels. Med J Aust 2:723

Lendvay PG, Owen ER (1970) Microvascular repair of completely severed digit: Fate of digital vessels after six months. Med J Aust 2:818

Lendvay PG (1973) Replacement of the amputated digits. Br J Plast Surg 26:398

Lister GD (1977) Personal communication

Lister GD, Kleinert HE, Kutz JE, Atasoy E (1977) Primary flexor tendon repair followed by immediate controlled mobilisation. J Hand Surg 2:441

Lu MM (1969) Successful replacement of avulsed scalp. Plast Reconstr Surg 43:231

Mandl H, Freilinger G, Holle J (1976) Replantationen im Handbereich mit ersten funktionellen Ergebnissen. Vortrag auf der 17. Tagung d. österr. Gesellschaft f. Chirurg, Salzburg 27.–29. Mai 1976, Veröffentlicht: Acta Chirurgica Austriaca, Steiner H, Zimmermann G, 1976/77

Mayer JE (1973) Dipyridamol and aspirin tested against an experimental model of thromboses. Ann Surg 178:108

McCullough DW, Frederickson JM (1973) Neovascularized rib grafts to reconstruct mandibular defects. Can J Otolaryngol 2:96

McGraw JB, Furlow LT Jr (1975) The dorsalis pedis arterialized flap. A clinical study. Plast Reconstr Surg 55:177

McGregor IA, Jackson IT (1972) The groin flap. Br J Plast Surg 25:3

McLean BH, Buncke HJ (1972) Autotransplant of omentum to a large scalp defect with microsurgical revascularization. Plast Reconstr Surg 49:268

Miller GDH, Anstee EJ, Snell JA (1976) Asuccessful replantation of an avulsed scalp by microvascular anastomoses. Plast Reconstr Surg 58:133

Millesi H (1976) Diskussionsbemerkung auf der 17. Tagung d. österr. Gesellschaft f. Chir., Salzburg, 27.–29. 5. 1976

Nicoladoni C (1897) Daumenplastik. Wiener Klin Wochenschr 28:663

O'Brien BMcC (1977) Microvascular reconstructive surgery. Churchill Livingstone, Edinburgh London New York

O'Brien BMcC, Hayhurst JW (1973) Metallized microsutures and a new microneedle holder. Plast Reconstr Surg 52:673

O'Brien BMcC, Miller GDH (1973) Digital reattachment and revascularisation. J Bone Joint Surg 55A:714

O'Brien BMcC, Shanmugan N (1973) Experimental transfer of composite free flaps with microvascular anastomoses. Aust NZ J Surg 43:285

O'Brien BMcC, Miller GDH, McLeod AM, Newing RK (1973a) Saving the amputated digit and hand. Med J Aust 1:558

O'Brien BMcC, McLeod AM, Hayhurst JW, Morrison WA (1973b) Successful transfer of a large island flap from the groin to the foot by microvascular anastomoses. Plast Reconstr Surg 52:271

O'Brien BMcC, McLeod AM, Miller GDM, Newing RK, Hayhurst JW, Morrison WA (1973c) Clinical replantation of digits. Plast Reconstr Surg 52:490

O'Brien BMcC, Morrison WA, Ishida H, McLeod AM, Gilbert A (1974) Free flap transfer with microvascular anastomoses. Br J Plast Surg 27:220

O'Brien BM, McLeod AM, Sykes PJ, Donahoe S (1975) Hallux-to-hand transfer. The Hand 7:128

Ohmori K (1977) Vortrag auf dem 3rd Congress of the European Section of the Int. Confederation for Plast

and Reconstructive Surgery, May 22.–27. 1977, The Hague
Ohmori K, Harii K (1975a) Transplantation of a toe to an amputated finger. The Hand 7:134
Ohmori K, Harii K (1975b) Free groin flaps: Their vascular basis. Br J Plast Surg 28:238
Olivari N, Olivari B (1975) Beeinflussung der Lappendurchblutung und Nekroserate nach Verschiebeschwenkplastiken durch Pentoxifyllin und Dextran 40. Med Welt 26:1973
Östrup LT, Fredrickson JM (1974) Distant transfer of a free, living bone graft by microvascular anastomoses. Plast Reconstr Surg 54:274
Östrup LT, Frederickson JM (1975) Reconstruction of mandibular defects after radiation, using a free living bone graft, transferred by microvascular anastomoses. Plast Reconstr Surg 55:563
Östrup LT, Tam CS (1975) Bone formation in a free, living bone graft transferred by microvascular anastomoses. Scand J Plast Reconstr Surg 9:101
Owen ER (1975) Replantation of amputated extremities. Langenbecks Arch Chir 339:613
Owen ER (1976) Personal communication

Reimann R, Fritz G (1975) Der Leistenlappen – anatomische Untersuchungen zum axialen Gefäßverlauf. Handchirurgie 7:109
Reuter H (1970) Hemmung der Plättchenaggregation durch Acetylsalicylsäure. Dtsch Med Wochenschr 95:14
Rigg BM (1975) Transfer of a free groin flap to the heel by microvascular surgery. Plast Reconstr Surg 55:36
Robinson DW (1976) Microsurgical transfer of the dorsalis pedis neurovascular island flap. Br J Plast Surg 29:209

Scharrer J (1969) Thromboseprophylaxe mit Aspirin. Der Einfluß von Acetylsalicylsäure auf die Thrombozytenaggregation in vitro und in vivo. Klin Wochenschr 47:1318
Schmidt-Tintemann U (1970) Chirurgische Operationslehre IV. 8. Ergänzung, Urban & Schwarzenberg, München Berlin Wien
Schmidt-Tintemann U, Biemer E, Duspiva W (1976) Replantationen abgetrennter Finger, Daumen und Hände durch Mikrogefäßchirurgie. Dtsch Ärztebl 20:1367
Serafin D, Rios AV, Georgiade N (1976) Fourteen free groin flap transfers. Plast Reconstr Surg 57:707
Six peoples hospital, Shanghai (1976) Persönliche Mitteilungen
Six peoples hospital Shanghai. Research laboratory for replantation of severed limbs (1976) Free muscle transplantation by microvascular neurovascular anastomoses. – Report of a Case. Chin Med J 2:47
Snyder CC, Knowles RP, Mayer PW, Hobbs JC (1960) Extremity replantation. Plast Reconstr Surg 26:251
Snyder CC, Batemann JM, Davis CW, Warden GD (1970) Mandibulo-facial restoration with live osteocutaneous flaps. Plast Reconstr Surg 45:14
Snyder CC, Stevenson RM, Browne EZ (1972) Successful replantation of a total severed thumb. Plast Reconstr Surg 50:553
Stranc MF, Labandter H, Roy A (1975) A review of 196 tubed pedicle. Br J Plast Surg 24:54
Strauch B, Murray DE (1967) Transfer of composite grafts with immediate suture anastomoses of its vascular pedicle measuring less than 1 mm in external diameter using microsurgical techniques. Plast Reconstr Surg 40:325
Strauch B, Bloomberg AE, Lewin ML (1971) An experimental approach to mandibular replacement: Island vascular composite rib grafts. Br J Plast Surg 24:334

Tamai S (1974) Present status and prospect of limb and finger replantation. Surg Diag Treat 6:547
Tamai S (1977a) Personal communication
Tamai S (1977b) Paper at Third Congress of the European Section of the Int. Confederation for Plastic and Reconstructive Surgery, 22.–27. May, 1977, The Hague
Tamai S, Komatsu S, Sakamoto H, Sano S, Sagaushi N, Hori Y, Tatsumi Y, Okuda H (1970) Free muscle transplants in dog with microsurgical neurovascular anastomosis. Plast Reconstr Surg 46:219
Tamai S, Nakamura Y, Motomiya Y (1977) Microsurgical replantation of a completely amputated penis and scrotum. Plastic Reconstr Surg 60:287
Taylor GI, Daniel RK (1975) The anatomy of several free flap donor sites. Plast Reconstr Surg 56:243
Taylor GI, Miller GDH, Ham FJ (1975) The free vascularized bone graft. Plast Reconstr Surg 55:533
Taylor GT (1979) Vortrag: Fifth International Symposium on Microsurgery Guarujá, Brasilien, 15.–18. Mai
Tschopp HM (1976) Microsurgical neuro-vascular anastomoses for transplantation of composite bone and muscle grafts. Springer, Berlin Heidelberg New York

Webster M (1977) Photoelektrischer Pulsfühler zur Überwachung von freien Transplantaten. Persönliche Mitteilungen
Wells JH, Edgerton MT (1977) Correction of severe hemifacial atrophy with a free dermis-fat flap from the lower abdomen. Plast Reconstr Surg 59(2):223
Werber KD, Biemer E (1978) Eigene Erfahrungen mit Replantationen von Fingern im Bereich der Zone I (Fingerkuppen). Vortrag auf der Tagung der Deutschsprachigen Arbeitsgemeinschaft für Handchirurgie, Budapest, 14.–17. Juli 1978
Werber KD, Biemer E (1978) Erfahrungen mit der percutanen Sauerstoffpartialdruckmessung in der Lappenplastik. Vortrag auf der 9. Tagung der Vereinigung der Deutschen Plastischen Chirurgen, 18.–21. Okt., Köln

Subject Index

accessories 7
accident surgery 58
acetyl-salicylic acid 48, 69, 109
adaptation 19, 40
adaptor 8
adjacent joints 65
adjustment speed 6
adventitia 18, 21, 30, 33, 41, 45, 46
age
– indications 61
– limit 61
– replantation 61
ampicillin 70
amputated part 56
– condition of 63
– disinfection of 63
amputation 33, 59
– classification 59
– definition 56
– level 63, 70
– mechanism 70
– subtotal 33, 56, 57, 98
– total 56, 87, 98
anaesthesia 16
– duration of 16
– for experimental animals 16
anaesthetic 108
anastomosis 18, 19, 21, 24, 32, 33, 37, 41, 45
– end to end 3, 18
– end to side 3, 28
– microvascular 3
– patency 30
– site 19, 30, 31, 43, 44, 45
– vicinity 45
angiography
– indication 107
– post-operative 110
– pre-operative 107
angle of vision 6
animal trials 3, 16
anoxaemic time 56, 63, 67, 68
anterior iliac spine 130
anterior (front) wall 19, 21, 24, 25
anticoagulants 47
anticoagulation 69
anuria 58

approximating clamp 25
approximator clamp 11, 13
arm-rests 9, 63
arterial defect 35
– grafts 37
– palmar arch 73
arteries 3, 19, 40, 63, 67
artery 38, 119
– anterior tibial 122, 135
– arcuate 122, 135
– carotid 28
– common digital 59
– deep circumflex iliac 117, 121, 130
– dorsal digital 135
– dorsal metatarsal 122, 135
– dorsalis pedis 117, 121, 122, 135
– facial 122
– femoral 26, 32, 33, 40, 41, 42
– labial 100, 103
– lateral tarsal 135
– medial circumflex femoral 129
– palmar digital 59
– posterior auricular 128
– posterior tibial 112, 135
– profunda femoris 129, 133
– radial 57, 137
– subscapular 117, 128
– superficial circumflex iliac 105, 117
– superficial epigastric 112, 117
– temporal 100, 102, 117, 121, 128
– thoracodorsal 117, 128
– ulnar 57, 75
arthrodesis 67, 82, 85, 95
assistant 6, 7
assistant microscope 6, 7
associated injuries 63
asymmetric biangulation 19
attachments 4, 5, 7
automatic film adaptor 8
avulsion injuries 33, 37, 79, 80, 81, 82, 98
"axial pattern flap" 105, 118
axillary flap 117, 128

back wall 18, 19, 21, 25, 28, 30
background material 13
basic instrumentation 10, 13
beam splitters 7
bifurcation 17
bilobed flap 119
binocular eyepieces 8
– tube 6, 8
bleeding 17, 19
blister formation 114
blistering 89
blood 5
– clots 18, 21
– coagulation 47
– flow 40
– grouping 63
– loss 19, 69
– viscosity 48
bone 57, 64
– shortening 33, 64
– transplantation 110, 131
burning injury 125
bypass (carotid artery) 28

calcification 33
calibre differences 18, 33, 109
camera, 35 mm 8
cannulisation 3
capillary filling 89, 110
– tubes 3
care
– of amputated part 62
– of instruments 10
carpal tunnel 75
carrying ring 7
ceiling-mount 6
central venous line 108
centralisation 108, 109
circular saw 75
clamping 21, 40
clamps 11, 12, 13, 21
– closing pressure 11
– closing strength 12
classification 57
cleaning 63
– amputated part 63
– instruments 10
"climbing thread technique" 19

clips 3, 13, 19, 63
closing strength 12, 13
– calculation 12
coaxial illumination 6
cold sensitivity 97
collagen 33
colour 110
colour TV 9
combined skin flap with bone transplantation
– see also osteo-cutaneous flaps 130
comminuted fractures 65
complications of microvascular suture 30
composite graft 70
compressed fracture 66
continuous oversew 67
contrast 22
co-observer tubes 7, 8
– monocular 7
– stereo 7
cooling 40, 62, 108
– "dry cooling" 62
– in replantation 58
co-ordinated coupling 6
counterloop 13
cross-facial nerve graft 133
cross leg flap 105
crude grip 98
crushing 33, 76, 98
– area 78
– injuries 75
– severe 76, 78, 98
– total 78
"cuffing" technique 19
cutting plane 18

dacron prosthesis 38
damage to cables 7
degloving injuries 79, 83, 84, 98, 127
delto-pectoral flap 123, 127
dextran 48, 69, 109
diameter 19
digit amputation 55, 59
digital artery 27, 67
– nerves 65
– vein 31
dilatation 18
dipyridamol 47, 48, 69, 109
disinfectant solution 16
disinfection in replantation 63
distal phalanx 61
distance release 8
documentation 7, 8
donor area 108, 118
– defect, donor site 108, 116, 117, 119
– site 113
– flaps 118
– micro-vein grafts 35, 36
– vessel 28
Doppler equipment 14, 89, 110
dorsalis pedis flap 117, 121, 122, 123
dressing change 89
– in free flap transplantation 110
– in replantation 69
dressings 69
dual microscope 7

elasticity 35
electrolytes 63
electronic flash-gun 7
"en-bloc" amputation 75, 99
end to end anastomosis 17, 18, 21, 30, 35, 41, 108, 111
end to side anastomosis 17, 27, 28, 30, 109, 111
endothelium 45
extensor tendon 57, 65, 68

fascia lata 119
fat flap 118
fibre-optic 5, 7
fibrin 19, 41
fibrin-glue 3, 19
fibrinolysis 41, 45, 48
– autography 45, 46
fibula transplant 131
field of vision 3, 8
film 7
– adaptor 8
finger joints 85
– reconstruction 134, 142
– tip 117
– transplantation 88
fish-mouth incision 137, 138
flap transplantation
– advantages 116
– disadvantages 116
– free 105, 116
– special requirements 117
flexor tendons 57, 63
– superficial 65, 67
– suturing 65, 67
floor support 6
flushing liquids 47
flushing out 13, 23, 47
focussing 5
Fogarty catheter 30, 114
foot control 9
– pedal 5, 6
forceps 9
forefoot stump 121
forehead flap 117
foreign body 3, 63

Galilei
– alternator 5
– change 6
– exchange 7
gracilis flaps 129
graft 33, 35, 37, 38
grindstone 13
grips 10
groin flap 105, 111, 114, 117, 118, 119
guanethidin 48
guillotine amputation 75, 98

haematocrit 63
haemoglobin 63
halogen lamps 5, 8
hand 54, 61
– amputations 59, 68, 70, 73, 78
– zones 59, 70
heparin 47, 48, 69
heparinisation 47, 69
heparinised Ringer's lactate 13, 18, 19, 21, 23, 47
high performance lighting 5
histology 34, 40
holding sutures 3, 17, 19, 21, 24, 25
hospital stay 116
hyperaemia 109
hyperextensibility 136
hyperplasia
– subintimal 40, 42

iliac crest 121, 130
– flap 121
incapacity to work 59, 62
indication for replantation
– age 61
– children 59
– distal phalanx 61
– hand 59, 61
– mechanism of injury 61
– middle hand 59, 61
– multiple amputations 59
– replantation 59, 61
– thumb 59, 61
insertion 20
instruction manuals 5
instrumental knotting 19
instruments 3, 4, 9, 10, 13, 40
insurance, compensation 59
interchangeable objective 5
– optics 8
intercostal artery 117, 130
interdigital fold flap 121
interrupted sutures 18, 19, 21, 28, 29
intima 18, 42, 45, 46
– defects 40
irrigators 13
ischaemic time (see anoxaemic time) 56

jewellers forceps 9
joint prosthesis 72, 85, 86, 141
– replacement 85

Kirschner wire
– central 65
– crossed 65, 66
knots 17, 19, 21
knotted sutures 17

lamps 5
large toe pulp flap 117
– – transplantation 134, 135
late results
– functional 97
lateral thoracic vessels 123
latissimus-dorsi flap 129
layer of thrombus 21, 40
lens attachment 7
light requirements 9
loupe magnification 63
loupe spectacles 4, 16
loupes 4
lumen 18, 23, 40, 43, 45
– contriction 3
– dilated 23
– flushed 23
– stretching 13

macro-replantation 58
magnesium sulphate solution 47
magnification 4, 6, 7
– range 6
management post-operative 89
mandible reconstruction 131
manufacturers 5
marking 63, 64, 108
measure 12, 13
media necrosis 3, 19, 40, 41
medicinal treatment 47, 48, 68
– in replantation 68
metal containers 10
metalosis 66
metatarsal, second 135, 136
micro-circulation 47, 48
– -forceps 13, 18, 30, 31
– -instruments 9, 10
micro-replantation 55, 58
– other parts of the body 99
micromorphology 40
microscope 4, 5, 19, 39
microsurgical operative techniques 3, 4
microthrombectomy 30
microvascular anastomosis 26, 40
– assessment of 30
microvascular surgery 38
– development of 3
– experimental 16
microvascular suturing 17, 28, 46
– complications of 30
micro-vein grafts 30, 37, 38, 39, 67
– donor site 35
– indication 33
– results 38
– rules 36
middle-hand amputation 55, 59, 68
mouth 107
multiple amputations 59
muscle
– anoxaemic time 58
– deltoid 123
– extensor hallucis brevis 122, 135
– extensor hallucis longus 122, 135
– flexor pollicis longus 137
– gracilis 129, 132, 133
– interosseus 135
– latissimus dorsi 128, 129
– pectoralis 123, 133
– rectus femoris 133
– sartorius 118
– transplantation 107, 110, 133
musculo-cutaneous flaps 129

nail bed 99
– growth 99
neck contracture 122
necrosis 76, 114
needle 15, 18, 28
– holder 11, 13, 18
neo-intima 40
nerve 63
– deep peroneal 135
– facial 133
– fibular 125, 137
– median 75
– obturator 129, 133
– radial 137
– superficial peroneal 123
– trigeminal 133
– ulnar 75
nerve suturing 68
neurovascular bundle
– identification of 63, 67
nylon 3, 15
– suture 15, 43, 45

occupational therapy 94
ocular 8
omentum transplantation 105, 134
operating courses 4, 9
operating field 6, 7, 8, 17, 19
operating microscope 3, 4, 5, 7, 9
– schematic diagram 5
– zoom 6
operating seat 9
operating technique
– microscopic 3, 4
operating time 116
operative field 4
operator 6
optical extensions 9
osteo-cutaneous flaps 130
osteosynthesis 64
– methods 65
oxacillin 70
papaverin 47
patency 27, 30, 33, 40, 47
– test 30
penile amputation 100
percutaneous PO_2 measurement 89, 110
perfusion 65
persantin 69
photo
– adaptor 7
– automatic 8
– camera 8
– cell 8
– lenses 7
– magnification 7
photo-attachments 7
photography 8
physiotherapist 94
picture transmission 9
pinch grip 98
plasminogen 41, 45
– activator 40, 41, 45, 46
plastic bag 5, 62
plateau forceps 13
platelet aggregation 47, 48
(see also thrombus formation)
– inhibitor 48
porta caval shunt 28
post-operative analysis 38
– bleeding 47
– investigation 40
– management 59, 94
– results 98
pre-operative examination
– in replantation 63
preparation 17, 22, 135
pressure bandage 62
primary treatment of amputation injuries 62
procain 47
pseud-arthrosis 95
pulse meter, photoelectric 89, 110
push-button 6

rabbit 16, 32, 33, 34, 55, 105
radial fossa 137
"random pattern flap" 105, 118
rat 16, 41, 42
– aorta 17, 42, 43, 44, 46
re-anastomosis 30, 31, 114
recanalisation 40
re-endothelialisation 40, 44
reflux, venous 67, 68
renal damage, toxic 58
re-operation
– indication 89
replant 36
replantation 3, 4, 33, 35, 37, 38, 42, 47, 55, 56, 69, 70, 71, 72, 79
– in children 59
– definition 56

replantation development 55
- experimental 3, 55
- functional 97
- indications 58, 59, 61
- macro- 58
- micro- 55, 58
- nomenclature 56
- of single digits 59
- technique 58, 63, 65
- without venous anastomosis 69
replantation centres 4
- feasibility 58, 62
- service 38, 104
- surgery 38, 48
re-sensitivity 117
residual blood flow 56
respiratory depression 16
results 97
- survival 97, 98
- replantation 97, 98
- vein grafts 33
retro-auricular flap 128
revascularisation 56, 57
- definition 57
reversion prism 8
rheomacrodex 69
rhesus monkey 55
rib and chest wall transplant 130
rib transplantation 131, 132
rings 3
rotation 65
- error 95
- stability 65
round body needles 15

scalp flap 105
scalping injury 100, 102
scanning electron-microscopy 40, 43
scarification 69
scintigraphy 110
scissors 9, 13, 14
screw 66
sealing 21
seat
- height 17
- position 9, 17, 62
second toe transplantation 135
secondary amputation 99
secondary operations 95
sensitivity 98
shock treatment 69
shortening 33, 36
side branches 36
silicon photo diode 8
skin bridges 56, 57
- closure 65, 68
- flaps 48
- temperature 89
small finger 90
small fragment instruments 66
smoking 89
soft tissue defect 105
spasm 37, 47, 109
split thickness skin graft 93, 110, 114, 123, 125
spring scissors 11
stability 65, 66
stereo beam splitter 6
stero-optic 6
stereoscopic double microscopes 4
- camera 8
- co-observer tube 7, 8
- view 6, 8
sterilisation 10
sticking plaster 3
stretching 13, 40
stricture 18
subcutaneous fatty tissue 110
subintimal hyperplasia 40, 42
supervision, post-operative 108, 110
support after replantation 69
support ring 6
surface compression 12
surgeon 7
survival results 97, 98
suture dehiscence
- in tendons 95
suture devices 3
suture material 15, 19, 40
- nerves 68
- tendons 67
- tendon sheath 67
suture site 30, 44
suture technique 17, 33
- continuous 16
suturing 18, 19
- arteries 67
sympathetic blockade 48

table microscope 5
table stand 4, 5
technique
- replantation 58, 63
- tissue transplantation 108
temperature monitoring 110
temporal flap 117, 123
- region 105
tendon 63
- sheath 65, 67
tenolysis 95
tensile strength 3
tension 17, 33, 40, 63
tetanus prophylaxis 63
thinning 110, 119
thoraco-dorsal vessels 123
thoracotomy 131
thread 15, 19
thrombectomy 30, 89, 90, 92, 114
thrombin 19
thrombosis 18, 30, 31, 35, 47, 67, 76, 89, 90, 92, 93, 114
- prophylaxis 47, 48
- rate 38
thrombus 30, 37, 40, 45
- formation 28
- material 30
thumb 3, 36, 55, 87
- amputation 55, 80, 82, 87
- reconstruction 134
tissue transplantation 4, 16, 33, 47, 105
- complications 110
- contra-indications 107
- definition 106
- development 105
- free 4, 16, 33, 47
- indications 106
- medicinal treatment 109
- nomenclature 106
- planning 108
- post-operative supervision 110
- preparation 107
- technique 108
toe pulp flap 121, 123, 126, 127
- replantation 99, 123
- transplantation 134
total amputation 56
- oblique 36
totocillin 70
tourniquet 63
transplantation 16
- immunology 16
transporting 7
transposition flap 105
trauma 40
turbulence 17, 18
TV adaptor 7, 8
TV camera 8
TV transmission 9
two toes "en bloc" transplantation 140

ulceration 111, 112
ultrasonic cleaner 10

vascular spreader 13
- surgery 30
vein graft 32, 33, 35, 36, 37, 38, 47, 78, 79, 81, 89
veins 3, 19, 33, 36, 40, 63
- cephalic 123
- long saphenous 135
- posterior tibial 111
- short saphenous 135
- superficial epigastric 112
- superficial temporal 121
vein scissors 14
vein spreader 13, 14
vein transplant 3, 38
vena cava 22
venous anastomosis 28, 63, 68
- obstruction 89

vessel anastomosis 13, 26, 30
- clamp 11, 12, 13, 25
- clips 9, 19
- defect 30, 33, 65
- grafts 38
- lumen 3, 19, 28
- shortening 37
- spasm 47, 48
- stumps 3, 13, 17, 18, 33, 47

vessel suture 25
- continuous 3
vessel wall 13, 18, 29, 45
- changes in 33
- damage of 30, 47
- thickening of 33

wall-mounted microscope 4
web space 117, 123

wire-sutures 65
wound debridement 64

X-ray 63
xero-arteriography, intravenous 32
XY coupling 6

zone division of the hand 59, 70
zoom microscope 6

Microsurgery

By Cheng Zhong-wei, Yang Dong-yue, Chang Di-sheng, Chao Yu-lin
1982. 366 figures, approx. 9 tables. Approx. 500 pages
ISBN 3-540-11281-2
Distribution rights for the People's Republic of China: Shanghai Scientific and Technical Publishers

Microsurgery for Cerebral Ischemia

Editors: S. J. Peerless, C. W. McCormick
Reprint. 1981. 282 figures. XVII, 372 pages
ISBN 3-540-90495-6
Distribution rights for Japan: Igaku Shoin Ltd., Tokyo

Microsurgery for Stroke

Editor: P. Schmiedek
Co-editors: O. Gratzl, R. F. Spetzler
1977. 133 figures, 63 tables. XVII, 291 pages
ISBN 3-540-90250-3
Distribution rights for Japan: Igaku Shoin Ltd., Tokyo

Microvascular Anastomoses for Cerebral Ischemia

Editors: J. M. Fein, O. H. Reichmann
1978. 197 figures including 12 four-color plates. XV, 324 pages
ISBN 3-540-90240-6

W. Seeger

Microsurgery of the Brain

Anatomical and Technical Principles

1980. 351 figures. XI, IV, 727 pages
In two volumes, not available separately
ISBN 3-211-81573-2
Distribution rights for Japan: Nankodo Co. Ltd., Tokyo

H. M. Tschopp

Microsurgical Neuro-Vascular Anastomoses

for Transplantation of Composite Bone and Muscle Grafts
An Experimental Study
With a Foreword by M. Allgöwer

1976. 50 illustrations, some in color. V, 52 pages
ISBN 3-540-07517-8

E. J. Wylie, R. J. Stoney, W. K. Ehrenfeld

Manual of Vascular Surgery

Volume 1
1980. 557 figures, 471 in full color. XII, 264 pages
(Comprehensive Manuals of Surgical Specialties)
ISBN 3-540-90408-5

Springer-Verlag Berlin Heidelberg New York

MIX
Papier aus verantwortungsvollen Quellen
Paper from responsible sources
FSC® C105338

If you have any concerns about our products,
you can contact us on
ProductSafety@springernature.com

In case Publisher is established outside the EU,
the EU authorized representative is:
Springer Nature Customer Service Center GmbH
Europaplatz 3, 69115 Heidelberg, Germany

Printed by Libri Plureos GmbH
in Hamburg, Germany